Handbook of
NONINVASIVE
DIAGNOSTIC
TECHNIQUES
in VASCULAR
SURGERY

Handbook of
NONINVASIVE DIAGNOSTIC TECHNIQUES *in* VASCULAR SURGERY

BOK Y. LEE, M.D., F.A.C.S.
Chief, Surgical Service
Principal Investigator in Surgical Research
Veterans Administration Medical Center
Castle Point, New York
Associate Professor of Surgery
New York Medical College
Valhalla, New York

FRIEDA S. TRAINOR, Ph. D.
Research Physiologist
Veterans Administration Medical Center,
Castle Point, NY.

WILLIAM R. THODEN, B.S., M.A.
Research Assistant
Surgical Service and Research Service
Veterans Administration Medical Center,
Castle Point, NY.

DAVID KAVNER, D. Eng.
Chief, Biomedical Engineer
Veterans Administration Medical Center,
Castle Point, NY.

Appleton-Century-Crofts / New York

81 82 83 84 85 / 10 9 8 7 6 5 4 3 2 1

Prentice-Hall International, Inc., London
Prentice-Hall of Australia, Pty. Ltd., Sydney
Prentice-Hall of India Private Limited, New Delhi
Prentice-Hall of Japan, Inc., Tokyo
Prentice-Hall of Southeast Asia (Pte.) Ltd., Singapore
Whitehall Books, Ltd., Wellington, New Zealand

Library of Congress Cataloging in Publication Data
Main entry under title:

Handbook of noninvasive diagnostic techniques in vascular
    surgery.

    Bibliography: p.
    Includes index.
    1. Blood-vessels—Surgery.   2. Diagnosis, Surgical.
3. Diagnosis, Ultrasonic.   4. Electrodiagnosis.
I. Lee, Bok Y., 1928–   II. Title: Noninvasive
diagnostic techniques in vascular surgery. [DNLM:
1. Vascular diseases—Diagnosis.   WG 500 H236]
RD598.5.H36   617'.41307543   81-10870
ISBN 0–8385–3620–4   AACR2

Text design: Alan Gold
Cover design: Gloria J. Moyer

PRINTED IN THE UNITED STATES OF AMERICA

We dedicate this handbook to Dr. John L. Madden, a truly outstanding teacher and surgeon, in grateful appreciation for the education, teaching, and support that he has given us. He has been and continues to be a driving force and inspiration to us all.

Contents

Foreword I

Surgeons must be careful
When they take the knife
For beneath their fine incisions
Stirs the culprit. Life!
EMILY DICKINSON

This admonition was written long before the technical wonders of vascular surgery broke out of the dog laboratories and into the clinical arena. The breakthroughs in sutures and prosthetic vascular conduits combined with an aging population have made vascular surgery the fastest growing surgical specialty. This field of surgery is most unforgiving in regard to clumsy handling of tissues and inept technique. Successful vascular surgeons pride themselves on the importance of virtuoso dexterity and careful planning for their operative procedures. But Emily Dickinson suggested that although deft cutting and sewing are essential, the ultimate surgeon must also take life possessions into account. As a career-long teacher of surgery it has been my experience that virtuoso technicians are born, not made but that physiology can be taught even to the most noncerebral mechanic.

Nowhere in modern medicine is the payoff of good applied physiology better demonstrated than in vascular surgery. Radiologic advances have provided superb roadmaps and some quantitation of flow patterns but assessment of function based upon the noninvasive wonders of the biomedical engineering revolution has added true science to the art and craft of vascular surgery.

For the past 20 years Dr. Lee's clinical biomedical engineering team has been responsible for many fine research reports based upon skilled use of electromagnetic flowmetry and later noninvasive vascular diagnostic instruments. The publications as well as the teaching symposia in vascular surgery organized by Dr. Lee over the years resulted in many inquiries regarding the planning, instrumentation and operation of the modern vascular laboratory. This book combines the most current physiological knowledge of systemic blood flow with detailed and practical methodology for clinical assessment.

Dr. Bok Y. Lee and his group at Castle Point Medical Center have recognized from the beginning the impact that the clinical vascular laboratory would have on the results of surgery in this field and have become leaders in applied vascular physiology. The unique Veterans Administration environment at Castle Point has also permitted the ultimate application of the team approach to difficult clinical problems. Superb clinical surgery combined with dedicated engineering and basic science have produced a remarkable series of clinical successes and contributions to vascular physiology.

The modest title "Handbook of Noninvasive Diagnostic Techniques in Vascular Surgery" conceals the fact that this is a milestone on the way toward the true science of surgery. The material in this book is as important to the vascular surgeon as his ultimate goal—the perfect anastomosis.

LOUIS R. M. DEL GUERCIO, M.D., F.A.C.S.
Professor and Chairman
Department of Surgery
New York Medical College
Valhalla, New York 10595

Foreword II

Tremendous progress has been made in recent years in vascular surgery, both in diagnostic and therapeutic modalities. The monumental advances of arteriography alone are indicative of the value of the procedure as a diagnostic medium. With the increase in the older age groups in the population requiring vascular surgery has come a similar increase in numbers of diagnostic instruments and procedures. The growth of the noninvasive diagnostic vascular laboratory has led to the development of a number of noninvasive devices utilizing transcutaneous ultrasound, electrical impedance, and electromagnetic measurements for diagnostic purposes.

The ultimate goal of the vascular surgeon is the restoration of a pulsatile blood flow. He frequently needs an evaluation capability intraoperatively and postoperatively as well as preoperatively to assure the success of the procedure. In support of these needs Dr. Lee and coauthors have developed this handbook of vascular test procedures which should help the surgeon select and become familiar with evaluative procedures for specific problems. Dr. Lee and coauthors have prepared this handbook based on their broad clinical and research experience. It contains a wealth of information for the vascular surgeon, for surgical residents and interns as well as for nurses and technicians working in vascular laboratories or with vascular patients. It is equally valuable as a reference for cardiologists and internists treating patients with vascular disease.

CARL W. HUGHES, M.D.
Assistant Chief Medical Director
for Professional Services
Veterans Administration
Washington, D.C. 20420

Preface

The everincreasing number of persons with peripheral vascular disease emphasizes the need for precise methods for the assessment of the vascular system and for the evaluation of a course of surgical-medical treatment. In response to this need, the last seven years have seen a flood of new diagnostic procedures made available to the physician. The 1976 Report of the Inter-Society Commission for Heart Disease Resources—Medical Instrumentation in Peripheral Vascular Disease states that ". . . considerable confidence can now be placed in instrumentation and in the procedures which can be utilized for the objective study of the peripheral vascular system. Proper application of these techniques in a well supervised vascular laboratory or in the physician's office will result in a more precise definition of vascular systems, better identification of patients who may benefit from surgical or medical therapy, and ultimately, a reduction in medical costs." The Commission goes on to say that these procedures ". . . are most important as part of the preoperative, intraoperative, and postoperative management of patients undergoing arterial reconstructive surgery."

The instrumentation available to the physician ranges from being relatively simple and applicable to use in the physician's office to extremely complex and expensive instrumentation that is realistically limited to major referral medical centers. With this abundance of instrumentation, how is the physician to choose what is most appropriate for his office or hospital setting? Where can the physician find, without hours of searching, descriptions of principles, techniques, applications, and interpretations of results in order to make a decision as to which instrumentation is best for the individual physician? And, once one decides on a particular instrumention, who are the suppliers, and who are the most experienced in the field on whom one can rely to make comparisons? These are some of the more frequent questions that have been asked of us. We have unfortunately had to reply that there is currently no one resource that clearly responds to these inquiries. Our collective dissatisfaction with this necessarily negative response led us to the preparation of this manuscript.

We have endeavored to present material in such a manner as to permit the physician at least a basic knowledge of principles, techniques, and application of the available instrumentation. It is our hope that such basic knowledge will allow the physician to make an intelligent decision as to what instrumentation and what tests are most applicable for any particular situation. In doing so, we have made an effort to emphasize the importance of the physician's own senses in carrying out a careful, thorough physical examination that will provide the initial clues as to the patient's problems. We feel that the new, sophisticated instrumentation that has become available should not be taken as a replacement for the qualities that make a good physician, and we have made a concerted effort not to give that impression. The reciprocity of understanding and personal experience is the mainstay for the acquisition of knowledge.

In Chapters 1 and 2 we have attempted to present an expansive dissertation on the taking of a patient history, the initial physical examination, and the more detailed subsequent initial clinical examination of the patient. Our belief in the importance of this aspect of the management of a patient is reflected in its detail. In Chapter 3 we have presented the instrumentation and testing procedures from a mechanical point of view to allow an understanding of how these techniques and instrumentation provide information. In Chapter 4, the step-by-step techniques and the normal results obtained from these techniques are presented. Chapter 5 details the use of the techniques in the evaluation of the systems, discusses what type of results are abnormal, and what such abnormal results mean in terms of associated pathology. Chapter 6 reviews and attempts to place in perspective the traditional techniques of contrast angiography for the visualization of vessels, and the newer noninvasive or semi-invasive techniques for visualization, scanning, and sounding of the vascular system. Chapter 7 presents a discussion of the principles and use of thromboelastography in the evaluation of coagulation dynamics. This technique has important implications in the detection of and management of hypercoagulability, management of heparin administration, and so forth. Chapter 8 details the effect of risk factors on the development of peripheral vascular disease. An understanding of the risk factors associated with vascular disease and their possible elimination or control can provide measures for the prevention of disease. Chapter 9 is most important, as it presents selected case reports showing the use of the previously presented instrumentation in the management of actual disease states.

It is our hope that this text will provide immediate practical information on some of the more useful systems in the laboratory-clinic setting. One of our main objectives is the stimulation of a more generalized use of the currently available techniques in order to provide a more standardized approach to the diagnosis and management of the dysvascular patient.

Acknowledgments

It is with a great deal of pleasure that we the authors express our gratitude to a number of people whose efforts have significantly contributed to the publication of this manual.

Appreciation must be extended to John L. Madden, M.D., for his myriad professional achievements that have inspired us and many of our colleagues and for his ever present support and encouragement during the period of establishing our Clinical Vascular Laboratory and during our continuing quest to provide our patients with state-of-the-art care. Inspiration to pursue this endeavor has also come from our affiliation with New York Medical College and our association and work with Louis R. M. Del Guercio, M.D., Professor and Chairman, Department of Surgery. We also thank Henry M. Dratz, M.D., Medical Center Director, and J. Warren Toff, M.D., Chief of Staff, for their support and their sharing with us the belief in the importance of noninvasive diagnostic techniques in vascular surgery.

A special note of gratitude is due John Vazquez who is in the unenviable position of shouldering the burden of responsibility for maintaining and adapting our noninvasive vascular instrumentation and the preparation of medical illustrations. Also deserving a special note of appreciation is Teresa Geelan for her superb secretarial skills in typing the manuscript and maintaining the project in some degree of order. The work and dedication of these two people have been exemplary and they have consistently produced excellent results even under the most difficult of circumstances. Without their efforts, the completion of the manual would have been a most difficult task.

We also appreciate our vascular technicians, Ouk Chhnor, Bernard Mazer, Janice Roman, Phyllis Berkowitz, and Jane Lewis.

Under the outstanding leadership and guidance of William J. McCann, Jr., M.D., Director of Surgery, New Rochelle Hospital Medical Center, many surgical residents have rotated through the Surgical Service during this time and all have made special contributions for which we are grateful.

Last, but not least, we wish to thank Appleton-Century-Crofts. We are particularly indebted to Robert E. McGrath, David Stires, and Stanley George for their confidence and patience, and to other members of their excellent staff for their efforts in bringing this manual to publication.

Handbook of
NONINVASIVE
DIAGNOSTIC
TECHNIQUES
in VASCULAR
SURGERY

CHAPTER 1

EXAMINATION OF THE PATIENT

GENERAL CONSIDERATIONS

A complete demographic background, history, and physical examination are required for all patients before a diagnosis is made. This is especially important for individuals with vascular disease. No vascular problem is ever a complete and separate entity; attention must be given to any general health problems, particularly in concurrent conditions such as hypertension and diabetes mellitus. The patient's background data should indicate occupation, family history, health habits, and how these factors may have influenced or determined the patient's current status.

1

MEDICAL AND SOCIAL HISTORY

The technique of history taking must be developed. Listen to the patient and learn to pursue clues. Be sure to differentiate information supplied by the patient from the observations made by the examiner. Bear in mind the importance of time-related factors and their relationship to the patient's symptoms. The accuracy of information on events and symptoms and their sequence must be carefully evaluated.

PATIENT BACKGROUND AND DEMOGRAPHIC INFORMATION

This information is important to the total assessment of the individual. It is expected to provide a framework with respect to the patient's lifestyle and the potential effect that it may have had or continues to have on the etiology of the patient's symptoms. It should be made clear to the patient that this information is essential for evaluation and treatment (see Figs. 1-1–1-3).

Date: _____

Name: _____

Address: _____

Telephone Number: _____

Date of Birth: _____ SSN: _____

SOURCE OF INFORMATION

Patient ( )

Relative ( )   Indicate relationship: _____

Friend ( )   Medical Record ( )

Other ( ) _____

INFORMATION ABOUT PERSON CLOSEST TO PATIENT

Relationship: _____

Name: _____

Address: _____

Telephone Number: _____

FIGURE 1-1.   Patient information.

1. Race: White ( )   Black ( )   Oriental ( )   Other: _____
2. Marital Status: Single ( )   Married ( )   Separated ( )   Divorced ( )
   Widowed ( )   Other: _____
3. Religion: _____
4. Living Arrangements: Spouse ( )   Parents ( )   Alone ( )
   Relatives ( )   Friends ( )   Institution ( )   Other: _____
5. Education (number of years): _____
6. Employment: Working ( )   Number of hours/week: _____
   Sick leave ( )   Unemployed ( )   Student ( )   Retired ( )
   Volunteer ( )
7. Housing: Own home ( )   Rented home ( )   Apartment ( )
   Rented room ( )   Mobile home ( )   Health facility ( )
   Other: _____
8. Community: Urban ( )   Suburban ( )   Rural ( )
9. Occupation: _____

FIGURE 1-2.   Demographic data.

FAMILY HISTORY AND MEDICAL HISTORY

A detailed and thorough medical history is required of the patient and of his family. There is a great value in knowing which question to ask and which physical signs to seek. What information is the patient capable of giving? How reliable is this information? How pertinent is it? How useful will it be? Answers to these questions are determined by the manner in which the information is sought. What does the patient have to say? The family history does not necessarily require as much detail as does the patient's own medical history (see Figs. 1-4–1-5).

PRESENT ILLNESSES, COMPLAINTS, SYMPTOMS

Time relationships are most important in making an assessment of a patient's current illnesses, complaints, and/or symptoms. Dates of onset, progression, and/or changes should be carefully documented. All symptoms should be itemized and characterized as to type and severity, and the exact location and factors that aggravate or alleviate the

1. Occupational Physical Activity:

    Sedentary ( ) Regular ( ) Rigorous ( )

2. Daily Exercise Program:

    None ( ) Occasional ( ) Regular ( ) Rigorous ( )

3. Kind of diet: _____ Who prepares food: _____

    Problems with food and meals: _____

4. Alcohol Ingestion: Yes ( ) No ( ) Seldom ( ) Occasional ( )

    Beer ( ) Wine ( ) Hard liquor ( )

5. Current smoking: Yes ( ) No ( )

    Cigarettes ( ) Years ( ) Packs/day _____

    Pipe   ( ) Years ( ) #/day   _____

    Cigars   ( ) Years ( ) #/day   _____

6. Past smoking: Yes ( ) No ( )

    Cigarettes ( ) Years ( ) Packs/day _____

    Pipe   ( ) Years ( ) #/day   _____

    Cigars   ( ) Years ( ) #/day   _____

7. Drug use: Never ( ) Past ( ) Present ( )

8. General lifestyle

    Hobbies: _____

    Recreation: _____

    Sleep cycle: _____

FIGURE 1-3. Health habits.

	Yes	No	Relative
CEREBROVASCULAR			
Insufficiency	( )	( )	_____
Psychiatric disorder	( )	( )	_____
Organic brain syndrome	( )	( )	_____
Stroke	( )	( )	_____

(continued)

FIGURE 1-4. Family history.

	Yes	No	Relative
CARDIOPULMONARY			
Angina pectoris	( )	( )	_____
Arrhythmia	( )	( )	_____
Cardiomegaly	( )	( )	_____
Heart disease	( )	( )	_____
Myocardial infarct	( )	( )	_____
Obstructive pulmonary disease	( )	( )	_____
Pulmonary embolism disease	( )	( )	_____
Pulmonary embolism	( )	( )	_____
Pneumonia	( )	( )	_____
Tuberculosis	( )	( )	_____
Other	( )	( )	_____
VASCULAR DISEASE			
Arterial occlusive disease	( )	( )	_____
Aneurysm	( )	( )	_____
Collagen disease	( )	( )	_____
Hypertension	( )	( )	_____
Hypotension	( )	( )	_____
Neuropathy	( )	( )	_____
Thrombophlebitis	( )	( )	_____
Varicose veins	( )	( )	_____
Other	( )	( )	_____
OTHER DISEASES			
Allergy	( )	( )	_____
Bone and joint	( )	( )	_____
Chronic infection	( )	( )	_____
Endocrine	( )	( )	_____
Diabetes mellitus	( )	( )	_____
Thyroid	( )	( )	_____
Other	( )	( )	_____

(continued)

FIGURE 1-4.   Family history *(continued)*.

	Yes	No	Relative
OTHER DISEASES (cont.)			
Eye	( )	( )	_____
Ear	( )	( )	_____
Nose	( )	( )	_____
Throat	( )	( )	_____
Gastrointestinal	( )	( )	_____
Hematological	( )	( )	_____
Hepatic	( )	( )	_____
Malignancy	( )	( )	_____
Neurological	( )	( )	_____
Renal-genito-urinary	( )	( )	_____
Other	( )	( )	_____
GENERAL			
Major surgical procedures	( )	( )	_____
Injury and disability	( )	( )	_____
Alcohol abuse	( )	( )	_____
Drug abuse	( )	( )	_____
Other	( )	( )	_____

COMMENTS:

FIGURE 1-4.   Family history *(concluded).*

CEREBROVASCULAR DISEASE	Never	Prior	Now	Duration *(Years/Months)*
Insufficiency	( )	( )	( )	_____/_____
Psychiatric disorder	( )	( )	( )	_____/_____
Organic brain syndrome	( )	( )	( )	_____/_____
Stroke	( )	( )	( )	_____/_____

(continued)

FIGURE 1-5.   Medical history.

	Never	Prior	Now	Duration (Years/Months)
CARDIOPULMONARY				
Angina pectoris	( )	( )	( )	_____/_____
Arrhythmia	( )	( )	( )	_____/_____
Cardiomegaly	( )	( )	( )	_____/_____
Heart disease	( )	( )	( )	_____/_____
Myocardial infarct	( )	( )	( )	_____/_____
Obstructive pulmonary	( )	( )	( )	_____/_____
Pulmonary embolism	( )	( )	( )	_____/_____
Pneumonia	( )	( )	( )	_____/_____
Tuberculosis	( )	( )	( )	_____/_____
Other	( )	( )	( )	_____/_____
VASCULAR DISEASE				
Arterial occlusive disease	( )	( )	( )	_____/_____
Aneurysm	( )	( )	( )	_____/_____
Collagen disease	( )	( )	( )	_____/_____
Hypertension	( )	( )	( )	_____/_____
Hypotension	( )	( )	( )	_____/_____
Neuropathy	( )	( )	( )	_____/_____
Thrombophlebitis	( )	( )	( )	_____/_____
Varicose veins	( )	( )	( )	_____/_____
Other	( )	( )	( )	_____/_____
OTHER DISEASES				
Allergy	( )	( )	( )	_____/_____
Bone and joint	( )	( )	( )	_____/_____
Chronic infection	( )	( )	( )	_____/_____
Endocrine	( )	( )	( )	_____/_____
Diabetes mellitus	( )	( )	( )	_____/_____
Thyroid	( )	( )	( )	_____/_____
Other	( )	( )	( )	_____/_____
Eye	( )	( )	( )	_____/_____

(continued)

FIGURE 1-5. Medical history (*continued*).

OTHER DISEASES (cont.)	Never	Prior	Now	Duration (Years/Months)
Ear	( )	( )	( )	_____/_____
Nose	( )	( )	( )	_____/_____
Throat	( )	( )	( )	_____/_____
Gastrointestinal	( )	( )	( )	_____/_____
Hematological	( )	( )	( )	_____/_____
Hepatic	( )	( )	( )	_____/_____
Malignancy	( )	( )	( )	_____/_____
Neurological	( )	( )	( )	_____/_____
Renal-genito-urinary	( )	( )	( )	_____/_____
Other	( )	( )	( )	_____/_____
GENERAL				
Major surgical procedures	( )	( )	( )	_____/_____
Injuries	( )	( )	( )	_____/_____
Disabilities	( )	( )	( )	_____/_____
Alcohol abuse	( )	( )	( )	_____/_____
Drug abuse	( )	( )	( )	_____/_____
Other	( )	( )	( )	_____/_____

COMMENTS: Brief description of any medical problems now present.

FIGURE 1-5.   Medical history (concluded).

symptoms should be identified. The effects of prior and current treatment and the rate and degree of progression should be determined. Evaluation of the disability imposed by the symptoms and an analysis of associated conditions or complaints will facilitate decisions.

To document the nature and the duration of the patient's complaints and symptoms, a checklist should be completed (Fig. 1-6). A more detailed information sheet can then be completed for each complaint and/or symptom (Fig. 1-7).

Suggested Checklist: Does the patient complain of _____?

Does the patient have symptoms of _____?

	Yes	No	Mild	Moderate	Severe
GENERAL					
Chills	( )	( )	( )	( )	( )
Depression	( )	( )	( )	( )	( )
Drowsiness	( )	( )	( )	( )	( )
Insomnia	( )	( )	( )	( )	( )
Libido increase	( )	( )	( )	( )	( )
Libido decrease	( )	( )	( )	( )	( )
Nervousness	( )	( )	( )	( )	( )
Pain	( )	( )	( )	( )	( )
Weakness	( )	( )	( )	( )	( )
Weight gain	( )	( )	( )	( )	( )
Weight loss	( )	( )	( )	( )	( )
HEAD AND NECK					
Blurred vision	( )	( )	( )	( )	( )
Headache	( )	( )	( )	( )	( )
Hearing defect	( )	( )	( )	( )	( )
Nasal congestion	( )	( )	( )	( )	( )
Scotoma	( )	( )	( )	( )	( )
Tinnitus	( )	( )	( )	( )	( )
Vertigo	( )	( )	( )	( )	( )
CHEST AND ABDOMEN					
Abdominal discomfort	( )	( )	( )	( )	( )
Constipation	( )	( )	( )	( )	( )
Diarrhea	( )	( )	( )	( )	( )
Dyspnea	( )	( )	( )	( )	( )
Nausea	( )	( )	( )	( )	( )
Orthopnea	( )	( )	( )	( )	( )
Palpitations	( )	( )	( )	( )	( )
Vomiting	( )	( )	( )	( )	( )

(continued)

FIGURE 1-6.   Present complaints/symptoms.

	Yes	No	Mild	Moderate	Severe
LEGS AND ARMS					
Burning	( )	( )	( )	( )	( )
Coldness	( )	( )	( )	( )	( )
Cramps	( )	( )	( )	( )	( )
Discoloration	( )	( )	( )	( )	( )
Gangrene	( )	( )	( )	( )	( )
Muscle atrophy	( )	( )	( )	( )	( )
Nail changes	( )	( )	( )	( )	( )
Numbness	( )	( )	( )	( )	( )
Pallor	( )	( )	( )	( )	( )
Pain	( )	( )	( )	( )	( )
Rest pain	( )	( )	( )	( )	( )
Rubor	( )	( )	( )	( )	( )
Sensitivity	( )	( )	( )	( )	( )
Swelling	( )	( )	( )	( )	( )
Tenderness	( )	( )	( )	( )	( )
Ulceration	( )	( )	( )	( )	( )
Varicose veins	( )	( )	( )	( )	( )
SKIN AND OTHERS					
Ataxia	( )	( )	( )	( )	( )
Atrophic shiny skin	( )	( )	( )	( )	( )
Epistaxis	( )	( )	( )	( )	( )
Gynecomastia	( )	( )	( )	( )	( )
Mens irreg.	( )	( )	( )	( )	( )
Muscle spasm	( )	( )	( )	( )	( )
Nicotine stains	( )	( )	( )	( )	( )
Petechiae	( )	( )	( )	( )	( )
Photosensitivity	( )	( )	( )	( )	( )
Rash	( )	( )	( )	( )	( )
Other	( )	( )	( )	( )	( )

FIGURE 1-6.   Present complaints/symptoms (*concluded*).

To obtain further details relating to the patient's complaints and symptoms, the following information should be obtained for each:

1. Complaint/Symptom: _____

2. Location: Right ( )   Left ( )

      Medial ( )   Lateral ( )   Dorsal ( )   Ventral ( )

      Finger ( )   Toe   ( )   Head ( )

      Hand   ( )   Foot ( )   Neck ( )

      Wrist   ( )   Ankle ( )   Back ( )

      Forearm ( ) Leg   ( )   Other _____

      Elbow   ( )   Knee ( )

      Arm   ( )   Thigh ( )

      Shoulder ( ) Hip   ( )

3. Onset: Sudden ( )   Gradual ( )

4. Duration: Days _____.   Weeks _____.   Months _____.

      Years _____.

5. Frequency: (times per)   Day _____.

      Week _____.   Month _____.   Year _____.

6. Temporal pattern:

      Continuous ( )   Intermittent ( )   Day ( )   Night ( )

      None ( )

7. Course: Static ( )   Improved ( )   Worse ( )   Fluctuates ( )

8. Interferes with: Sleep ( )   Work ( )   Exercise ( )   Other _____.

9. Factors which influence (aggravates/relieves/no effect):

      Activity _____

      Cold _____

      Dependency _____

      Elevation _____

      Emotions _____

      Exercise _____

      Heat _____

      Menses _____

      Pressure _____

      Rest _____

(continued)

FIGURE 1-7.   Details of complaints and symptoms.

9. Factors which influence (aggravates/relieves/no effect (*cont.*):

    Vibration _____

    Weather changes _____

    Other (including Rx) _____

10. Descriptive comments:

FIGURE 1-7.   Details of complaints and symptoms *(concluded)*.

PHYSICAL EXAMINATION

For a thorough systematic physical examination, appropriate work conditions are important. A comfortable, well-lighted working area should be provided with adequate work space and privacy for the patient. A well-organized program with appropriate data forms and personnel can mean the difference between success or failure (see Figs. 1-8–1-13).

In preparing the patient for examination, establish when the last food and alcoholic beverages were ingested; when the last cigarette, cigar, or pipe had been smoked; what form of exercise had been undertaken during the past week; what mode of transportation was used, and how far the patient walked to arrive at the clinic or office; and whether the patient is apprehensive or anxious.

Name: _____ Date: _____ Time: _____

Room temperature _____°C

Height: _____cm Weight: _____kg Temp. _____°C

Pulse Rate: _____/min.   Respiratory rate: _____/min.

Blood Pressure (mm Hg):

    Right arm: _____ Left arm: _____

General Appearance and Mental Status: (Describe with respect to orientation, memory, mood consciousness. Give initial impression of patient's physiologic age, coordination, and cooperation.)

FIGURE 1-8.   Vital signs, general appearance, and mental status.

	Normal	Abnormal	Not Examined	Explanation of Abnormalities
HEAD				
Skull	( )	( )	( )	_____
Scalp	( )	( )	( )	_____
NECK				
Appearance	( )	( )	( )	_____
Masses	( )	( )	( )	_____
Range motion	( )	( )	( )	_____
Thyroid	( )	( )	( )	_____
Trachea	( )	( )	( )	_____
EYES				
Eyelids	( )	( )	( )	_____
Conjunctivae	( )	( )	( )	_____
Cornea	( )	( )	( )	_____
Sclera	( )	( )	( )	_____
Lens	( )	( )	( )	_____
Pupils	( )	( )	( )	_____
Fundi	( )	( )	( )	_____
Movements	( )	( )	( )	_____
Vision	( )	( )	( )	_____
EARS				
Acuity	( )	( )	( )	_____
External ear	( )	( )	( )	_____
Canals	( )	( )	( )	_____
Drums	( )	( )	( )	_____
NOSE				
External	( )	( )	( )	_____
Mucosa	( )	( )	( )	_____
Septum	( )	( )	( )	_____
Turbinates	( )	( )	( )	_____

(continued)

FIGURE 1-9.   Systems examination.

	Normal	Abnormal	Not Examined	Explanation of Abnormalities
MOUTH – THROAT				
Lips	( )	( )	( )	_____
Breath	( )	( )	( )	_____
Teeth	( )	( )	( )	_____
Gums	( )	( )	( )	_____
Tongue	( )	( )	( )	_____
Mucosa	( )	( )	( )	_____
Tonsils	( )	( )	( )	_____
Pharynx	( )	( )	( )	_____
Glands	( )	( )	( )	_____
Speech	( )	( )	( )	_____
CHEST – BREAST				
Thorax	( )	( )	( )	_____
Movements	( )	( )	( )	_____
Masses	( )	( )	( )	_____
Nipples	( )	( )	( )	_____
Chest x-ray	( )	( )	( )	_____
PA	( )	( )	( )	_____
Lateral	( )	( )	( )	_____
LUNGS				
Percussion	( )	( )	( )	_____
Sounds	( )	( )	( )	_____
Inspiration	( )	( )	( )	_____
Expiration	( )	( )	( )	_____
HEART				
Impulse	( )	( )	( )	_____
Palpation	( )	( )	( )	_____
Rhythm	( )	( )	( )	_____
Auscultation	( )	( )	( )	_____

(continued)

FIGURE 1-9. Systems examination (continued).

	Normal	Abnormal	Not Examined	Explanation of Abnormalities
VASCULAR				
Pulses	( )	( )	( )	_____
Carotid	( )	( )	( )	_____
Radial	( )	( )	( )	_____
Femoral	( )	( )	( )	_____
Popliteal	( )	( )	( )	_____
Posterior tibial	( )	( )	( )	_____
Dorsalis pedis	( )	( )	( )	_____
Neck veins	( )	( )	( )	_____
Peripheral veins	( )	( )	( )	_____
ABDOMEN				
Wall	( )	( )	( )	_____
Distension	( )	( )	( )	_____
Tenderness	( )	( )	( )	_____
Liver	( )	( )	( )	_____
Spleen	( )	( )	( )	_____
Kidneys	( )	( )	( )	_____
Hernia	( )	( )	( )	_____
GENITALIA				
Male:				
Penis	( )	( )	( )	_____
Scrotum	( )	( )	( )	_____
Testes	( )	( )	( )	_____
Epididymis	( )	( )	( )	_____
Inguinal canal	( )	( )	( )	_____
Female:				
External	( )	( )	( )	_____
Urethra	( )	( )	( )	_____
Vagina	( )	( )	( )	_____
Cervix	( )	( )	( )	_____

(continued)

FIGURE 1-9.   Systems examination (continued).

	Normal	Abnormal	Not Examined	Explanation of Abnormalities
GENITALIA (cont.)				
Female (cont.):				
Uterus	( )	( )	( )	_____
Adnexa	( )	( )	( )	_____
RECTUM AND PROSTATE				
Anus	( )	( )	( )	_____
Sphincter	( )	( )	( )	_____
Rectum	( )	( )	( )	_____
Prostate	( )	( )	( )	_____
BACK				
Configuration	( )	( )	( )	_____
Mobility	( )	( )	( )	_____
Tenderness	( )	( )	( )	_____
EXTREMITIES				
Muscles	( )	( )	( )	_____
Joints	( )	( )	( )	_____
Edema	( )	( )	( )	_____
Ambulation	( )	( )	( )	_____
Coordination	( )	( )	( )	_____
Amputation	( )	( )	( )	_____
Deformities	( )	( )	( )	_____
NEUROLOGICAL				
Cranial nerves	( )	( )	( )	_____
Peripheral nerves	( )	( )	( )	_____
Reflexes	( )	( )	( )	_____
Biceps	( )	( )	( )	_____
Triceps	( )	( )	( )	_____
Patellar	( )	( )	( )	_____
Achilles	( )	( )	( )	_____
Plantar	( )	( )	( )	_____

(continued)

FIGURE 1-9.   Systems examination (*continued*).

	Normal	Abnormal	Not Examined	Explanation of Abnormalities
SKIN				
Texture	( )	( )	( )	_____
Turgor	( )	( )	( )	_____
Lesions	( )	( )	( )	_____
Hair	( )	( )	( )	_____
Nails	( )	( )	( )	_____
LYMPHATICS				
Nodes	( )	( )	( )	_____
Cervical	( )	( )	( )	_____
Axillary	( )	( )	( )	_____
Inguinal	( )	( )	( )	_____

Signature: _____ Title: _____

FIGURE 1-9. Systems examination (concluded).

	Absent		Mild		Moderate		Severe	
	Right	Left	Right	Left	Right	Left	Right	Left
Intermittent claudication	( )	( )	( )	( )	( )	( )	( )	( )
Cramp	( )	( )	( )	( )	( )	( )	( )	( )
Tightness	( )	( )	( )	( )	( )	( )	( )	( )
Tiredness	( )	( )	( )	( )	( )	( )	( )	( )
Pain	( )	( )	( )	( )	( )	( )	( )	( )
Coldness	( )	( )	( )	( )	( )	( )	( )	( )
Paresthesia	( )	( )	( )	( )	( )	( )	( )	( )
Trophic skin changes	( )	( )	( )	( )	( )	( )	( )	( )

(continued)

FIGURE 1-10. Initial evaluation of signs/symptoms of vascular disease.

	Absent		Mild		Moderate		Severe	
	Right	Left	Right	Left	Right	Left	Right	Left
PULSES								
Carotid	( )	( )	( )	( )	( )	( )	( )	( )
Subclavian	( )	( )	( )	( )	( )	( )	( )	( )
Brachial	( )	( )	( )	( )	( )	( )	( )	( )
Radial	( )	( )	( )	( )	( )	( )	( )	( )
Ulnar	( )	( )	( )	( )	( )	( )	( )	( )
Abdominal	( )	( )	( )	( )	( )	( )	( )	( )
Aorta	( )	( )	( )	( )	( )	( )	( )	( )
Iliac	( )	( )	( )	( )	( )	( )	( )	( )
Femoral	( )	( )	( )	( )	( )	( )	( )	( )
Popliteal	( )	( )	( )	( )	( )	( )	( )	( )
Dorsalis pedis	( )	( )	( )	( )	( )	( )	( )	( )
Posterior tibial	( )	( )	( )	( )	( )	( )	( )	( )
Elevation rubor	( )	( )	( )	( )	( )	( )	( )	( )
Elevation pallor	( )	( )	( )	( )	( )	( )	( )	( )
Delay in return of color to the skin	( )	( )	( )	( )	( )	( )	( )	( )
Skin appearance	( )	( )	( )	( )	( )	( )	( )	( )
Venous filling time	( )	( )	( )	( )	( )	( )	( )	( )

FIGURE 1-10. Initial evaluation of signs/symptoms of vascular disease *(concluded)*.

It is especially important for the patient to be aware that for an initial examination which will include a careful examination of the vasculature, there should be little or no food and alcohol for eight hours, and no smoking for at least two hours prior to the examination; if it is cold he should dress warmly and acclimate to the room temperature before the examination.

The role played by the examiner is very important and should include the careful use of one's eyes, ears, and fingers in examining the patient. Observations should be accurately reported by all persons coming in contact with the patient (physician, assistant(s), nurse(s), technician(s), and trainee(s).

CURRENT: Yes ( )   No ( )

	Name	Dose	Schedule	Duration	Reason for Treatment
1.	___	___	___	___	___
2.	___	___	___	___	___
3.	___	___	___	___	___

PRIOR: Yes ( )   No ( )

	Name	Dose	Schedule	Duration	Reason for Treatment
1.	___	___	___	___	___
2.	___	___	___	___	___
3.	___	___	___	___	___

COMMENTS:

FIGURE 1-11.   Current treatment and medication schedule.

OPHTHALMIC EXAMINATION

	Left Eye 20/		Right Eye 20/	
VISUAL ACUITY	Normal	Abnormal	Normal	Abnormal
Visual fields	( )	( )	( )	( )
Fundi	( )	( )	( )	( )
Ophthalmoscopy	( )	( )	( )	( )
Ophthalmodynamometry	( )	( )	( )	( )
SPLIT LAMP EXAMINATION				
Anterior chamber	( )	( )	( )	( )
Posterior chamber	( )	( )	( )	( )
Iris	( )	( )	( )	( )

(continued)

FIGURE 1-12.   Ophthalmic and auditory examinations.

OPHTHALMIC EXAMINATION (cont.)

	Left Eye 20/		Right Eye 20/	
	Present	*Absent*	*Present*	*Absent*
Pupillary light reflex	( )	( )	( )	( )
	None	*Present*	*None*	*Present*
Corneal opacity	( )	( )	( )	( )
Lens	( )	( )	( )	( )

AUDITORY EXAMINATION

AUDITORY ACUITY

EAR	*500*	*1000*	*2000*	*3000*	*4000*	*6000*
Right						
Left						

Tinnitus: absent   ( )   present   ( )

Hearing: normal   ( )   abnormal   ( )

COMMENTS:

FIGURE 1-12.   Ophthalmic and auditory examination (*concluded*).

HEMATOLOGY

	Value	Unit
Hemoglobin	_____	gm%
Hematocrit	_____	%
RBC ($\times 10^6$)	_____	mm^{-3}
WBC ($\times 10^3$)	_____	mm^{-3}

DIFFERENTIAL:

Segmented neutrophils	_____	%
Lymphocytes	_____	%
Monocytes	_____	%

(continued)

FIGURE 1-13.   Clinical laboratory examination.

HEMATOLOGY (cont.)

DIFFERENTIAL (cont.)	Value	Unit
Eosinophils	_____	%
Basophils	_____	%
Bands	_____	%
Other:	_____	_____
	_____	_____

BIOCHEMISTRY

	Value	Unit
Calcium	_____	mg%
Phosphorus	_____	mg%
Glucose (fasting)	_____	mg%
BUN	_____	mg%
Uric acid	_____	mg%
Total protein	_____	G%
Albumin	_____	G%
Total bilirubin	_____	mg%
Direct bilirubin	_____	mg%
Alkaline phosphatase	_____	u/L
LDH	_____	u/L
SGOT	_____	u/L
SGPT	_____	u/L
CPK	_____	u/L
CO_2	_____	mEq/l
Na	_____	mEq/l
K	_____	mEq/l
Cl	_____	mEq/l
Creatinine	_____	mg%
Cholesterol	_____	mg%
LDL	_____	mg%
HDL	_____	mg%
Triglycerides	_____	mg%
Other:		

(continued)

FIGURE 1-13.   Clinical laboratory examination (continued).

URINALYSIS

Specific gravity

pH	Acid ( )	Neutral ( )	Alkaline ( )
Protein	Neg ( )	Trace ( )	Positive ( )
Sugar	Neg ( )	Trace ( )	Positive ( )
Ketones	Neg ( )	Trace ( )	Positive ( )

MICROSCOPIC EXAMINATION OF SEDIMENT

	None	Rare	Occa-sional	Few	Moder-ate	Many	Count
WBC/hpf	( )	( )	( )	( )	( )	( )	( )
RBC/hpf	( )	( )	( )	( )	( )	( )	( )
Epithelial cells	( )	( )	( )	( )	( )	( )	( )
CASTS							
Hyaline	( )	( )	( )	( )	( )	( )	( )
Granular	( )	( )	( )	( )	( )	( )	( )
Red cell	( )	( )	( )	( )	( )	( )	( )
White cell	( )	( )	( )	( )	( )	( )	( )
Bacteria	( )	( )	( )	( )	( )	( )	( )
Other:							

FIGURE 1-13.   Clinical laboratory examination (*concluded*).

CHAPTER 2

INITIAL CLINICAL EVALUATION

GENERAL APPEARANCE
INSPECTION AND OBSERVATION
- Size, Symmetry, Atrophy
- Skin Color and Texture
- Ulceration and Gangrene
- Edema
- Peripheral Pulsations
- Peripheral Sounds
- Surface Temperature
- Pain and Fatigue
FUNCTIONAL TESTS
- Position Tests
- Assessment of Skin Surface Temperature
- Compression Maneuvers
- Walking Tests
- Palpation of Arteries and Veins

It is essential that clinical skills be developed by which the examiner can identify and evaluate patients with vascular disorders.

The physician's diagnosis of a patient's disorder depends upon an accurate collection of data and its analysis. Errors leading to a mistaken diagnosis may occur in either step: the correct analysis of a faulty set of data leads to an erroneous conclusion as does a faulty analysis of an accurate set of data.

A physician's clinical evaluation of a patient does not lend itself to quantification as does the physical examination. For example, in a physical examination, height, weight, and blood pressure can be easily measured. In a clinical evaluation, however, pain, changes in skin color or texture, or body sounds are not quantifiable. Even in evaluating arterial pulses, which can be assigned numbers, a 4$^+$ pulse evaluation by one physician may be interpreted as a 3$^+$ pulse by another. In most instances the patient's clinical manifestations are dimensionless. Frequently, however, facts from the physical examination that can be expressed numerically are of less diagnostic significance than facts from the clinical evaluation that cannot be expressed numerically.

Data obtained from a clinical evaluation are of two types: symptoms, which are the patient's personal observations of his condition as related to the physician; and signs, abnormalities detected by the physician. In the interpretation of a patient's symptoms or signs, the physician should follow three steps: (1) listen to and understand the patient's symptoms or signs; (2) specify the symptom or sign as to location and character; and (3) give a name to the patient's complaint. For example, a patient may present to the physician with the symptom of a headache. The physician specifies the patient's complaint of a headache as being a throbbing pain in the right side of the head. With these facts in mind the physician can name the patient's complaint as a migraine.

As with more general disease states, it is essential that the physician carefully develop his skill in clinically evaluating a patient for peripheral vascular disease.

GENERAL APPEARANCE

In the initial evaluation, general impressions should be acquired in a systematic way. The examiner should obtain clues (by seeing, hearing, feeling, and sensing) which will be guidelines for decision-making with respect to the individual's signs, symptoms, and/or complaints.

The functional test procedures are utilized to provide information with respect to the nutritional blood supply available to the skin and muscle. This information complements and supplements that obtained through the medical history and physical examination and helps justify the decision to seek further laboratory tests.

All observations should be accurately recorded. The first question to be asked is the individual's physiologic age. The examiner should be able to determine this based on a general impression of the individual's alertness, eye appearance, facial and hair texture, and body size, structure, and posture.

INSPECTION AND OBSERVATION

The initial inspection involves: (1) carefully documented observations of the skin and extremities, and (2) critical assessment of temperature, pulsations, audible blood flow sounds, and degree of pain and fatigue.

SIZE, SYMMETRY, ATROPHY

The relative size of the extremities and any evidence of asymmetry should be noted. Signs of atrophy are generally evident as follows:

1. The *nails* may be brittle, deformed, stunted and thickened
2. The *hair* may be lusterless, thin, and totally absent from areas of the extremities
3. The *skin* may be tight and waxy, or scaly and dry with fine cracks and wrinkles
4. The *muscles* of the extremities may be flabby and wasted

In making these observations, the site and location of signs and symptoms should be clearly indicated.

SKIN COLOR AND TEXTURE

Careful observations of skin color, especially that of the extremities, can furnish important clues with respect to peripheral circulation. Skin color is ultimately determined by the status of the major arteries and veins and the oxygen saturation of the microvascular beds. The capillary beds are influenced by neuromuscular control of arterioles and veins, that is, normal sympathetic tone. In a warm environment, blood to normal light skin will produce a healthy pink color, whereas that of more pigmented skin will produce various shades of healthy gold and brown hues. Inspection of the skin should be done in well-lighted, comfortable surroundings free of drafts and temperature changes. Final evaluation of skin color should be made relative to the information obtained during the physical examination.

A number of terms are used in describing skin color that are of significance in distinguishing the specific disease entity. *Pallor* is associated with blanching, which occurs when the microvessels constrict, and is a common finding in vasomotor and vascular disorders.

Cyanosis describes a bluish, dusky discoloration of the skin resulting from insufficient oxygenation of the blood and tissues. A careful distinction should be made with respect to the characteristics of cyanosis. *Generalized cyanosis* can occur in the presence of subnormal arterial oxygen saturation often present during respiratory and/or cardiac failure. *Localized cyanosis* reflects slowed circulation to an area resulting from vasospasm, drainage impairment, and local pooling in the minute vessels. *Transient cyanosis* is often observed as one of a sequence of color changes occurring in occlusive vascular disease. *Persistent localized cyanosis* is frequently associated with a severe vascular disturbance, and the combination of *rapidly developing, persistent cyanosis* plus a *cold extremity* generally implies impending gangrene.

Myriads of discrete dilated venous channels of varying widths and lengths present a *cyanotic or blue discoloration* typical of venous disease.

Rubor is a deep reddish hue that develops when the affected foot is maintained in a dependent position.

Erythema refers to redness. Like cyanosis, it can be observed in varying shades and patterns both in the upper and lower extremities; e.g., pallor may be observed when a limb is elevated, may persist for a few seconds when the limb is in a dependent position, and then a redness appears which may deepen to a purple hue, indicating a pooling in the minute vessels. Other patterns of redness can occur that are not due to vascular disease and note should be made of associated incidences related to strictly a skin condition.

Stasis pigmentation is a characteristic sign of chronic venous insufficiency; the skin below the knees and especially about the ankles will bear a constant light-brown or very dark discoloration.

Certain characteristic skin features are also associated with disturbances of the venous circulation. Especially in light-skinned individuals, the superficial veins are generally quite evident below the skin surface. Determine whether there are increased numbers of veins. These may be evident especially in the groin, the lower anterior and lateral aspects of the abdomen, the pectoral region, and over the shoulders. The increased number of vessels in these regions indicates occlusion of main vessels.

With the patient in a standing position, a careful inspection can determine the presence or absence of varicose veins. Primary varicose veins, which develop in the branches of the long and short saphenous veins, are visible as dilated, tortuous venous channels. Secondary varicose veins appear in atypical locations as short distended venous segments, and are the result of deep venous occlusion or arteriovenous fistula. The skin should also be inspected for discoloration, pigmentation, and ulceration, usually in areas of *cord-like veins*. Dilation of small skin vessels, microvarices, may often be evident in the region of the medial malleolus.

Assessment of the texture and consistency of the skin and subcutaneous tissues helps to determine the status of the peripheral circulation. Generally firm, elastic skin and subcutaneous tissues indicate good nutrition, whereas large areas of soft, flabby tissues imply impaired blood supply. Poor arterial flow for long periods of time leads to trophic changes.

Check the nails of the fingers and toes. Characteristic of chronic arterial disease is a pile-up of debris under the nails with evidence of poor growth, deformity, and brittleness. Remember that fungal infections, bacteria, drugs, nicotine, systemic disorders, and trauma can produce changes in nail color and texture.

The feet should be inspected for the presence of calluses over weight-bearing regions and corns in areas subjected to friction. The skin of the toes, soles, and heels should be checked for the presence of fissuring, since this can lead to areas of infection and ulceration.

ULCERATION AND GANGRENE

Once the skin has been inspected for trophic changes, look for old scars, lost digits, and healed ulcers, which often are covered by thin, parchment-like skin. Look for evidence of superficial patches of ulceration, gangrene, or more extensive involvement. Although most ulcerations are secondary to peripheral vascular disease, some are secondary to dermatologic, endocrine, hematologic, and other systemic diseases.

Three common types of chronic ulceration (ischemic, stasis, and neuropathic) are frequently encountered in the lower extremities. Generally a series of five sets of observations permits an accurate determination of the etiology of the ulcer: (1) *location*—dorsum of the foot, on the toes, under a callus, at a pressure point, some other location on the extremity; (2) *characteristic features*—shape of the ulcer, appearance of the edges, presence of granulation tissue, depth of the ulcer and color of the tissues; (3) *pain*—no pain, mild, severe, relieved when limb is elevated, occurs especially at night and prevents sleep, is relieved when limb is placed in a dependent position; (4) *manipulation*—movement does or does not cause bleeding, how much and what is its appearance; and (5) *associated findings*—trophic changes, stasis dermatitis, or neuropathy.

Gangrene is obvious if the skin is black, shriveled, dry, and hard. Prior to these changes there may have been a deep purple-black cyanosis. Gangrene progresses from the distal to proximal tissues. Thermal injury, pressure necrosis, sensitization to medications applied to the skin and hypertension can cause superficial gangrene.

Ulceration and gangrene should be accurately documented. This is best done by using a standard format for describing the lesion, making a diagram including measurements, and obtaining a color photograph. An accurate history should be taken including time and manner of occurrence, duration, and prior treatment.

EDEMA

The term *edema* usually refers to an excessive accumulation of fluid in the tissues. High venous pressure is the most frequent cause of edema. This increase in pressure can be caused by one or more of the following: intrinsic venous obstruction due to external compression of iliac veins or peripheral vein thrombosis, incompetent venous valves that allow an unopposed transmission of gravitational pressure, right-sided heart failures, and venous hypertension secondary to arteriovenous fistula. In fact any event that increases capillary permeability or interferes with removal of fluid by lymphatic vessels will cause edema. During motionless standing an ankle venous pressure of 80 to 100 mm Hg can be measured; however, as long as the venomotor pump mechanism is competent, intermittent shifting of body weight can reduce this pressure to 20 to 30 mm Hg.

Four types of regional edema are most often encountered in the clinics: edema due to chronic venous insufficiency, orthostatic edema, lymphedema, and lipedema.

An accurate description of the swollen limb or portions of the extremity and the patient's complaints is necessary for a clinical diagnosis.

In evaluating the edema, six categories of observations can be utilized:

1. *Consistency of the swelling*—browny, spongy, pitting, or noncompressible
2. *Location and distribution of the swelling*—diffuse or marked in one or more areas of the feet, hands, ankles, legs, arms
3. *Effect of elevation on the swelling*—completely relieves it, mild relief, or none
4. *Associated skin changes*—none, atrophic, trophic, pigmented, shiny, fibrotic, ulcerated
5. *Pain accompanying the edema*—a heavy ache, a tight, almost bursting feeling, dull ache, little or no pain, sensitive skin
6. *Bilateralism*—both extremities equally or unequally affected

PERIPHERAL PULSATIONS

An essential step in vascular evaluation is a systematic bilateral examination of peripheral pulses. Pulses detected at the periphery represent the rhythmic expansions of elastic arteries which are synchronous with the heart beat. Application of light pressure by the fingers to the surface of the body, which is called palpation, provides a means for determining the characteristics of the structures beneath the surface.

Visual pulsations are often observed along the course of main arteries (Fig. 2-1). When pulsations are observed in the extremities, flexion of the limb may cause the visible artery to assume a tortuous path. Aneurysmal dilations, if present, are often palpated in the neck and groin areas and behind the lower thigh and knee. The peripheral pulses generally accessible for palpation are: (1) *carotids* in the neck; (2) *brachial, radial,* and *ulnar*, in the upper extremities; and (3) *femoral, popliteal, posterior tibial*, and *dorsalis pedis* in the lower extremities. Peripheral arteries are evaluated with respect to the presence or absence of pulsation, the force of the pulsation, the degree of vessel elasticity, and the presence or absence of beating of the arterial wall.

A strong pulsation generally means good circulation at the site of palpation, whereas a diminished pulsation indicates a possible obstruction. When a previously forceful pulsation appears diminished, development of an occlusion can be suspected. Absence of a palpable pulse can be interpreted as diminished perfusion of an artery due to proximal obstruction, actual obstruction at the site of palpation, or the presence of an anatomical anomaly or malformation. Sudden disappearance of a previously palpable pulse can mean an embolic or thrombotic occlusion present at or proximal to the site of palpation.

Thus, when evaluating pulses it is essential to keep in perspective the medical history and total physical examination, since lack or diminution of a palpable pulse in an accessible artery can mean one or more of the following:

1. The artery is obstructed at or proximal to the site of palpation
2. A diminished palpable pulse can disappear following exercise and the time for return of the pulsations indicates the degree of proximal obstruction
3. Palpable pulses can disappear due to vasoconstriction secondary to hypovolemia and inadequate cardiac output
4. Previously palpable pulses can disappear as a result of either obstructive trauma to arteries or through possibly inappropriate use of vasoactive drugs

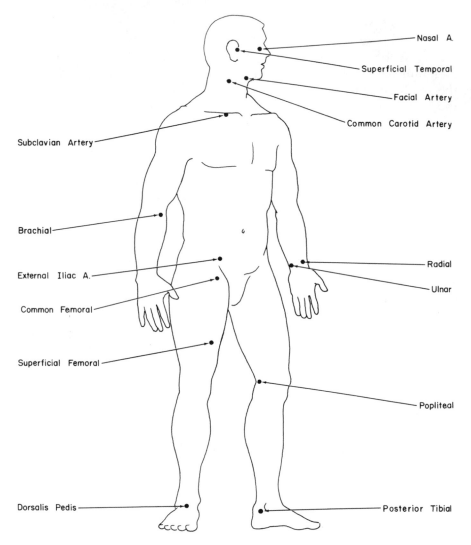

FIGURE 2-1. Arteries generally accessible for palpation.

5. Detection of a palpable pulse in an unusual location can indicate presence of collateral vessels that have developed around a slowly developing occlusion

6. Abnormal pulsations can be associated with arteriovenous fistulae and arterial aneurysms

PERIPHERAL SOUNDS

Auscultation is a term derived from the Latin *auscultatis*, from the verb *auscultare*, to listen to. It is most often done with the aid of a stethoscope. The placement of the bell of the stethoscope at the same sites on the periphery as those for palpation of arteries and veins allows the detection of sounds, if present, identified as bruits, hums, murmurs, and thrills.

A *bruit* may be a soft, short "whishing" or blowing sound often heard over an aneurysm. A *systolic bruit* is an abnormal sound occurring with systole of the heart. A bruit that is noisy and extends through the cardiac cycle with emphasis on systole most often indicates an arteriovenous fistula. With compression of the proximal vein the sound will be heard only in systole.

A *murmur* is usually characterized as a gentle blowing sound. A continuous murmur or bruit is often heard in partially obstructed arteries where there is a continuous flow through the partially obstructed segment during diastole. *Systolic murmurs* may be heard at the point of partial obstruction, as in thoracic outlet syndrome with external compression to the subclavian and axillary arteries. Systolic murmurs are usually heard in partially obstructed carotid, femoral, iliac, and renal arteries.

A *hum* is an indistinct, low, prolonged sound. *Venous hum* is a continuous, blowing, singing, or humming murmur heard over the right jugular vein in anemia, chlorosis, and occasionally in good health. This hum is also called *bruit de diable* or *humming tap* sound. Compression of the veins diminishes the intensity of the hum.

Thrill is a tremor or vibration both heard and felt. An *aneurysmal thrill* is a vibratory sensation felt on palpation of an aneurysm. *Systolic thrill* is felt on systole over the precordium in aortic stenosis, pulmonary stenosis, and aneurysm of the ascending aorta.

SURFACE TEMPERATURE

The temperature of the skin surface varies depending on the heat brought by the blood and the heat lost from its surface. Systemic temperature remains relatively constant. The skin surface temperature can vary several degrees from one area to another, with the widest variations occurring in the most peripheral parts. Changes in the caliber of the blood vessels of the digits permit a wide range of blood flow, thus, the temperature of the digits can vary from that of air to nearly that of the body core temperature.

Exposure to ambient temperatures, the presence of layers of fat over capillary areas, and local circulation patterns all influence the distribution of skin surface temperature. Since the heat reaching the skin surface is dependent on the rate of local cutaneous blood flow. the skin surface temperature can provide a qualitative index of cutaneous circulation.

PAIN AND FATIGUE

A painful extremity is perhaps the most common symptom that brings the patient to the physician. Vascular disease can cause several types of pain and it is essential to differentiate them. Initially the examiner should establish the patient's pain threshold and through a series of questions obtain an accurate description of the pain (Fig. 2-2). The conditions contributing to the pain and those situations in which the pain persists should be determined. An important point to remember is that an individual may not seek help if the pain is not too severe and/or sustained. Thus, the diminution and lack of pulses are not determined until much later when pain is more acute or the individual is examined for other reasons.

---

1. Do you never/usually/always tolerate a great deal of pain?

2. Does the distress described disable you? If yes, how does it disable you?

3. What activities have you had to decrease or stop?

4. Is your job affected by the distress and discomfort? Describe.

5. Would you characterize the distress as annoying rather than disabling? Or both?

6. In order to alleviate the discomfort or pain do you shift your weight or do you get off your feet?

7. Do you experience the same discomfort or pain at rest/sitting/at night in bed?

8. Does the discomfort or pain appear as soon as you exercise or after a period of time? How long?

9. Does the pain or discomfort persist for longer than 10 minutes after stopping the exercise?

FIGURE 2-2.   Typical questions used to determine the patient's pain threshold.

Some characteristic features of the pain of vascular disease help to differentiate the pain and to determine its source.

1. *An acute arterial occlusion* presents a pain that often occurs abruptly, is severe, and may cause the extremity to be weak; if it is a leg it might actually "give way." This pain may subside rather quickly, especially when collateral vessels are mobilized, or it may become

2. *The pain of chronic arterial insufficiency.* A combination of symptoms, such as numbness, coldness, tingling, and even total paresis, may be described; gradually these merge into the pain of ischemic neuropathy, pretrophic, or rest pain. For the lower extremity, the degree of arterial insufficiency will determine the type of pain (intermittent or persistent).

3. *Intermittent claudication* (from the Latin *claudicatio*, to limp) is the most frequent symptom presented for arterial insufficiency of the lower extremity. It is brought on by exercise and relieved by discrete rest. The term is used to classify aching, cramping, tiredness, and tightness. This distress is always induced by exercise and completely relieved by standing with weight on both feet. A constant amount of exercise at a constant rate will reproduce the symptoms. If the rate of exercise is increased the distress occurs sooner and if the walking distance that is required to bring about the distress becomes less, progression of the disease is indicated. A rapid and sudden increase in distress implies acute occlusion of a main or collateral arteries.

The level and degree of arterial occlusion will determine the location of the pain, which can appear in the buttock, thigh, calf, and/or ankle. The pain described for the calf is usually a cramp brought on by exercise and relieved by a few minutes of rest. It is generally caused by a block in the superficial femoral artery. Buttock and thigh claudication does not produce severe cramping muscle pain as often as a sensation of aching discomfort and weakness, and numbness when sitting. Foot claudication may exist alone if only distal arteries are involved. It also occurs in thromboangiitis obliterans. A cramp in the forefoot when walking, a wooden sensation, numbness, or cold feet at night are terms frequently used to describe foot claudication. These symptoms may also be associated with ischemic rest pain.

4. *Ischemic rest pain* can be a demoralizing type of pain for which even large amounts of narcotics produce no relief. This pain is confined to the more distal parts of the extremity and can be localized or centered about an ulcerated or gangrenous toe or area. Pain is constant and is often aggravated by elevation of the part and by cold. This persistent type of pain prevents sleeping and even eating becomes a chore. Painful toes may be relieved by placing the foot in the dependent position; however, this position can produce edema of the extremity, compounding the problem.

5. The pain of *ischemic neuropathy* is more diffuse and paroxysmal. The pain can extend from the toes to the mid-calf and is described as sharp and shooting from one end of the extremity to the other. It is usually asymmetric depending on the site of occlusion and is less influenced by position and temperature changes. *Diabetic neuropathy* differs from ischemic neuropathy in that it is bilaterally symmetrical and always associated with diabetes mellitus. Peripheral pulses are usually absent and rubor and trophic skin changes are evident.

6. Patients with *primary varicose veins* often complain of pulling, pricking, burning, and tingling sensations associated with the veins as well as a diffuse sensation of heaviness and fatigue. These complaints are usually relieved when the limbs are elevated. *Venous thrombosis* in the lower extremity may cause no pain unless there is inflammation, which produces localized tenderness along the course of the involved vein. At some time in the postphlebitic period, swelling may occur accompanied by an aching discomfort and a tight, heavy sensation aggravated by standing and relieved by elevation.

7. The pain of lymphatic disease, *lymphangitis*, is usually associated with edema. A pressure-like distress or bursting sensation gradually occurs as the edema accumulates. The edema is usually minimal in the early part of the day and reaches a maximum level by the end of the day. This is usually reduced by rest.

8. Pain in *aneurysmal disease* is manifested as pressure on neighboring structures, and by rupture or embolization distally. If marked adventitial inflammation is present the aneurysm will be painful and tender.

9. The pain of *Raynaud's disease* is generally expressed as numbness, stiffness, and tingling during pallor and cyanosis, and of tingling during rubor of the digits. When the pain is severe, this is generally characterized as *Raynaud's phenomenon* as a secondary manifestation associated with thromboangiitis obliterans, cryoglobulinemia and thoracic outlet compression syndrome.

10. The pain of *erythermalgia* is described as the pain of a burn or intense sunburn. It is associated with the ball of the foot, the tips of the toes, or corresponding parts of the hand. This pain is dependent on the warmth of the skin and is absent when the skin is cool.

To determine the patient's problem accurately it is essential to differentiate the pain of various vascular disorders from the pain due to other causes. Frequently misinterpretations occur; for example, in aortoiliac disease, back strain, lumbar disc, and arthritis of the hip are often suspected; in femoropopliteal disease, fallen arches, myositis, and arthritis of the knee are often suspected; and when branches of the popliteal artery are involved, plantar neuroma, foot strain, tight shoes, and osteoporosis are suspected. In patients who complain of distress or discomfort in their extremities but whose pulses appear to be normal or only slightly reduced at rest, it is essential to exercise the patient to the point of complaint and then to reexamine him immediately. Should the arterial pulsations be present but greatly reduced, occlusive disease is suspect. *Fatigue* usually associated with effort and which persists during activity is interpreted as inadequate perfusion. It generally precedes the pain of claudication and it will gradually increase as the disease progresses and will ultimately give way to the pain of intermittent claudication. Keep in mind, however, that fatigue can be secondary to mechanical factors such as flat feet, hard floors, and ill-fitting shoes, and that systemic disorders and/or neurologic diseases as a cause of fatigue must also be evaluated.

FUNCTIONAL TEST PROCEDURES

Much information regarding circulation to the extremities can be obtained by (1) observing skin color changes produced by placing the limbs in elevated and dependent positions, (2) applying pressure to the skin, (3) occluding arterial circulation for a short period of time, (4) palpating the skin, subcutaneous tissues, and peripheral arteries and veins, and (5) listening to blood flow through peripheral vessels.

POSITION TESTS

Changes in the color of the skin of the extremities that occur with changes in the position of the extremities provide important clues with respect to the presence or absence of vascular disease. Any abnormal changes in the color of the skin that occur with the placement of the extremities in the elevated and dependent positions can indicate the presence of occlusive arterial disease. Difference in skin color between comparable portions of the lower and upper extremities and comparable digits with respect to these changes in position can be significant.

Observation of the Lower Extremities

The Elevation Test.   Elevation of the extremities above the level of the heart will intensify the *pallor* of an ischemic limb; in a normal limb with good circulation, little or no change in color is noted. In the elevated position blood is drained from the cutaneous vessels and arterial inflow is slowed by hydrostatic pressure.

1. The patient is placed in the supine position and both limbs are elevated to a vertical position with a 90° angle at the hips (Fig. 2-3a). This maneuver can be facilitated by having the patient clasp hands behind the knees or thighs (Fig. 2-3b). The examiner may assist the patient by supporting the calves (Fig. 2-3c). The 90° angle and vertical positioning of the limbs may be difficult for some patients to assume or maintain. The position can be modified by elevating the limbs to a 45° angle and providing support for the limbs while in this position (Fig. 2-3d).

2. It is important to make note of which angle the patient assumes, how it is assumed, whether support was required, and the length of time the position was maintained. The use of a pocket stop watch is recommended for determining the time required for changes to occur.

3. With the limbs in an elevated position, the examiner presses the blood out of the skin by firmly stroking the plantar surface. For a foot with good circulation, the skin will remain pink. If pallor is evident in the distal portion of the limb(s), this is good evidence of reduced arterial circulation.

4. If little or no change is observed, the reaction is intensified by asking the patient to exercise both feet in the elevated position. The exercise may be either dorsiplantar flexion of the feet (30 times per minute for 3 minutes) or rotation of the ankles (30 times per minute for 3 minutes). Make note of which form of exercise the patient could do, the manner in which it was done, and the period of time for which it was done.

5. While the patient exercises, observe the skin of the soles and dorsum of the feet and corresponding digits. Normally there should be little or no change in the color of the skin when the limbs are elevated and when the feet are exercised in the elevated position. However, in the presence of arterial occlusive disease, patchy or diffuse areas of blanching occur. Pain may also occur and, in severe cases, the legs may be lowered in a very short time and all reactions will occur even before the ankle movements are begun.

6. When the extremities are returned to the supine position, the return

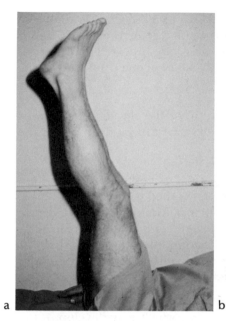

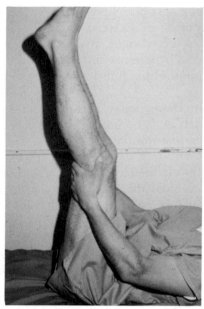

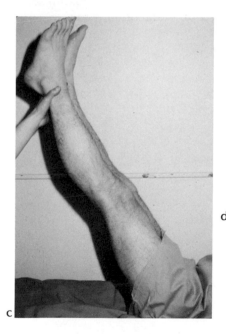

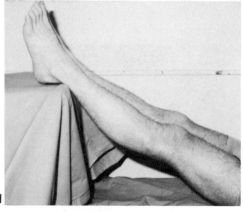

FIGURE 2-3a-d. The elevation test. (See text for discussion.)

of color to a blanched extremity may take 15 to 30 seconds or longer in the presence of arterial occlusion. As the color returns to the ischemic foot or feet a bright, livid red or purple color may appear. This is termed reactive hyperemia and is associated with the ischemia produced by the elevation of the limbs.

The Dependency Test.   The last step (6) of the elevation test can be omitted and the limbs that have been elevated can be dropped to the dependent position.

1. The elevated limbs are lowered; the patient comes to a sitting position and dangles the limbs over the edge of the bed or plinth (Fig. 2-4). Within 3 to 5 seconds the pink color of normal skin with good circulation will become slightly more intense. In a patient with arterial impairment who shows pallor of a foot or feet on elevation, there may be a delay of 45 to 60 seconds or more before color returns. Usually color returns as an irregular patchy discoloration rather than a uniform pink.

2. Leave the limb in a dependent position for 3 to 5 minutes, noting the presence or absence of intense *cyanotic rubor*, which may develop in the foot or feet. Rubor will generally occur in an extremity that manifests a delay in return of color when first placed in a dependent position.

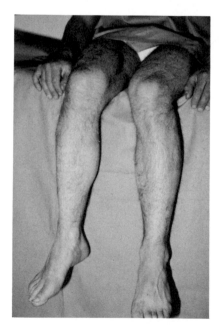

FIGURE 2-4.   The dependency test. (See text.)

3. Make note of time for development of *cyanosis* on dependency, since several factors can affect this response. A rapid development of cyanosis can indicate a decrease or absence of tone in the microvasculature and an immediate pooling of blood in the minute vessels. Changes in room temperature, a prior sympathectomy, the presence of varicosities, venous insufficiency, venous stasis, inflammatory skin changes, edema, and postsympathectomy pain can all affect the response to dependency.

When varicosities are present, color changes in the dependent position will occur rapidly due to the retrograde flow of blood into the subpapillary venous plexuses from proximal veins with incompetent valves. The impaired arterial circulation is masked by the rapid retrograde filling from the venous circulation.

Venous Filling Time

1. With the patient in the supine position, observe one or more of the prominent superficial veins on the dorsum of the foot.

2. Elevate the limbs to drain the veins and then lower the limbs to the horizontal position and note the time for refilling of the vein(s).

Normally this refilling takes 5 to 15 seconds. A delay indicates impaired arterial inflow and a venous filling time greater than 20 seconds can be considered abnormal. When varicose veins are present it is necessary to rule out presence of venous reflux since the superficial vessels will fill immediately when venous reflux is present. Fibrous changes in the walls of the superficial veins will also give misleading information since these changes will keep the veins from collapsing.

The examiner may choose to determine venous filling time at the same time as return of color is observed. The elevated limbs may be swung into the dependent position and the time noted for the superficial veins on the dorsum of the foot to fill (Fig. 2-5).

While observing venous filling time, venous pressure can also be approximated. Slowly elevate the feet from the supine position and note the position at which the veins on the dorsum of the feet collapse. The vessels normally collapse when the feet are elevated just a few centimeters above the level of the right atrium. Should the vessels not collapse when the feet are elevated above the heart level, increased venous pressure is assumed (Fig. 2-6).

Observation of the Upper Extremity

The patient may stand or be seated facing the examiner. The upper extremities are raised above the head with palms open. The changes in

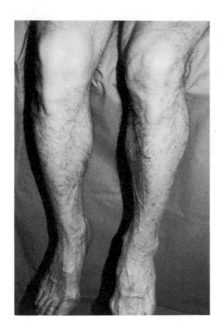
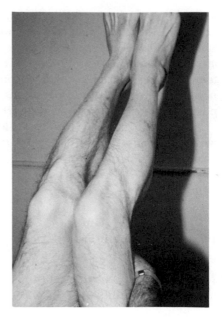

FIGURE 2-5. Determining venous filling time. (See text.)

FIGURE 2-6. Approximating venous pressure. (See text.)

color will be noted in the same manner as for the lower limbs. A potential for pallor of the palms and fingers may be determined by having the patient clench and open the fists 30 times a minute for at least 2 minutes. The palms are then held open and arms are lowered to the eye level of the examiner. The examiner may exercise along with the patient, so that skin color may be compared, thereby permitting a somewhat more accurate evaluation.

If there is significant generalized impairment of the arterial circulation, the skin of the palms and fingers will uniformly blanch. Nonuniform involvement will result in a patchy, irregular blanching pattern. When one or more fingers blanch while others appear normal, occlusion of the digital arteries is indicated.

When positioning the upper extremities to assess arterial circulation, the examiner can determine the status of venous pressure. With the upper extremities in a dependent position, the arms are raised gradually until the veins on the dorsum of the hands collapse. This should occur when the hands are about 10 cm above the level of the right atrium or about the level of the suprasternal notch. If the vessels do not collapse, increased venous pressure is indicated.

ASSESSMENT OF SKIN SURFACE TEMPERATURE

During the initial examination, skin temperature may be estimated by using the dorsum of the hand or the ventral surface of the fingers to palpate the patient's hands, feet, and proximal portions of the limbs.

1. Room temperature and the time that the patient arrives in the test area are recorded. This is important especially when the patient has come from the cold outdoors. After the patient removes shoes and socks allow approximately 30 minutes to elapse before assessing surface temperature.

2. Compare the skin surface temperature of one extremity with that of the opposite side and make similar comparisons for the hands, feet, and digits. Temperatures of symmetric parts should not vary more than 2C.

The most important clinical sign when palpating coolness relates to asymmetric limb temperatures. If the cold extremity is the symptomatic limb, this can be interpreted as an indication of arterial insufficiency.

Patients frequently use characteristic terms to describe limb temperatures. If *coldness* is described for bilaterally symmetrical areas it is not necessarily abnormal, since it can relate to increased sympathetic tones. *Transient bilateral symmetrical coldness* can be associated with vasospastic disorders. *Persistent bilateral symmetrical coldness* can indicate occlusive vascular disease especially if it accompanies color changes symptomatic of vascular insufficiency. When one extremity is described as *cold* with respect to the opposite limb the cold limb invariably manifests vascular involvement. *Localized warmth* usually implies inflammation. *Warm and hot* especially with dependent redness indicates obliterative disease plus inflammation. However, when *abnormal warmth* is expressed in the absence of inflammation, arteriovenous fistula or erythermalgia is suspected.

COMPRESSION MANEUVERS

Application of pressure to the skin surface by means of digital pressure and/or a compression cuff can give important clues to the status of the circulation in the area of application of digital pressure and in the limb to which the compression cuff has been applied.

Subpapillary Venous Plexus Filling Time

Apply firm digital pressure to the skin for 5 to 10 seconds. Observe color changes produced by sudden removal of the finger. In the presence of good circulation, the finger pressure will cause pallor of the skin due to displacement of blood from the local subpapillary venous plexus and deeper surrounding tissues. Release of the pressure should return the original color within 1 to 2 seconds.

Return of color will be delayed in the case of decreased arterial flow, excessive vasospasm, reduced or absent venous tone, or venous stasis. A filling time of more than 4 to 5 seconds is considered abnormal; color may return in an irregular manner with slow filling of the pale area from the outer edges inward. This simple test can also indicate skin turgor and tissue viability. Firm digital pressure to an already cyanotic area that produces transient pallor indicates potentially irreversible changes.

Reactive Hyperemia Response

Anoxia can be produced by the application of arterial occlusion pressure to a limb for several minutes. Rapid release of the compression cuff produces a series of color changes termed the hyperemic response to temporary anoxia. An appropriately sized compression cuff is wrapped firmly around the thigh or arm. The limb is elevated for 3 minutes to facilitate the drainage of blood and the cuff is then inflated to a pressure greater than the patient's arterial pressure. Time is noted and the extremity returned to a horizontal position. At the end of 3 minutes the pressure is released immediately and resultant color changes observed.

In the presence of good circulation, with release of pressure, a bright pink flush appears at a level just distal to the cuff. The pink flush will progress rapidly and uniformly down the extremity and should flush the digits within 10 to 15 seconds. The pink flush should continue for 10 to 40 seconds and then recede in same order as it advanced. The total response should be complete within 2 minutes.

When occlusive disease or marked vasospasm are present, the flush may by cyanotic instead of bright pink. There will be a delay in its appearance, the spread will be slow and patchy, and 2 to 3 minutes may elapse before the digits are flushed; some may take longer than others. The timing of the response and the characteristics of the flush should be noted.

Compression or Tourniquet Tests
to Assess Dilated and Varicose Vessels

Several compression or tourniquet tests are available for distinguishing varicose and dilated vessels in the superficial venous system. These procedures permit identification of the sites of incompetency in the great and small saphenous veins and in the communicating veins that connect the superficial and deep venous networks at various levels of the thigh and leg.

Single Tourniquet (Trendelenburg Test)

This test provides a means of differentiating between dilated and varicose veins of the lower extremity and determining patency of communicating vessels.

The patient lies in a supine position. The limb is elevated to empty the superficial veins, and a tourniquet is placed around the thigh just below the level of the fossa ovalis. Compression applied with the tourniquet is sufficient to occlude the great saphenous vein. With the tourniquet in place the patient assumes an upright position. The examiner waits 10 seconds and then releases the tourniquet. The manner in which the vessels fill is observed and recorded. *Immediate reflux filling* of the great saphenous vein and tributaries indicates incompetent valves in the main vessel, possibly at the level of the fossa ovalis with reflux filling into the superficial venous system through the saphenofemoral junction. *Slow filling* (30 seconds or more) is the normal response, since this is due to the movement of blood from the capillary system.

The examiner may elect to wait more than 10 seconds before removal of the tourniquet. A rapid appearance of dilated vessels in one or more areas at the level of the tourniquet indicates reflux flow from the small saphenous system or from the communicating branches.

The small saphenous vein system is tested in the same way with the tourniquet placed just below the level of the popliteal space. All observations are recorded at each site and competency or incompetency indicated.

Multiple Tourniquet Test

With the patient in a supine position, the limb is elevated to empty the superficial veins, and the examiner places four tourniquets around the extremity: upper, middle, and lower thigh and just below the knee. The patient then stands upright and the rate of filling of the superficial veins is noted. Rapid filling (less than 30 seconds) in the leg segment distal to the below-knee tourniquet indicates incompetent communicating veins. If there is no filling and no change the below-knee segment is released. If rapid filling occurs then the small saphenous vein is incompetent. If the same response is obtained with removal of the above-knee and middle-thigh tourniquets it is likely that vessels other than the great saphenous are incompetent. If with release of the last tourniquet there is rapid filling of the leg and thigh veins, the site of inadequacy is localized to the saphenofemoral junction.

Thumb Compression—Tourniquet Test

This test further aids in differentiating the involvement of the small saphenous vein. The leg is elevated and a single tourniquet is placed around the lower thigh to prevent reflux through the great saphenous system. The popliteal space is compressed with the thumb as the fingers press against the knee. The patient stands and the compression is maintained for 20 to 30 seconds. A normal response is absence of sudden filling of veins in the lower leg. If there is immediate filling the site of reflux is the communicating veins joining the veins of the lower leg. If filling from above downward occurs when the pressure in the popliteal space is removed, incompetency in the small saphenous vein is indicated.

Pratt Test for Localizing Incompetent Valves of Communicating Veins

The leg is elevated and a high-thigh tourniquet and an elastic bandage from the toes to the groin are applied. The patient stands with the tourniquet in place while the elastic bandage is unrolled from high-thigh to toes. At each level at which the bandage is unwound, the examiner looks for the sudden appearance of distended veins. If they appear, the examiner uses the fingers to press the veins and collapse them. With removal of the pressure the examiner looks for an immediate reappearance of the dilated vessels. This is further evidence of incompetent communicating vessels. The test is repeated with the tourniquet placed at a level just below the distended vessels. At each level that dilated vessels appear the examiner carefully marks each group of incompetent veins.

Compression Maneuver (Tourniquet Tests) for Patency and Competency of the Deep Venous System

The result of thrombosis of a deep vein channel is either permanent occlusion of the vessel or recanalization with local destruction of the valves. In assessing the postphlebitic syndrome it is important to determine which situation is present.

Perthes' Test

The patient stands and the examiner places a tourniquet around the thigh to compress the great saphenous vein. The patient exercises the limb by alternately flexing and extending the knee ten times, or else the patient is asked to walk. (1) In the presence of patent and competent deep veins, blood flows into the deep veins during the exercise and the superficial vessels collapse and remain collapsed. (2) In the presence of incompetent deep veins, the superficial veins empty during the physical effort and refill immediately on stopping the exercise. (3) The tourniquet is applied at different levels to determine the sites of incompetency. (4) In the presence of nonpatent deep veins, with increased pressure, the superficial veins will become more distended during the exercise.

Tourniquet Plus Evaluation

The patient stands and a tourniquet is placed around the thigh so that the superficial veins distend. The patient lies down and elevates the extremity. The superficial vessels should collapse. If they remain distended a block in the deep venous system is implied. However, since blood may still be pooled in the deep vein system, the patient stands again with the tourniquet still in place. A sudden distension of the superficial veins implies nonpatent deep veins.

An Elastic Bandage Test

The extremity is elevated to collapse the superficial veins and a series of circumferential measurements are made of the lower leg. Then starting at the toes, the leg is wrapped snugly with an elastic bandage up to the knee and the patient is asked to walk at 1.5 to 2.5 mph for 10 to 20 minutes. The calf measurements are then repeated with the limb in the elevated position. (1) In the presence of a deep venous system block, discomfort is experienced during walking and increases as walking continues. Removal of the bandage relieves the symptoms immediately and at the end of the walk the calf circumference will have increased. (2) In the presence of patent deep veins and competent communicating channels, walking with the bandage in place should produce no discomfort. The compression collapses the superficial veins and shunts blood into the deep vessels via the perforators.

WALKING TESTS

There is no simple objective clinical test for completely evaluating the circulation in the muscles of the extremities. The patient's subjective response to some form of exercise must be used to obtain an estimate of the degree of involvement.

Claudication Time and Distances

A simple walking test that can be controlled by the examiner can supply some measure of the patient's capacity to walk before experiencing symptoms in the exercising muscles. Before the patient is asked to walk, he should indicate how far, how fast, and how often during a day he usually walks.

The examiner walks with the patient and sets the pace (e.g., 100 to 120 steps per minute) on a level surface such as a long corridor. With the examiner holding the patient's arm, the patient should be able to assume the pace set. A stopwatch should be used to determine the time for symptoms to appear. The patient may indicate this verbally, may favor the affected limb, or may slow the pace. The time at which the patient is compelled to stop because of pain is recorded as the absolute walking time. The length of the walk can be expressed in standard city blocks and indicates the claudication distance. The length of time for the pain to disappear while the patient remains in standing position is termed the pain disappearance time. These responses are usually quite reproducible, though they may vary with the patient's sense of well-being, a possible "training" effect, or progression of the disease.

Palmar or Plantar Flexion —Extension or Wrist–Ankle Rotation

With the patient in a supine position and the limbs elevated, he exercises by alternately flexing and extending ankles and toes (wrists and fingers) or by rotating the wrists and ankles. It is important to note the number of times each exercise is done, when the blanching appears (plantar-palmar ischemia) and the character of pain if present. In the presence of marked arterial insufficiency both pallor and pain will appear.

PALPATION OF ARTERIES

To palpate the peripheral vessels accurately, compare the *amplitude* and *force of pulsation* in a vessel with that of its corresponding vessel on the opposite side. The following points should be remembered: (1) The *amplitude* of peripheral pulses is influenced by cardiac rhythm, cardiac output, environmental temperature, and the degree of stenosis or occlusion. (2) A weak or indistinct pulse may be difficult to distinguish from the pulse in the tips of the examiner's fingers. (3) When this occurs, the examiner can place the middle finger of the left hand over the right radial artery pulse and then palpate the patient's pulse with the middle finger of the right hand. Pulsations in the examiner's fingertips are generally more subdued and more diffuse as compared with more localized pulsation(s) of the patient's artery (arteries). (4) It may be simpler to palpate, using some pressure, about 1 cm lateral to the patient's pulse; if the pulse first sensed was the patient's it will no longer be felt. (5) Another alternative is for the examiner to exercise in order to increase his pulse rate, and so that it will be different from the patient's.

Grading Pulsations

It is customary to assign a grade to each pulsation. Although considerable subjectivity is involved, grading permits an initial critical evaluation. A useful practice is to grade on the basis of 0 to 4, with 0 indicating no pulsation; 1—marked impairment of arterial pulsations, a barely palpable pulse, or present but markedly reduced pulse; 2—moderate impairment, palpable but weak, present, and moderately decreased or reduced; 3—slight impairment, diminished pulsation, or present and slightly decreased, or reduced; and 4—normal strong pulse (Table 2-1).

Extracranial Arteries of the Head and Neck

The *common carotid artery* is palpated low in the neck adjacent to the trachea (Fig. 2-7a). The examiner may prefer to stand behind the patient and to press gently against the transverse process of the cervical vertebrae (Fig. 2-7b). Palpation in the region of the bifurcation can produce reflex bradycardia or release an embolus from an arteriosclerotic plaque. Bilaterally palpate along the course of the artery and compare and grade. It is often possible to feel a thrill over the bifurcation, indicating a narrowed lumen. This artery can be tucked behind the sternomastoid

TABLE 2-1. PULSES

Location	Artery	Right	Left	Comments
Head	Common Carotid			
	Superficial Temporal			
	External Maxillary			
	Subclavian			
Arm				
	Axillary			
	Brachial			
	Radial			
	Ulnar			
Abdomen				
	Aorta			
	Iliac			
Leg				
	Common Femoral			
	Superficial Femoral			
	Popliteal			
Foot				
	Anterior Tibial			
	Posterior Tibial			
	Dorsalis Pedis			

0 = absent; 1 = markedly reduced; 2 = moderately reduced; 3 = slightly reduced; 4 = normal

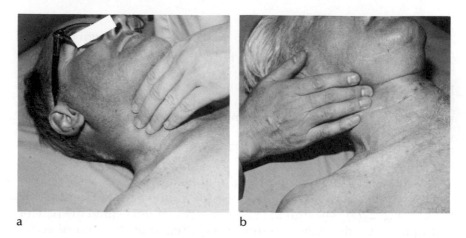

a   b

FIGURE 2-7a, b.   Palpation of the common carotid artery from the front (a) or from behind (b). (See text.)

muscle, which requires deep probing. Very prominent carotid pulsations can indicate a tortuous vessel due to an aneurysm.

Light pressure is applied to the *superficial temporal artery* with two or three fingers against the temporal bone just in front of the ear above the zygoma (Fig. 2-8). The external maxillary artery can be palpated as it crosses the midportion of the mandible. Absence of pulses in these arteries infers possible occlusion of the external carotid artery.

The *subclavian artery* continues into the arm as the *axillary artery*. It is somewhat difficult to palpate in heavy-set individuals, but can usually be felt at the base of neck above the clavicle (Fig. 2-9a, b). Bilateral arm

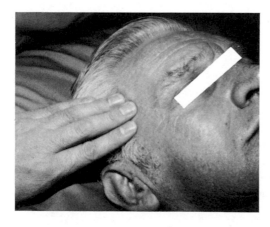

FIGURE 2-8.   Palpation of the superficial temporal artery. (See text.)

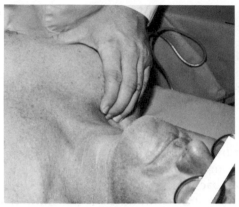

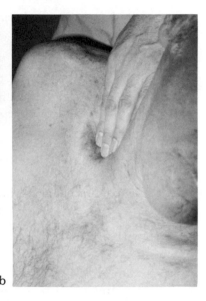

FIGURE 2-9a, b. Palpation of the subclavian artery from the front (a) or from behind (b).

pressures should be done with the physical examination since a difference between the two arms suggests a block of the proximal portion of the subclavian artery. In the presence of a complete block, a weak pulse may be due to the presence of collaterals providing flow to the arm via a *vertebral artery*. Thus blood is diverted from the *basilar artery*, giving rise to cerebral vascular insufficiency, which results in *subclavian steal syndrome*.

The subclavian artery can be compressed by structures near it, the scalenus anticus muscle and thoracic outlet. Note the effect on the radial pulse of different positions of the shoulder girdle relative to the rib cage. These position effects are determined following palpation of the radial and ulnar arteries.

To *palpate the radial artery* the patient takes a deep breath, braces his shoulders, and turns his head to one side and then the other.

To perform *hyperabduction* the arm is raised to the level of and above the shoulder. Pull the arm downward at the elbow against the resistance of the patient. Note the position when the pulse disappears and evaluate the patient's symptoms and complaints. Be sure to have the radiographer reproduce these positions.

Costoclavicular Syndrome Test. The patient sits facing the examiner and the radial artery is palpated. The patient pulls the shoulders back and raises the arm(s) to shoulder level. If the pulse(s) disappear or decrease sharply, or if paresthesia and pain occur in the arm, the test is positive.

Hyperabduction Syndrome Test.   The patient faces the examiner, who palpates the radial artery. The arm is raised above and behind the head and the fist clenched several times. A sharp decrease or disappearance of the pulse and the presence of paresthesia and pain indicate a positive test.

Scalenus or Cervical Rib Syndrome (Adson test).   The patient sits with arms abducted to the thorax and the examiner palpates the radial artery. The patient bends the head backwards, holds a deep breath, and turn the head to the side. A positive test is indicated if the pulse decreases markedly or disappears and paresthesia and pain occur.

Arteries of the Arm

The *axillary artery* is palpated in the axilla (Fig. 2-10a, b). As this artery passes down the arm it becomes the brachial artery.

The *brachial artery* is palpated by encircling the upper arm in the lower third with the hand and pressing the tissues on the medial aspect of the arm against the bone (humerus) (Fig. 2-11a). The artery may also be palpated at the *antecubital space* where it bifurcates into the radial and ulnar arteries (Fig. 2-11b).

The *radial artery* is palpated at the wrist on the radial side of the forearm. It is located near the proximal volar carpi skin crease and medial to the styloid process of the radius. The patient may be sitting or

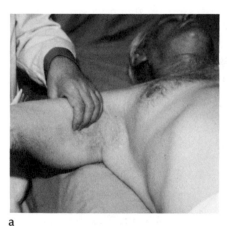
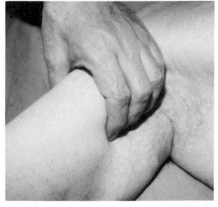

a   b

FIGURE 2-10a, b.   Palpation of the axillary artery. (See text.)

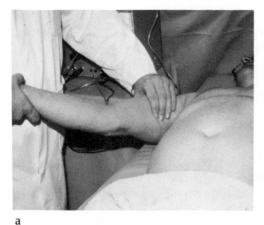

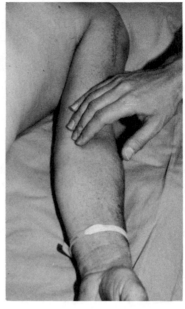

a

FIGURE 2-11a, b. Palpation of the brachial artery on the inside of the upper arm (a) or at the antecubital fossa (b). (See text.)

b

standing with the hands slightly pronated. The examiner faces the patient and with the patient's right hand in the examiner's right hand, the examiner's left fingers curl around the lateral aspect of the wrist and pressure is applied gradually over the radial artery with the second, third, and fourth fingers. This procedure is reversed for the left radial artery (Fig. 2-12).

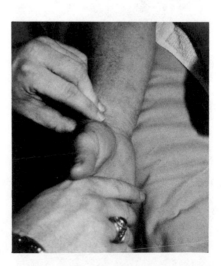

FIGURE 2-12.   Palpation of the radial artery.

It is also possible to palpate both radial arteries at the same time. This is an important maneuver if there is a difference in the arterial supply to the two arms. The examiner faces the patient placing the left hand around the patient's right arm above the wrist and the right hand around the patient's left arm above the wrist. The tips of the second, third, and fourth fingers are pressed laterally against the volar aspect of the flexor tendons.

A similar procedure is followed to evaluate the *ulnar artery*. The patient's hands are supinated and the artery is palpated from the volar aspect down the middle of the extensor tendons on the ulnar side. When the artery is located beneath the flexor carpi ulnaris tendon, the wrist must be flexed and the tendon pushed medially in order to pick up arterial pulsations (Fig. 2-13). Very frequently this artery is not present.

Once the radial and ulnar arteries have been graded several other maneuvers can be done while the patient and the examiner continue to face each other. If it has been difficult to palpate these arteries and to evaluate the circulation to the hand, Allen's test is done.

Allen's Test.   The patient's arm is raised above heart level to increase drainage of the small cutaneous vessels of the palm. Both the ulnar and radial arteries are compressed and the patient opens and closes the fist several times for further venous outflow, thus blanching the palmar surface (Fig. 2-14a). The examiner maintains the compression on the arteries and the patient's hand is brought back to the level of the heart; the fist is relaxed and compression on the ulnar artery is released. The re-

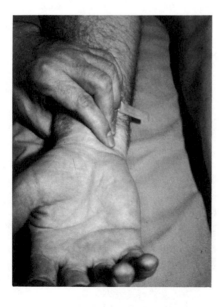

FIGURE 2-13.   Palpation of the ulnar artery. (See text.)

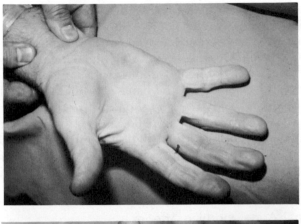

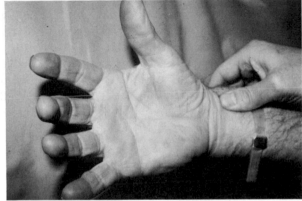

FIGURE 2-14a, b.   Allen's test. (See text.)

turn of color to the palm and digits is observed and timed (Fig. 2-14b). With a patent ulnar artery, the skin may flush immediately or within several seconds and the skin of the thumb and thenar eminence may remain pale. But if the entire palmar surface remains blanched as long as the radial artery is compressed and if color returns immediately on release the indications are that the artery may be occluded due to disease or that an anatomical anomaly exists between the artery and the volar arches.

The same steps are repeated while maintaining compression of the ulnar artery in order to determine the contribution of the radial artery to the circulation of the hand. The deep branch of the radial artery forms the deep volar arterial branch. With the ulnar artery compressed and the radial compression released, the appearance of a faint flush and a delay of more than 5 seconds indicates a radial obstruction, and faint and delayed flushing to one or more digits implies local obstruction.

Should the examiner prefer not to compress both arteries simultaneously, the patient's arm is raised above heart level and firm digital pressure applied first to the radial artery, while the patient opens and closes his fist several times to promote venous drainage and pale skin. With radial compression maintained the hand is brought to the level of the heart and the fist relaxed. The skin should flush promptly if the ulnar artery is patent. Continued palmar pallor and return of color only when the radial compression is released indicates ulnar artery occlusion or anatomic anomaly. This procedure can be repeated with compression of the ulnar artery in order to evaluate the contribution of the radial artery to the circulation of the hand.

Abdominal Aorta and Iliac Arteries

The *abdominal aorta,* which is the largest artery to be palpated, can be felt distal to the renal arteries in most patients except the obese. When palpating from the right side of the patient, both hands, which are placed at the level of the umbilicus and immediately cephalad to it, are moved from the side towards the midline. Whenever a dilated aorta is felt the width of the expansile pulsation should be estimated. Both hands are used to approach the aorta from the opposite side in order to differentiate a *tortuous aorta* from an *aneurysm* (Fig. 2-15).

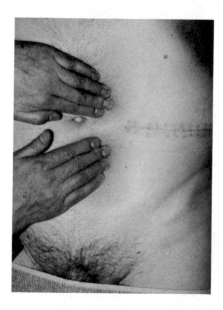

FIGURE 2-15.   Palpation of the abdominal aorta. (See text.)

In many instances complete occlusion of the terminal aorta can be so gradual that there may be few or no symptoms and the occlusion can be extended proximally to the renal arteries. In such cases, collateral vessels have developed and a weak pulse may be felt in the groin.

The *external iliac arteries* are palpated by moving the hands into the right and left quadrants and running the fingertips of both hands along a line from the middle of the inguinal ligament towards the umbilicus.

Arteries of the Lower Extremity

The *common femoral artery*, which is the main artery to the lower extremity, can be palpated in the area where it passes under the inguinal ligament. Under normal conditions, this vessel has the strongest pulsations of all palpable vessels.

The patient is placed in a recumbent position and the examiner stands facing the patient's head at the side to be examined. The second, third, and fourth fingers are placed along the course of the artery directly below and medial to the inguinal ligament. By applying pressure with the fingertips and pressing gently towards the ileopubic eminence, the artery can be felt (Fig. 2-16). A pulse that is graded as 3 indicates proximal stenosis in the aorta and/or the iliac arteries.

The *deep femoral artery* (profunda femoris), which arises from the common femoral artery a very short distance below the groin level, supplies the muscles of the thigh. This artery is situated too deep in the muscles to be palpated.

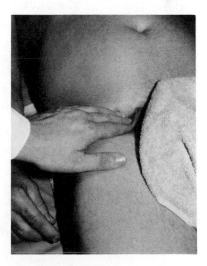

FIGURE 2-16.   Palpation of the common femoral artery. (See text.)

During the examination of the pulses in the lower extremities a rectal examination can help to determine an aneurysm of the hypogastric arteries, to evaluate congenital A-V fistulas involving these arteries and their branches, and to detect a large elongated abdominal aneurysm palpated with the fingertips.

It should be kept in mind that an acute obstruction (embolus) of the bifurcation of the major artery can result in increased pulsations immediately proximal to the site of the occlusion. This augmented pulse occurs because all of the energy of the pulse is in a lateral direction at the site of the obstruction. Thus, soon after an embolus to the bifurcation of the femoral artery, an abnormally strong pulse may be felt.

As the common femoral courses the thigh, it becomes the *superficial femoral artery*. This artery can be palpated only in very thin patients. This artery is very frequently occluded at the point where it branches off from the profunda femoris. Another site of occlusion is low in the thigh in the *adductor canal*.

Accurate palpation of the *popliteal artery* in particular requires practice. As the superficial femoral artery enters the popliteal fossa at the back of the knee, it becomes the popliteal artery. There are three ways to palpate the artery: (1) the patient lies face down on a plinth or bed. The examiner stands at the side to be examined and faces the patient's feet. The patient's leg is flexed at the knee. The examiner palpates the leg below the ankle or the foot at the arch with the opposite hand. Using the thumb of the examining hand, the examiner applies gradually increasing pressure into the popliteal space in order to palpate the artery (Fig. 2-17a and b). (2) The patient may be seated facing the examiner. The thumbs of both of the examiner's hands are placed against the patella and the fingers pressed into the popliteal space. The fingers of the right hand palpate the artery while the fingers of the left hand force the artery and tissues against the right fingers, thus compressing the artery between the two sets of fingers (Fig. 2-17c). (3) The following method is a modification of the above procedure. The patient assumes a recumbent position, flexes the knees, and remains relaxed. The examiner uses the hands as above. Should pulsations be felt with both hands while they are slightly separated, an aneurysm is suspected. If no pulsations are felt, blockage of the lower superficial femoral artery and the popliteal artery is implied.

Arteries of the Foot

The three main branches of the popliteal artery are the *anterior tibial*, *posterior tibial*, and *peroneal arteries*, which are not palpable in the calf area. These arteries course closer to the periphery in the region of the ankle and the *dorsalis pedis artery*, which is a continuation of the anterior tibial

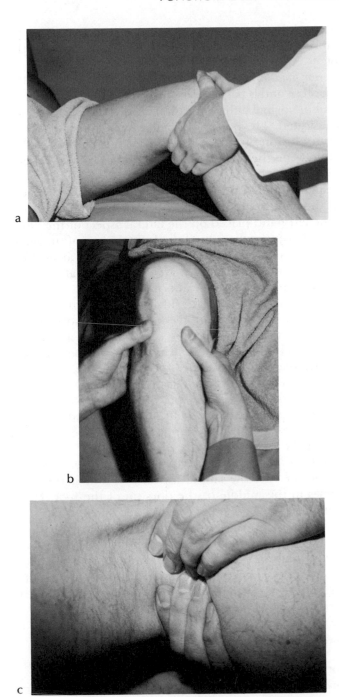

FIGURE 2-17a, b, c.   An approach for palpation of the popliteal artery. (See text.)

artery, nears the surface on the dorsum of the foot. The pulsations, which are termed *pedal pulses*, are detectable at the ankle and the dorsum of the foot.

The *posterior tibial artery* is considered the most anatomically constant artery on the foot and is palpated at the level of the ankle. A pulse is very rarely absent in normal individuals; if it is not palpable, occlusive arterial disease is indicated. The posterior tibial artery extends down the medial and posterior portion of the leg deep in the calf muscles and it surfaces in the foot between the medial malleolus and calcaneus, where it is palpated easily.

With the patient in a sitting or supine position, the examiner supports the heel of the patient's foot (right heel in the right hand), and with the thumb of the left hand placed on the lateral aspect of the ankle and the palm extended over the dorsum of the foot, the tips of the second, third, and fourth fingers palpate the right posterior tibial artery (Fig. 2-18a). The procedure is reversed for the left posterior tibial artery.

The examiner may choose an alternate position. For the right posterior tibial artery stand at the right side facing the patient's feet. Cup the fingers of the left hand over the medial malleolus with the left thumb placed on the lateral malleolus. The second, third, and fourth fingers slide slightly distal to and somewhat posterior to the medial malleolus (Fig. 2-18b). Reverse the procedure for the left side.

Firm pressure is required since this artery may not course close to the surface. Slight dorsiflexion of the foot places stretch on the artery making it easier to palpate. In the presence of obesity and edema the artery may be difficult to palpate. Visible pulsations may be evident if there is calcification of the artery.

The *dorsalis pedis artery* is a continuation of the anterior tibial artery. It is generally located on the lateral aspect of the first metatarsal as the artery courses in the middle of the dorsum of the foot. However, this artery often varies its course, making it necessary to palpate the total dorsum of the foot before deciding that it is not present.

The approach to this artery is similar to that for the posterior tibial artery, except that the thumb of the examining hand is placed on the plantar surface of the patient's foot and the flexor surfaces of the terminal phalanges of the second, third, and fourth fingers palpate the artery. The fingers are moved from side to side to locate the artery and at the same time the applied pressure is varied in order to pick up weaker pulses (Fig. 2-19a,b,c).

Anterior Tibial and Peroneal Arteries

The *anterior tibial artery* is palpated at the site where it reaches the ankle (Fig. 2-20). The *peroneal artery* courses deep in the lower leg and

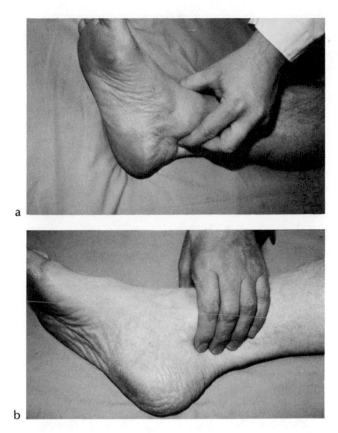

FIGURE 2-18a, b.   Alternate positions for palpation of the posterior tibial artery.

is difficult to palpate. The anterior branch of this artery may be located just anterior to the lateral malleolus. With complete occlusion of the posterior tibial artery a perforating branch of the peroneal artery may enlarge and produce a prominent pulsation on the superior aspect of the external malleolus.

PALPATION OF VEINS

The Superficial Veins

A systematic examination of the skin and subcutaneous tissues of the limbs should be done to determine the status of the superficial veins. By palpating the skin and subcutaneous tissues areas of tenderness, thicken-

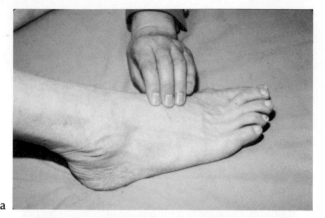

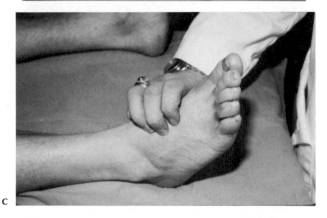

FIGURE 2-19a, b, c. Palpation of the dorsalis pedis artery. (See text.)

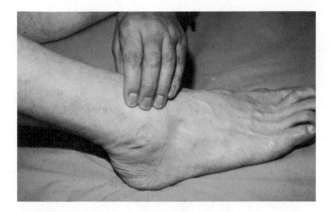

FIGURE 2-20. Palpation of the anterior tibial artery. (See text.)

ing and possible thrombosis can be detected. Potential venous involvement is indicated by the presence of one or more of the following signs: inflammation, marked prominences, distensions, abnormal pulsations, reflux flow, and thrombophlebitis.

When inflammation is evident by the presence of red skin in small zones or narrow strips along the superficial veins, the area is palpated to detect differences in temperature between the reddened area(s) and the immediate surrounding tissues. Palpation along the course of the veins is done to detect any card-like masses that may or may not be tender to pressure. By elevating the limb it can be determined whether the vessel is dilated or thrombosed. A prominent dilated vein can be expected to collapse and become imperceptible to the fingers when the limb is elevated, whereas a thrombosed vessel will remain unchanged.

The two most prominent superficial venous systems, the great saphenous and small saphenous veins, are the most probable sites for superficial thrombophlebitis. The great saphenous vein is palpated on the medial aspect to the thigh and leg, and the small saphenous vein is palpated over the lateral and posterolateral surfaces of the lower leg up to the level of the popliteal space. It is difficult to palpate deeper veins but thrombi, if present, can be felt in proximal portions of the femoral vein and sometimes in a popliteal vein. It is easy to palpate the jugular, axillary, and brachial veins (Fig. 2-21).

With the patient in a standing position, the hydrostatic effect of the column of blood dilates vessels, making distended and prominent superficial veins more evident. In these vessels, the valves are still competent and there should be no evidence of backward flow.

During palpation of varicose veins, the site(s) of incompetent valves is

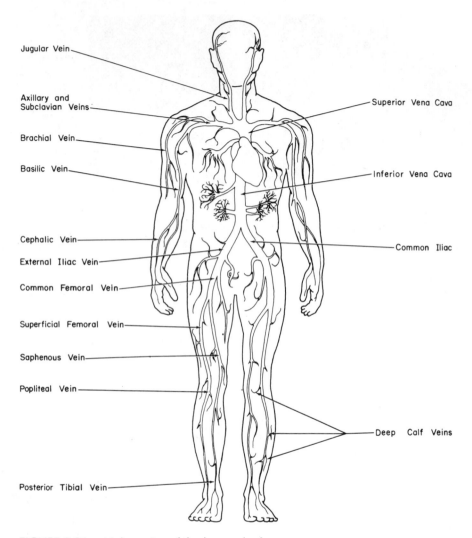

Jugular Vein

Axillary and
Subclavian Veins

Brachial Vein

Basilic Vein

Cephalic Vein

External Iliac Vein

Common Femoral Vein

Superficial Femoral Vein

Saphenous Vein

Popliteal Vein

Posterior Tibial Vein

Superior Vena Cava

Inferior Vena Cava

Common Iliac

Deep Calf Veins

FIGURE 2-21.   Major veins of the human body.

initially determined by some simple techniques: (1) Compress a vein at a proximal site with the fingers of one hand and use the fingertips of the other to perceive the distal impact of movement of the column of blood. This procedure can be done along the course of the vein. If an impulse is palpated 20 cm or more distally, incompetency is indicated. (2) The upper portion of the long saphenous vein is palpated while the patient is asked to cough. When valves are incompetent, the cough impulse will be transmitted distally in the thigh. (3) The presence of thickened subcutaneous tissues due to edema and fat necrosis produces fascial defects. These defects, if palpated along the course of a prominent or varicose vein, imply incompetency of valves of the perforator veins.

When increased numbers of veins are observed spreading across junctional areas, such as the groin, the shoulder, and the trunk, the direction of blood flow in these vessels is determined in order to identify normal versus collateral vessels. With the patient in a supine position, the examiner collapses a vein with one index finger and strips the blood from the vein with the other index finger. The pressure from each finger is released alternately and direction of blood flow is determined by the speed with which the segment refills.

The Deep Veins

The main venous channels or deep veins of the extremities are located deep in the tissues and cannot be inspected or palpated easily. A silent thrombus of the deep veins of the calf and foot (phlebothrombosis) is one of the most difficult clinical entities to diagnose. However, some simple maneuvers are helpful in the initial clinical evaluations.

Dorsiflexion (Homan's Sign).   With the patient in the supine position, the examiner lifts the leg with one hand while forcibly dorsiflexing the foot with the other. The tissues of the posterior portion of the calf are stretched and in the presence of thrombosis of the local veins the increased stretch produces pain. Fullness and tension of the calf muscles may be present, as well as a tenderness of the sole of the foot evidenced by the compression. When foot symptoms are present, thrombi in the deep plantar veins may be implied. Many conditions other than the presence of thrombi in the veins can also produce pain or dorsiflexion; therefore, this maneuver alone should not be used for diagnosis of deep vein thrombosis.

Palpating to Detect Infiltration in the General Region of the Calf Veins (Neuhof's Sign).   The patient is placed in the supine position, the heels rest on the bed, the knees are flexed, and the calf muscles relaxed. The examiner palpates the entire posterior portion of the upper leg. Detection of thickening and infiltration deep in the calf muscles and the presence of tenderness is considered good evidence for deep vein thrombosis. Often these signs are present when dorsiflexion produces no response. The examiner also palpates for tenderness in the lower third of the thigh and especially at the junction of the superficial femoral and popliteal veins.

Palpating to Detect a Thrombus in the Deep Veins of the Anterior Muscles of the Leg.   With the patient in the supine position, the examiner passively extends the leg 45° or less. If no pain is elicited, the toes are plantar-flexed as the foot is held extended. Evidence of pain anywhere lateral to the anterior crest of the tibia indicates a possible thrombosis. The vena comitantes of the anterior tibial veins are superficial at this level. Contraction of the anterior group of muscles by foot extension produces compression, which elicits a pain response.

Palpating for Changes in Skin Temperature.   Palpate in the area of the suspected deep vein thrombosis for differences in skin temperature. The temperature differences can be either increased warmth or cold and are especially significant if there are bilateral differences.

Calf Compression.   A sphygmomanometer cuff is placed around the calf and inflated to suprasystolic pressures. A normal calf can withstand pressure of 180 to 200 mm Hg without undue discomfort or pain. However, in the presence of a deep vein thrombosis, pressures as low as 100 to 200 mm Hg can produce severe pain. This procedure is not without some danger. In the presence of friable clot, a piece of the clot could conceivably dislodge and lead to a pulmonary embolism.

CHAPTER 3

INSTRUMENTATION

INTRODUCTION

The basic function of all biomedical instrumentation is to enable the clinical physician and/or researcher to obtain reliable and relevant measurements of physiologic parameters. This includes the gathering of information pertaining to a wide range of physiologic variables; the establishment of a diagnosis; the routine evaluation of a physiologic system to ascertain its functional integrity; and the monitoring of a physiologic system or systems (1) to provide information on the system's functional state, either on a periodic or continual basis; and (2) for control of a system whose functioning is automatically altered in response to changes in measured parameters of that system. Such instrumentation may be broadly divided into that used for clinical purposes specifically or that which is primarily research-oriented. Clinical instrumentation is typically easy to use and durable. It provides a restricted range of measurements that give the information necessary for decision making in the course of treatment. In contrast, instrumentation that is primarily research-oriented is of a higher degree of complexity and specialization and is characteristically designed for high accuracy, sensitivity, and specificity.

A number of factors are of importance in understanding medical instrumentation. The *range* of the instrumentation refers to the amplitude and frequency input over all levels in which the instrument is anticipated to function. Ideally, the instrument should be capable of providing the operator with usable measurements over a range of smallest to largest anticipated values.

An instrument's *stability* refers to its capability to return to a steady state rather than oscillating uncontrollably following an input variation. Stability varies with the degree of amplification and feedback. It is imperative that the system of instrumentation be sufficiently stable over the most useful range. An instrument's *baseline stability* refers to maintaining an unchanging baseline value without drift.

Linearity is the extent to which variations in input to the instrument are followed by variations in the instrument's output. In a linear system, the sensitivity of the system is the same for all absolute levels of input. It is essential that an instrument has linearity over the most important range of measurements.

The *sensitivity* refers to how small a variation in a parameter can be effectively measured. While the term *range* refers to the measured parameter's absolute value, sensitivity is concerned with the minute changes that can be detected and directly determines an instrument's resolution, i.e., the minimal variation that can be detected accurately. If an instrument has too great a sensitivity, instability or nonlinearity results.

The term *hysteresis* refers to the phenomenon where, when measuring a given parameter, one obtains different readings when the value is approached in a descending direction and in an ascending direction. An example would be in a meter where the presence of a mechanical friction causes a lag in response, thus leading to an error in reading secondary to hysteresis.

An instrument's variation in sensitivity present over the frequency range of the measurement is referred to as its *frequency response*. The instrument should have the capability of a response rapid enough to permit a reproduction of all frequency components with the same sensitivity. Such a phenomenon is referred to as a *flat response* for a given range of frequencies.

The measurement of systemic error is referred to as *accuracy*. Systemic errors may be secondary to a number of factors: the presence of component errors due to drift or thermal variation or tolerance; mechanical errors secondary to meter movements; poor frequency response inherent in the instrumentation; atmospheric pressure and/or temperature alterations; operator errors in reading the measurements due to parallax or poor lighting; or errors arising from the influence of the technique on the parameter being measured.

The *signal-to-noise ratio* of an instrument should be as high as possible. The presence of noise may be due to interference from power lines, particularly where long leads are being used, or may be due to electrostatic, electromagnetic, or other sources.

Another important factor is the instrument's *isolation*, i.e., the instrument does not yield an electrical connection directly between the test subject and the ground. This prevents interference between several instruments being used simultaneously, and, more importantly, ensures the safety of the patient.

Biomedical instrumentation should be simple to operate, to allow widespread use and reduce the possibility of error. However, certain problems may arise. It may not be possible to place a measuring instrument so as to make direct measurements of a particular variable. In such cases, one must resort to indirect measurements, using a more easily measured variable to extrapolate a useful estimate of an unmeasurable variable. The limitations and validity of the "substitute" variable must be carefully assessed.

In a system as complex as the human body, the variability of data is considerable. Different values may be obtained for a given variable under the same conditions, even for the same patient. Physiologic variables are thus represented by a probable range of values rather than a precise measurement.

Biomedical instrumentation may be classified in one of four ways.

1. By the quantity that is being measured, e.g., temperature, pressure, flow. This allows rapid comparison of different instrumentation that can be used for measuring the same parameter. This method is used in this chapter where instrumentation is discussed for measuring pressure, flow, volume (plethysmography), temperature, and sound.

2. By the principle applied in the measurement, e.g., ultrasonic, resistive, electromagnetic. This facilitates the introduction of new applications.

3. By physiologic systems, e.g., cardiovascular, neurological, etc. This classification is advantageous for the specialist interested in the instrumentation available for a particular field of study.

4. By clinical speciality, e.g., pediatrics, cardiology, etc. Such a classification is valuable for the medical field.

This chapter presents basic physical principles and a rationale for how the biomedical instrumentation that will be presented in application and use in subsequent chapters accomplished its particular function. It is hoped that this relatively basic review will give the reader an understanding of how such instrumentation works and not just how to use it.

PRESSURE MEASUREMENTS

The measurement of arterial blood pressure is the most frequently performed of all cardiovascular measurements. Blood pressure is influenced by a number of factors including the force, frequency, and magnitude of the heart's contractions; the elasticity of the arteries; and the state of the arterioles. Arterial blood pressure is thus an excellent indicator of the functional status of the cardiovascular system.

Arterial blood pressure can either be measured directly (invasive) or indirectly (noninvasive). Direct measurement requires a pressure sensor and a recording or display system. Indirect measurement is typically the familiar sphygmomanometric technique.

SENSORS

Different types of pressure sensors or manometers are available: the traditional mercury-filled U tube, modified aneroid devices, optical instrumentation for recording diaphragm displacement. and various electrical transducers—strain-gauge manometers, capacitance manometers, and inductance manometers. Electrical transducers are accurate and easily used; the most commonly employed is the strain-gauge, where changes in pressure displace a diaphragm and cause a change in electrical resistance. With this type of transducer, the stiffer the diaphragm, the more reliable the method. Such transducers respond rapidly to change in pressure, in contrast to the mercury manometer with its large inertia, which requires a large displacement.

A *manometer* can be considered analogous to an oscillatory system of a weight or mass on a string. If the weight or mass is moved and released, the system will oscillate with the amount of oscillation determined by the extent of damping. In the ideal state the system will oscillate at a constant or natural frequency expressed as:

$$\omega_0 = \sqrt{s/m}$$

where ω_0 is the system's natural frequency, s is the stiffness of the spring, and m is the mass.

Viscous damping is when the resistance to spring motion is proportional to the movement's velocity. This is expressed as:

$$\beta_0 = \frac{R}{2m}$$

where β_0 is damping, R is the viscous damping, and m is the mass.

From these two relationships, the damping of the oscillating system can be categorized as follows: (1) damping is equal to natural frequency ($\beta_0 = \omega_0$), referred to as critical damping. This is where the system will not oscillate but rather return to the position of equilibrium exponentially. (2) Damping is greater than the natural frequency ($\beta_0 > \omega_0$), referred to as overdamping, where the rate of return is slower. (3) Damping is less than the natural frequency ($\beta_0 < \omega_0$), referred to as underdamping, common for most manometers, where the system oscillates with exponential decay of its amplitude. In the presence of critical damping, a manometer's amplitude response will continuously decrease from zero frequency up. In contrast, with underdamping, a manometer's amplitude response increases as frequency increases to a point where it peaks at the manometer's natural frequency. With particular reference to response to amplitude, the optimal damping is seen at a point 0.707 of the critical damping.

Before choosing a system, its use must be determined, as both high-quality amplitude response and minimal phase distortion cannot be built into the same system. For example, if detailed accuracy of different frequencies' phase velocities were required, a system with minimal damping would be necessary.   A strain-gauge transducer is based on the fact that a fine wire being strained within its elastic limit will undergo a change in resistance secondary to changes in its diameter, length, and resistivity.

This can be shown as follows. The resistance of a wire is expressed as:

$$R = \frac{\rho L}{A}$$

where ρ is the wire's resistivity, L is its length, and A is its cross-sectional area. Differentiating this equation provides for the differential change in R:

$$dR = \frac{\rho dh}{A} - \rho A^{-2} LdA + L\frac{d\rho}{A}$$

If these two equations are then divided and incremental values introduced, the resultant formulation is representative of finite changes in parameters and is a function of standard mechanical coefficients:

$$\frac{\Delta R}{R} = \frac{\Delta L}{L} - \frac{\Delta A}{A} - \frac{\Delta \rho}{\rho}$$

The relationship between changes in diameter and changes in length is given by Poisson's ratio μ which, when substituted for the middle term in the above, gives:

$$\frac{\Delta R}{R} = (1 + 2\mu)\frac{\Delta L}{L} + \frac{\Delta \rho}{\rho}$$

which demonstrates that changes in a wire's resistance are a function of changes in its dimensional length ($\Delta L/L$) and area [$2\mu (\Delta L/L)$] as well as changes in the wire's lattice structure ($\Delta \rho/\rho$).

Strain gauges can be either banded or unbanded. An integrated strain gauge has a pressure transducer made using a silicone substrate for the structure of the diaphragm. Elastic-resistance strain gauges are those commonly used in plethysmographic studies. As the elastic strain gauge is stretched, one can see from the above equation that the resistance will increase due to a decreasing diameter and an increasing length.

Further details on strain gauges as well as other sensor devices can be obtained from the biomedical instrumentation texts listed in the selected references.

INSTRUMENTATION SYSTEMS

The measurement of blood pressure may be categorized into three groups: direct pressure measurements where there is a direct access to the blood vessel, either through a cutdown or percutaneous insertion and direct measurement of the pressure with a transducer; indirect pressure measurements where external pressure is applied to the circulatory system and its effect on the system is examined; and indirect relative pressure measurement using uncalibrated instrumentation to determine the presence of flow as an indication of pressure without measurements of absolute pressure.

Indirect Measurement

Indirect pressure measurements are standard determinations providing a noninvasive means for the determination of the intraarterial pressure. Typical of indirect measurements is the sphygmomanometer, consisting of an inflatable cuff for vessel occlusion, a bulb for cuff inflation, and a mercury or aneroid manometer for the detection of pressure. The appropriately sized cuff (see below) is applied to the upper arm. The cuff is inflated to over systolic pressure and then gradually released. A quick approximation of the systolic pressure can be made by feeling for the return of the pulse. This is referred to as the Riva-Rocci method. This method requires a sensitive touch and cannot be used to measure diastolic pressures. This technique is used in determining segmental Doppler systolic pressures when the Doppler probe detects the return of blood flow, which is taken to be the systolic pressure.

In the routine determination of arm blood pressure, a stethoscope is placed over the brachial artery as the cuff is inflated. When the cuff pressure is above systolic, the transmural pressure across the completely compressed artery is zero or a negative value. As the cuff is slowly deflated to a pressure just below systolic, there is a brief interval at the beginning of the systolic component of each cardiac cycle where the compressed artery can open against the surrounding tissue pressure. This allows a small spurt of blood to flow. In the remaining portion of the cardiac cycle the surrounding tissue pressure is too great and the artery remains compressed. This small spurt of blood has an increased velocity, as velocity varies inversely to cross-sectional area: $V = Q/A$. This increased velocity is of a magnitude that exceeds the criteria for turbulence and a sharp sound (best described as a tapping) of short duration is produced. This is the first Korotkoff sound and the pressure at which it is noted is taken to be the systolic pressure. As the cuff pressure is reduced further, the artery can open wider and for a longer period of time during an individual cardiac cycle. The velocity of the blood remains at a magnitude that gives turbulent flow. The sounds become louder and extended with further decreases in cuff pressure. The sounds finally reach a maximum intensity and then disappear when the vessel can remain open throughout the cardiac cycle.

At a point between where the sounds reach maximum intensity and where they diminish, the sounds become muffled. This point is very close to diastolic pressure measured directly, usually a few millimeters higher. As the cuff pressure is reduced, as long as it remains above the diastolic pressure there is a period during the cardiac cycle when the artery is momentarily compressed, giving a brief period of silence. When the cuff pressure goes below diastolic, the artery remains patent throughout the cardiac cycle. As the artery remains patent, there are no brief periods of silence and the sounds become muffled. This provides the physiologic basis for using the pressure at which the Korotkoff sounds become muffled as the diastolic pressure, and not the pressure at which the sounds disappear.

The Korotkoff sounds disappear at approximately 8 mm Hg below true diastolic. That the sounds disappear is due to the velocity of the blood having fallen to a point below the critical value for turbulent flow and as such has no physiologic basis for being indicative of diastolic pressure. Judging the disappearance of sound as the diastolic pressure can be very inaccurate. For example, at rest, a person's systolic pressure may be 130, diastolic (muffled sounds) of 85, and diastolic (sound disappearance) 80. After a period of exercise, the systolic may be 180, diastolic (muffled sounds) 90, and diastolic (sound disappearance) 40. The sounds disappear at extremely low pressure due to the increased flow through the arm following the period of exercise flowing at a velocity that is great enough to be above the critical value for turbulence even though the pressure in the occluding cuff is small. When recording the blood pressure obtained by this technique it is good practice to record both diastolic pressures—first when the sound becomes muffled and second when the sound disappears—120/80/75.

The diastolic pressure recorded as when the Korotkoff sounds disappear may be low due to the presence of a normal brachial artery that is narrower than usual. In such patients the reduced arterial radius lowers the critical value for turbulence as the velocity increases; thus, disappearance of the sounds occurs at a much lower pressure while the pressure that produces a muffled sound remains constant. A true diastolic pressure that is low is indicative of aortic incompetence.

The use of auscultation for the detection of blood pressure has a major drawback for use in peripheral vascular disease in that pressures cannot be recorded at sites distal to an area of atherosclerotic occlusion. In such instances, an indirect measure of pressure can be accomplished using a device sensitive to blood flow. With such devices, one can determine the exact pressure where blood flow returns following gradual release of a proximal occluding cuff. A variety of methods can be employed: mercury strain gauge, photoplethysmography, ultrasonic Doppler.

Automatic and semiautomatic devices are also available for the indirect measurement of blood pressure. Most of the instrumentation available involve the use of a pressure transducer that is affixed to a sphygmomanometer cuff, a microphone placed over the artery under the cuff, and a normal physiologic recording system. Such instrumentation works well in the normal patient at rest but is not useful for active patients or patients in circulatory shock.

In the indirect measurement of blood pressure, the basic assumption that is made is that the pressure placed on the artery is equal to the pressure in the occluding cuff. The pressure at the cuff is transmitted via the tissues to the artery. The equal distribution of the pressure is determined by the size of the cuff. Adequate cuff size width is approximately 40% of the extremity's circumference. There is no consensus about an adequate cuff length. If the cuff is short, the examiner should be sure it is placed properly over the area of interest. If a large cuff is used, placement does not present a problem. Whatever size cuff is used, it should be placed at heart level to negate any hydrostatic effects.

Direct Measurement

In direct measurement of blood pressure, the most commonly used arrangement involves an external transducer (also referred to as extravascular) connected to a liquid-filled catheter coupling the transducer with the blood vessel. Alternatively, the pressure transducer may be incorporated into the tip of the catheter. This is referred to as an internal or intravascular transducer system.

The *external* or *extravascular* transducer system consists of a catheter filled with heparinized saline solution (to aid in maintaining the system's patency) that is attached to a three-way stopcock that is attached to the dome of a pressure transducer. The catheter is inserted into the blood vessel either through a cutdown or percutaneously. The pressure wave is transmitted through the column of fluid in the catheter to the dome of the transducer and then displaces the diaphragm of the transducer. The recorded pressure is then either displaced on an oscilloscope or printed on a stripchart.   In this type of system, the catheter is important. The natural frequency of a catheter is expressed as:

$$\omega_0 = r\,(\pi E/\rho L)^{1/2}$$

where ω_0 is the catheter's natural frequency, r is the catheter's internal radius, E the stiffness of the catheter (equal to $\Delta P/\Delta V$), ρ is the density of the liquid, and L is the length of the catheter. The system is extremely sensitive to the compliance as the natural frequency drops quickly with increasing compliance. The compliance can be increased by the presence of leaks or air bubbles in the system, which additionally increase the damping.

Damping for the system can be expressed as:

$$\beta = \frac{\beta_0}{\omega_0} = \frac{4\eta}{r^3} (L/\pi E)^{1/2}$$

when η is the liquid's viscosity. It is easily seen that damping varies inversely with the third power of the catheter radius and inversely to the compliance of the system. It varies directly with the viscosity of the liquid and the square root of the system's length. Air bubbles in the system cause a fall in natural frequency and increase damping by causing marked decreases in the system's stiffness.

In view of the above, a system for the external or extravascular measurement of blood pressure should use catheters that are relatively stiff (polyethylene or Teflon) and as short a length as possible. To prevent leaks, wide-bore snugly fitting stopcocks should be used, and the use of several stopcocks in series should be avoided.

The *internal* or *intravascular* transducer system uses a transducer mounted at the tip of a catheter. This obviates the need for a fluid-filled catheter to couple the transducer with the blood vessel. Such a system allows high-frequency response and eliminates delay from transmission through a fluid-filled catheter. The major drawback of these systems is that they are extremely delicate and tend to break after a few uses.

BLOOD VELOCITY AND FLOW

Measuring the volume of blood in cc/second or ml/minute flowing in surgically exposed arteries and veins provides information for intelligent decision making in evaluation of surgical procedures and effect of drugs. Detecting the velocity of blood flowing in the vascular system by noninvasive methods and measuring changing electrical and physical properties of limbs by harmless procedures leads to informed understanding of blood flow in health and diseased states. The electromagnetic flowmeter, ultrasonic devices, impedance plethysmograph, and mercury-filled strain gauges are instrumentation techniques used to quantify blood flow phenomenon. Concepts in statistics and pattern recognition are used to analyze waveforms and numerical values obtained by direct measurement. Analysis of this data leads to a greater confidence and knowledge of vascular function. The data and waveforms herein are better comprehended if the reader is conversant with the instrumentation methods used.

ULTRASONIC DOPPLER FLOWMETRY

To a very large extent, the acceptance of noninvasive vascular testing and the proliferation of clinical vascular laboratories is due to the development of the ultrasonic Doppler flowmeter in the early 1960s. This device provided the medical community with a reasonably priced and easy-to-use tool that can provide quantitative information about the vascular system with a sensitivity heretofore unattained.

The principles of operation of the basic continuous-wave ultrasonic Doppler flowmeter are relatively straightforward. The key to its operation are two identical piezoelectric crystals that convert electrical energy into mechanical energy. These crystals of lead zirconate titanate respond to an oscillating electrical signal by expanding and contracting, thus creating a longitudinal compression wave. Similarly, when a compression wave of a certain frequency impinges on such a crystal, it is converted to an electrical signal with that frequency.

In practice the continuous-wave Doppler flowmeter operates as follows. The probe containing two crystals, a transmitting and a receiving crystal, is placed on the surface of the skin above a blood vessel. Coupling gel is employed to eliminate air between the crystals and the body. Air is a poor conductor of sound and the air-skin interface would reflect much of the sound waves. The transmitting crystal is activated by a radio-frequency between 5 and 10 MHz. Sound waves of this frequency (ultrasound) enter the body and are reflected and scattered from interfaces or sharp density variations. Some sound waves are intercepted and reflected from the moving erythrocytes in the moving blood stream. This causes a frequency shift between the transmitted waves and the reflected waves depending on the velocity of the blood cells. This shift in frequency is called the Doppler shift.

Some of the reflected ultrasonic waves are returned to the probe and hit the receiving crystal, activating it at that frequency. The velocity of the blood (μ) is related to the frequency shift (fd) according to the following formula:

$$\mu = \frac{fd \ C}{2f_0 \cos \theta}$$

Here C is the speed of sound in tissue (~ 1500 m/s), f_0 is the frequency of the transmitted wave, and θ is the angle between the sound beam and the direction of blood movement.

For velocities encountered within the blood stream, fd is in the audible frequency range. The more rapid the velocity the higher the pitch of the Doppler sound. We do not hear pure tones because at any one time, the ultrasound beam is reflected off cells at varying velocities; those near the wall moving relatively slowly compared with the center stream.

A frequency-to-voltage converter provides an analog voltage that can be used to record the Doppler output on a stripchart recorder. Some of the Doppler flowmeters have a zero-crossing detector to determine directionality of the blood movement. This is the continuous wave directional Doppler Flowmeter.   By no means has the Doppler flowmeter

By no means has the Doppler flowmeter reached a plateau of sophistication and application. Pulsed Doppler flowmeters are being developed that will determine blood velocity at known distances of penetration. These devices offer the promise of determining velocity profiles noninvasively and in real time. Recently, devices that provide a detailed analysis of the relative contribution of the various frequencies that make up the Doppler signal were introduced. These aid in determining the types of flow regime that is encountered such as turbulence that shows up as a broadening of the spectra. In addition, there are commercially available ultrasound devices that are coupled to positioners that can be used to "paint" a picture of where blood is flowing in the vessels. This technique has been extensively used at the bifurcation of the carotid arteries to visualize stenoses and obstructions.

ELECTROMAGNETIC FLOWMETRY

The electromagnetic flowmeter utilizes the principle of magnetic induction thus: an electrical conductor moving across the lines of force of a magnetic field generates an electrical potential. Since blood is a good conductor, appropriate alignment of blood vessel(s) across a magnetic field allows for the measurement of the induced electromotive force and determination of blood flow velocity. In application, the principle requires a magnetic field and properly oriented electrodes. All electromagnetic flowmeters detect flow velocity but when the cross-sectional area of fluid in the magnetic field is fixed and the device is calibrated, it is then used as a volume recorder. Two categories of electromagnetic flowmeters are used clinically: (1) the invasive EMF used around an exposed blood vessel in the operating room, and (2) the noninvasive EMF which utilizes a large magnet exterior to the body surface.

Several basic electromagnetic flowmeters are available, such as direct current, sinewave, and saw tooth. Small electrodes are mounted at a right angle to the magnetic flux and placed in contact with the outer surface of the vessel in order to detect the voltage induced across the resistance between electrodes. A moving conductor in a magnetic field and the voltage developed across a section of its resistance is expressed as follows:

$$V = vBd \times 10^{-8} \text{ volt}$$

where V is the electrode voltage induced by flow, v is the velocity of flow in centimeters per second, B the magnetic flux density in gauss, and d the inside diameter of the vessel measured in centimeters. When the inside diameter of the vessel and the magnetic flux density are constant, the electrode voltage induced by flow is proportional to velocity and the volume rate of flow.

Invasive Electromagnetic Flowmeter

1. The square-wave electromagnetic flowmeter provides a means for measurement of blood flow in surgically exposed but intact arteries and veins.
2. The flowmeter probe produces a magnetic field across the vessel.
3. Blood flow through the field generates an electrical current proportional to the velocity of the blood.
4. The signal is amplified and made available for presentation to the recorder.

The flow probes are constructed with various lumen sizes ranging from 3 to 125 millimeters in circumference. To obtain a good fit, the circumference of the vessel can be measured with suture material and then a somewhat smaller lumen probe is selected for use. To avoid trauma and to ensure ease of installation, the probes are kept as small and as light as possible. Probe size is important since accuracy and repeatability of measurement are dependent upon it. A vessel should always be slightly constricted to maintain good contact between the transducer electrodes and the walls of the blood vessel. A wise procedure is to always have on hand both large and small probes so that the right size probe will be available when the vessel is exposed.

When a probe is immersed in a volume conductor such as saline and body fluids, it has been noted that the detecting electrodes become polarized and gas forms at the electrode fluid interface. In the square-wave electromagnetic flowmeter, the magnetic field is reversed 240 times per second with an alternating square wave of current and the electrodes are gated ON after the start of the square wave and OFF before the square wave ends. Thus, a minimum artifact slow signal is detected in a uniform reversing magnetic field. By permitting only rapidly changing potentials to pass and by excluding DC polarization voltages by AC coupling of the amplifier, only true flow-generated signals are displayed.

Calibration of the electromagnetic flowmeter is obtained by passing a known volume of saline or blood through a section of an excised vessel in a given period of time. Flow transducers are calibrated at the time of production and all meters have probe factor sensitivity and balance controls in order to obtain standardization. Detection of zero flow or baseline is a problem in some flowmeters and is due mainly to polarization and the dynamic nature of blood flow. A zero baseline can be determined by occluding the vessel or removing the magnetic excitation and then balancing out any residual polarization potentials. The rapidly changing, pulsatile velocity signal and the electrical output are analogous to the instantaneous volume flow. Instantaneous values are utilized to define the pulsatile flow waveforms. The meter integrates the volume of blood flow for a time period including several cardiac cycles and mean flow is displayed on a meter in milliliters per minute. Significant information can be obtained from the characteristic of pulsatile or instantaneous blood flow volume. Pulsatile blood flow waveforms can be recorded on a tape and strip chart for subsequent quantitative analysis.

The electromagnetic flowmeter can be used effectively for ascertaining adequate flow levels and the probability of successful surgery is increased by using a quantitative evaluation at the time of the surgical procedure. An arteriogram cannot be expected to provide hemodynamic information as to flow within the arterial tree; thus, in the analysis of the causes of operative failure, intraoperative hemodynamics are relevant.

NONINVASIVE ELECTROMAGNETIC FLOWMETER

The operation of the noninvasive transcutaneous blood flowmeter is based on the same electromagnetic principle as the invasive flowmeter. Faraday's law of induction states that a moving conductor (blood) within a magnetic field generates a current perpendicular to both the magnetic field and the direction of conductor movement. In a limb, whose tissue's resistance is much greater than blood, the current can be translated into a voltage (Ohm's law) which can be measured at the skin using surface electrodes.

In order to be able to generate measurable skin voltages from the flowing blood, a relatively large magnetic field must be produced. This is accomplished using a motor-driven permanent magnet placed on tracks beneath the patient bed. The magnetic field in the vicinity of the blood vessels is approximately several hundred gauss.

Even with this large magnetic field, the voltages derived from the flowing blood and detected by the skin electrodes are only a few microvolts. These are of about the same magnitude as the local ECG potentials.

Random myoelectric and spurious amplifier noise may generate signals of even greater magnitude. In this linear system, all voltages are additive.

An essential aspect of this device is the extraction of the blood flow signal from the other voltage sources. This is accomplished in the following manner. Sources of voltages are classified as being either synchronous (ECG and blood flow) or random (EMG and noise). Random voltages are negated by averaging 16, 32, or 64 successive waveforms. These spike voltages are thus reduced to a constant DC output. Signals synchronous with the flow pulse are determined with the magnet withdrawn from its position beneath the patient. In this measurement mode, all voltage sources contribute with the singular exception of the blood flow signal. Subtraction of this signal from the total signal generated with the magnetic field in place yields the pure pulsatile component of blood flow.

Standard electrocardiogram leads are used to generate an ECG signal, which is utilized to trigger and time the acquisition of the blood flow data. In addition to these signal-processing aspects, an anomalous R-R interval rejection and large-noise rejection system are employed in the data reduction.

The actual blood flow in liters/minute is determined using the standard electromagnetic formula with values of limb geometry and local magnetic field at the site of measurement.

The acquisition of data including control of magnetic movement, waveform averaging, and flow computation is performed by the data control component of the flowmeter. A stripchart recording of the blood flow data and a printed output of the flow analysis are available within minutes of data sampling.

Components of the noninvasive electromagnetic flowmeter include a magnet on a movable cart. Two sets of electrodes are employed. The first is a standard electrocardiogram lead. The blood flow electrodes are placed on the area where the pulsatile blood flow measurements are desired.

The electrocardiogram and blood flow signals are fed into preamplifiers and then to the data acquisition section of the computer. The computer processes the data and controls the instrumentation system. Blood flow waveforms are continuously presented on a monitor scope. Data is preserved for permanent records on a stripchart recorder and also a printed teletype output.

Electrode placement determines the location of the flow measurement. Typical locations include the femoral, popliteal, and posterior tibial artery sites. For a complete blood flow profile a brachial artery measurement is also obtained and all data are obtained bilaterally.

The electrodes are standard Beckman silver-silver chloride floating electrodes. The skin is prepared by shaving and sanding with a fine sandpaper. When in position the electrodes are tested for electrical continuity and background noise.

Advantages of the noninvasive electromagnetic flowmeter are: patient safety and comfort, repeated measurement capacity, rapid testing and analysis of results, testing can be done in the vascular laboratory, and the instrument can be used as a monitoring device.

PLETHYSMOGRAPHY

Variations in limb volume or circumference can be accurately measured using one of several types of plethysmographic instruments. These devices are all noninvasive and very sensitive to small volume or girth changes that occur naturally or are induced by artificial means. The original plethysmographs were either water- or air-filled rigid containers that encapsulate a limb or digit. These early devices were bulky and awkward to use in a routine clinical setting. Problems, especially with sealing around the proximal portion of the limb and with temperature control, relegated these instruments to the physiology laboratory.

Segmental plethysmography has all but superceded these units in today's vascular clinic. The four most common types of these instruments measure volume changes by monitoring electrical impedance, pressure variations in an encirculating cuff, or the stretching of an elastic tube filled with mercury. The photoplethysmograph detects changes in reflectivity or opacity that result from the periodic filling and emptying of the underlying vessels.

Two origins of signals can be detected plethysmographically. The first concerns an amplification of naturally occurring waveforms that result from the passage of the pressure pulse through the segment being monitored. The increase and decrease of transmural pressure from systole to diastole and back again causes the vessels to expand and contract. This can be measured as a volume or girth variation on the limb and the recorded waveform corresponds closely to the arterial pressure waveform. The magnitude of these volume changes rarely exceeds 1% on the calf of a normal subject. The amplifier in such a system should have relatively high gain characteristics as well as suppression of the DC or steady state signal. A bandpass filter with sharp cutoffs at 0.2 Hz and at least 20 Hz is necessary to reduce low-frequency signals (such as breathing artifacts) and to allow the high-frequency components to be recorded.

Induced plethysmographic changes are often desirable for quantitation of the venous as well as the arterial flows. The widely used technique called venous occlusion plethysmography consists of monitoring the volume changes in a segment distal to a cuff inflated to about 40 mm Hg. The initial rate of volume increase represents filling of the venous bed and is the arterial perfusion. The decrease in calf volume following the sudden release of the cuff pressure allows the veins to empty. This rate of volume decrease is related to the patency of the venous system, a slow decrease being linked to the existence of a thrombosis in the deep veins.

PNEUMOPLETHYSMOGRAPHY

Of all the plethysmographs that are commercially available at present, the pneumoplethysmograph is the least technically sophisticated. At first glance, it appears a direct descendant from the earlier air-filled plethysmographs, but on more detailed examination it more closely resembles the oscillometer. In its simplest form, it consists of a blood pressure cuff connected to a pressure registering device. When the cuff is wrapped around an extremity or digit and inflated to a specified volume and pressure, waveforms, similar in shape to arterial pressure waves, can be detected and recorded.

The relationship between changes in cuff pressure (dP_c) and changes in the underlying arterial pressure (dP_a) is the following:

$$dP_c = K_1 K_c \frac{\bar{P}_c^2}{P_{atm} V_c} dP_a$$

The constant K_1 represents coefficient of gas compressibility, numercial unit conversions, and other variants. K_c is related to the elasticity of the cuff and depends not only on the material of construction, but the tightness of application. $\bar{P}_c$ is the average cuff pressure and V_c is the volume of air contained within the cuff. Assuming that during any one measurement procedure these parameters are constant we get

$$dP_c = K_T dP_a$$

Thus changes in the cuff pressure are proportional to changes in the arterial pressures and the resulting waveforms are similar. For routine noninvasive vascular diagnosis, this constant of proportionality is unknown and the actual arterial pressures are not determined.

Calibration of this system is performed by injecting a small volume of air into the cuff via a syringe and reading the pressure change as seen by a pen deflection on a stripchart recorder. Adjusting the sensitivity to obtain a 20 millimeter deflection when 10 cc of air (for example) is injected permits a degree of reproducibility of data and can be used for comparison of waveforms from patient to patient as well as following the progression of disease (or effectiveness of treatment) over the course of time.

Pneumoplethysmography is also suitable for venous occlusion techniques when used in conjunction with a proximal cuff. The venous engorgement that follows an inflation to about 40 mm Hg increases the monitoring cuff pressure and measurements of arterial inflow and venous outflow can be obtained.

Another type of pneumoplethysmograph is designed for analysis of the venous system by monitoring respiratory waves in various locations in the legs. Changes in intrathoracic pressure that occur during the respiratory cycle cause pressure waves that are propagated through the low-pressure venous system. These pressure waves can be detected in cuffs placed along the leg. This technique requires multiple cuffs along with appropriate transducers and stripchart channels. In the normal limb, the venous respiratory waveforms can be detected in the most distal segment of the legs. Venous thrombosis interferes with or prohibits transmission of these waves. By appropriately inflating cuffs at different segments, the degree and location of thrombosis can be identified.

The principle advantages of pneumoplethysmography lies in its relative simplicity and ease of use. These attributes should be carried over to a device that is relatively inexpensive and small in size. Unfortunately, appurtenances such as recorders and automatic cuff inflaters and deflaters tend to increase the initial cost and bulkiness of these devices. An additional drawback concerns the indirect cause-and-effect relationship between the vascular intraluminal pulsations and the pressure waves recorded in the cuffs. This difficulty is shared by many other indirect diagnostic devices and it is the price we pay for measurement techniques that are noninvasive.

IMPEDANCE PLETHYSMOGRAPHY

Limb volume changes, whether due to arterial pulsations or venous capacity variations, can be noninvasively and quantitatively measured using electrical impedance. This term refers to the measure of difficulty that an oscillating current has passing through matter. As a first approximation, the electrical impedance, Z, of a limb segment is related to the following three parameters: overall tissue resistivity ρ (ohm-centimeters), length of the segment ℓ (centimeters), and the cross sectional area S (square centimeters). These are related by the formula

$$Z = \frac{\rho \ell}{S}$$

We will make several simplifying assumptions to derive an operational relationship between measured impedance changes and computed limb volume changes. The limb segment can be represented by a right circular cylinder and the tissue is considered homogeneous with respect to resistivity and current flow.

Substituting the limb volume, $V = S\ell$, and differentiating, we obtain

$$dZ = -\rho \ell^2 \frac{dV}{V^2}$$

After some algebraic manipulation and using finite difference notation in place of differentials, we get

$$\frac{\Delta Z}{Z} = \frac{-\Delta V}{V}$$

This equation shows an equality between the fractional change in impedance and the fractional limb volume change. This can be expressed as percentage or equivalently, cc/100 cc.

To perform this measurement the impedance plethysmograph uses four electrodes that wrap around the limb. The outer two electrodes are the forcing electrodes and the inner ones are the measuring electrodes. The impedance plethysmograph provides a constant current of about 1 milliampere that flows through the outer electrodes. This current is oscillating at a high frequency of about 100 kHz. There are three reasons for employing this rapid cycling. It reduces capacitance effects, especially at the skin-electrode interface, and promotes a more even current distribution in the deep tissues. Also, this high-frequency current does not electrically activate either the muscle or nervous cells.

The current that is driven through the limb creates a potential drop or voltage difference that can be picked up by the inner electrodes and amplified. The impedance is electronically computed using a varient of Ohm's law, $Z = E/I$.

The output data from the impedance plethysmograph includes the base impedance, Z_0, and the change in impedance, ΔZ, or expressed as the fraction change $\Delta Z/Z_0$. This device can be calibrated by using suitable resistors (noninductive) of known values. This is usually done internally and expressed as voltage per impedance.

STRAIN-GAUGE PLETHYSMOGRAPHY

The third type of plethysmograph is the strain-gauge plethysmograph. This device employs a sensor that historically consisted of a thin tube of rubber filled with mercury. This tube is wrapped about a limb with a slight extension ($\sim 10\%$). The lateral expansion of the blood vessels as the pulse wave traverses a segment causes a small increase in size and circumference of the limb which stretches the elastic tube. This causes a small change in electrical resistance in the mercury, which is detected and amplified.

The relationship between the stretching of the elastic gauge and the volume changes in the limb can be simply derived as follows. We consider the mercury in the elastic tube to be a volume resistor. The resistance is expressed using the same equation as for the limb impedance

$$R = \frac{\rho \ell}{S}$$

In this equation the resistance, R, resistivity, ρ, the length, ℓ, and the cross-sectional area refer to the column of mercury. The volume of mercury is equal to the length times the cross section and remains constant upon stretching. Substituting this volume we get

$$R = \frac{\rho \ell^2}{V}$$

Differentiating this (holding the volume constant)

$$dR = \frac{2\rho \ell d\ell}{V}$$

or equivalently

$$\frac{dR}{R} = \frac{2d\ell}{\ell}$$

Now consider the limb segment with circumference, C. The volume of a length L is

$$V = \frac{C^2 L}{4\pi}$$

Differentiating this (keeping L constant) and rearranging terms, we obtain

$$\frac{dV}{V} = \frac{2dC}{C}$$

The length of the mercury column is equal to the circumference. Equating these two expressions, it follows that

$$\frac{dR}{R} = \frac{dV}{V}$$

That is, the fractional change in the resistance of the mercury equals the fractional change in limb volume. As with the impedance formulation, this is expressed as percentage change or, equivalently, cc/100 cc.

The standard method of calibrating the strain gauge plethysmograph is by stretching the tube to a known extension. This can be cumbersome for clinical use and most of the newer models have a built-in calibration signal. As with the pneumo- and impedance plethysmographs, the output is usually in analog form and requires a stripchart recorder to collect patient data for analysis.

PHOTOPLETHYSMOGRAPHY

The photoelectric plethysmograph has had an ubiquitous, yet almost unrecognized, presence in hospitals for many years. Almost all ECG monitors in ICU's and CCU's have a separate channel for a pulse monitor. This is the photoplethysmograph. This simple device is being used in an increasing number of applications, not only in the vascular clinic, but also in the private consumer market as a pulse or rate meter. Here its application is for a heart rate meter to help assess cardiac condition and physical fitness. A large variety of portable battery operated pulse meters are currently being sold for this purpose.

The primary difference between these devices and the photoplethysmograph used for vascular testing is the availability to record the pulse waveform. This waveform can be obtained from almost any area of the body and the overall shape of the curve is representative of the arterial pulse waveform. Unfortunately, no simple and direct relationship has been derived between the output of the photoplethysmograph and physiologic parameters of volume, pressure, or flow. Nevertheless, careful application of this device can yield important data on the vascular status of the patient.

The sensor of the photoplethysmograph consists of two units, a light source and a light-sensitive detector. The source of illumination is usually a miniature incandescent bulb or a light-emitting diode (LED). These emit light in various frequency ranges either naturally or by selective filters. The current state of application of the photoplethysmograph does not specify a particular portion of the spectrum for use. Essentially similar waveforms are recorded using lower-frequency LED's as well as the broad band of incandescent light.

The detector usually consists of either a phototransistor or, more commonly, a photoconductive cell, and should be matched with the illumination source with respect to frequency sensitivity. The photoconductive cell is a light-sensitive resistor whose electrical resistance decreases as a function of incident light.

Packaging the light source and detector adjacent to each other permits the measurement of light that is reflected from the outer few millimeters of skin tissue. The intensity of the reflected light is modulated by the volume of blood within the illuminated region. It is this variation of either the light absorption or reflection that occurs over a pulse cycle that yields the photoplethysmogram waveform.

Because of the small size of the sensor, and its sensitivity to cutaneous blood flow, this device sees much application in the analysis of perfusion of the digits and assessment of vasospastic disorders. It has recently been used in the evaluation of cerebral vascular disorders by measuring supraorbital area perfusion while the patient undergoes arterial compressive maneuvers. We have pioneered the use of the photoplethysmograph in the study of pressure sore etiology and for assessment of wound healing.

THERMOMETRY

A useful indication of the physiologic state of the patient is obtained through an examination of the individual's body temperature. For example, the presence of shock can be quickly determined by a drop in a patient's big toe temperature. Circulatory shock reduces blood pressure, which precipitates a reduction in peripheral blood flow, causing a decrease in the peripheral temperature. Measurements of systemic temperature and the temperature of the surface of the skin are the two most basic types of temperature measurements obtained from the patient.

Systemic temperature, which is the internal temperature of the body, may be determined by measurements at the mouth, axilla, or rectum. Although not frequently done, the most accurate measurement of the systemic temperature is obtained at the tympanic membrane, due to its close proximity to the temperature control center of the brain (the forepart of the hypothalamus).

The temperature of the surface of the skin varies in response to several factors: the circulation of the blood under the particular region being studied, the local metabolism of the area, thermal conductivity and the moisture of the skin, and the temperature gradient between the skin and the surrounding air. Variations in skin surface temperature may also be secondary to the presence of tumors or to changes in body structure.

The following sections will discuss the currently available instrumentation for temperature measurements: thermistors, thermocouples, radiation (infrared), and chemical (liquid crystals).

THERMISTORS AND THERMOCOUPLES

Thermistors and thermocouples can be categorized as nonmechanical transducers that have variable resistance. Their use in determining temperature is feasible by use of the thermoresistance effect and temperature-induced alterations in electrical resistivity of a semiconductor—the temperature coefficient. In practice, the thermistor is more commonly employed than the thermocouple for temperature measurements.

A *thermistor* is a semiconductor composed of ceramic materials. It is a thermal resistor with a high negative temperature coefficient. Most semiconductors have a negative temperature coefficient, while the temperature coefficient is positive for most metals. In contrast to metals, the thermistor, being composed of ceramic materials, has a resistance that decreases with increases in temperature and increases with decreases in temperature.

The following formula provides the empirical relationship that exists between R_t, the thermistor resistance, and T, the absolute temperature in Kelvin (K)

$$R_t = R_0 e^{[\beta(T_0 - T)/TT_0]}$$

where β is a material constant for the thermistor in kelvins and T_0 is the standard reference temperature in kelvins. Also referred to as the characteristic temperature, β ranges from 2500 to 5000 K and most frequently approximates 4000 K.

Manipulating the above equation by differentiation with respect to T and division by R_t, the temperature coefficient α can be determined in units of %/K:

$$\alpha = \frac{1}{R_t} \frac{dR_t}{dT} = \frac{-\beta}{T^2}$$

Linearity is seen in the voltage vs current characteristics up to the point where self-heating of the thermistor becomes a factor. Up to this point, in the linear portion of the curve, the current is directly proportional to the applied voltage on the basis of Ohm's law, and the temperature of the thermistor equals that of its surroundings.

Thermistors are available in various shapes (washer-shaped, rod, chip, bead). The small size of the thermistor allows for its easy attachment to the tips of catheters or needles.

The use of *thermocouples* (thermoelectric thermometry) is based on the fact that an electromotive force is present across the junction formed by two dissimilar metals. Contributing to this electromotive force are two independent processes—the Peltier electromotive force and the Thomson electromotive force. The Peltier electromotive force is secondary to the meeting of two unlike metals and the temperature at their junction. The net electromotive force of Peltier is approximately proportional to the difference between the temperatures found at the two junctions. The Thomson electromotive force is secondary to the gradient of temperature along each single conductor. The net electromotive force of Thomson is proportional to the difference of the squares of the absolute temperatures at the junctions of the metals. In order to determine an unknown temperature, one of the junctions is maintained constant at a known temperature.

INFRARED

The human skin is an almost perfect emitter of infrared radiation; it emits infrared energy in proportion to the surface temperature for any body location. Sources of heat or regions of coolness can thus be easily detected with an infrared thermometer. Expanding this simple application by incorporating an infrared thermometer into a scanner, one can scan the entire body with this technique referred to as thermography. Basically, infrared energy is measured and its magnitude modulates the intensity of a light beam, which produces a map of the infrared energy on photographic paper, the resultant image being referred to as a thermogram. Recently developed is a thermography unit that can display the thermogram in real time on a oscilloscope.

The basic premise of this technique is that there is a known relationship between the surface temperature of a body and its infrared emission or radiant power. The temperature of an object can thus be determined without contact. In the human, skin surface temperature varies in accordance with local factors such as cellular and circulatory process that are operating at each particular location. This has allowed the technique to be employed successfully in the early detection of breast cancer, in localizing and assessing the degree of arthritic involvement, in frostbite or burn patients to determine the degree of tissue destruction, and in peripheral vascular disease for detection of venous thrombosis and other vascular pathologies.

Planck's law, when multiplied by emissivity (ϵ), yields a measure of the radiation emitted by an object:

$$\omega_\lambda = \frac{\epsilon C_1}{\lambda^5 (e^{C_2/\lambda T} - 1)}$$

where C_1 is 3.74×10^4, C_2 is 1.44×10^4, T is the temperature of a black body, and ϵ is the emissivity, i.e., the extent to which a particular surface deviates from a perfect black body where the emissivity is considered to be a value of one.

By differentiating the above equation and setting it equal to zero and solving for λ, one obtains Wien's displacement law, which determines the wavelength (λ_m) for which ω_λ is a maximum

$$\lambda_m = \frac{2898}{T}$$

and by integrating the area under the curve, one determines the total radiant power of the body, ω_t, by means of the Stefan-Boltzmann law:

$$\omega_t = E\sigma T^4$$

where σ is the Stefan-Boltzmann constant (5.67×10^{-12}).

LIQUID CRYSTALS

Esters of cholesterol (a cholesteric liquid) exist as ordered molecular structures intermediate between a true three-dimensional solid and a liquid—a *liquid crystal.* The liquid crystals exist within a specific temperature range. Above this range, they are in the liquid phase and below this range they exist as three-dimensional solid crystals. These liquid crystals possess an unusually high sensitivity to temperature. When the liquid crystals are applied to a blackened surface, they give rise to iridescent colors the dominant wavelength of which is determined by small temperature alterations. The temperature sensitivity of the liquid crystals is 0.1 C and they have a spatial resolution of 1000 lines per inch.

The optical properties of solids and the mechanical properties of liquids are exhibited by the liquid crystals. A crystalline property that is an analog of circular dichromism arises from the molecular arrangement. This property gives maximal scattering of a specific light wavelength while other components of the light are transmitted through the material. The blackened surface to which the liquid crystals are applied absorbs the transmitted light and the maximally scattered light appears iridescent.

The wavelength of the maximally scattered light is a function of the molecular order. As there are weak intermolecular attractions in liquid crystals, the molecular order may be altered by small changes in internal energy, as by the change in temperature. A change in temperature would alter the internal energy, thereby changing the molecular order, which would precipitate a change in the wavelength of the maximally scattered light. One of the more significant properties of the color-temperature response of liquid crystals is its constancy, i.e., a given cholesteric liquid crystal will reliably show the same color at a given specific temperature. By altering the combination of esters in the liquid crystal, temperatures in the range of −20 C to 250 C can be measured. For example, a given liquid crystal mixture may show blue at 34 C, green at 31.4 C, and bronze at 29.9 C. This means that at a temperature greater than or equal to 34 C, the liquid crystal will exhibit a blue color; at temperatures between 34 C and 31.4 C, the liquid crystal will exhibit a green-blue color; at temperatures between 31.4 C and 29.9 C, the liquid crystal will be a bronze-green color; and at temperatures of 29.9 C or less, the liquid crystal will be a deep bronze.

The liquid crystals may be sprayed onto large areas or may be mounted onto a tape for determining temperature of smaller regions. The use of liquid crystals is helpful in locating veins and arteries, and in determining tumor size, vascularity, and response to treatment. It is also quite useful in peripheral vascular surgery for a rapid evaluation of skin temperature, for postoperative monitoring of graft patency, for evaluating the effect of lumbar sympathectomy or the response to vasodilator therapy, for determining amputation level, and for detecting potential areas of ischemic decubiti, pressure areas in amputated stumps, or localized regions of deficient circulation.

SOUND DETECTION

STETHOSCOPE

The stethoscope was first discovered in 1816 by René Théophile Hyacinthe Laënnec; the word is from the Greek *stethos*, "breast" and *skopien*, "to view." Since Laënnec's first use of a rolled piece of paper, many significant improvements have been made, and although many uses of the stethoscope have been replaced by more modern technology, it remains an indispensible tool to the modern physician.

The value of the stethoscope is dependent on the user. The sounds perceived by the user are greatly influenced by the way in which the stethoscope is applied to the patient and the interpretation of those sounds depends upon the examiner's acuity and training. The stethoscope additionally reflects the acoustics of the human ear. In this regard, the age of the user influences the response to the sounds heard through the stethoscope—the younger the user, the better the response.

The modern stethoscope is typically binaural with a single flexible tube attached to the chest piece. The contemporary chest piece usually contains two cups; one is bell-shaped without a diaphragm and is for the transmission of sounds of low pitch; the other side of the chest piece is a flatter cup that has a diaphragm and is for the transmission of sounds of high pitch.

There have been few acoustical studies of the stethoscope.* The stethoscope amplifies sounds due to a standing wave phenomenon. This phenomenon occurs at greater wavelengths of the transmitted sound. A stethoscope that is of single tubing design and with a chest piece as a shallow bell or trumpet bell shows attenuation of high frequencies. The presence of a single tubing gives an irregular distortion of the sound and considerable loss of high frequencies. In a stethoscope with double tubing and a deep trumpet-bell chest piece there is amplification of the higher frequencies. If one uses a stethoscope of double tubing and a shallow-bell chest piece, the amplification of high frequencies provided by the double tubing is negated by the use of a shallow-bell chest piece. With this variety in acoustic ability, depending upon which stethoscope type is being used, the physician may miss sounds that can be heard with a different type of stethoscope. If the stethoscope that is used attenuates the sound by as small an amount as 3 dB, those clinically significant sounds near the threshold of the examiner's hearing may be completely lost.

The quality of the sound perceived by the examiner is also influenced by the manner in which the chest piece is applied to the patient. If, when using a bell-shaped chest piece, it is firmly applied, there is greater attenuation of the low frequencies as compared with the high frequencies. In such instances, the skin of the patient functions as a diaphragm; with increasing pressure applied to the chest piece, the skin-diaphragm becomes taut, thus attenuating the low frequencies. Loose-fitting ear pieces may cause an air leak, thus reducing the contact between the examiner's ear and the patient's chest and lowering the examiner's perception.

As high-frequency sounds have harmonics or overtones that provide the distinctive characteristics of musical instruments, these same harmonics provide distinctive characteristics to the body's sounds that aid in the identification of lesions on the basis of sound alone, e.g., the murmur of a ventricular septal defect as compared with mitral insufficiency. High-frequency sounds are also important in localizing the sound's source, as they do not spread as far as or with the intensity of low-frequency sounds that radiate across the patient's chest. Some murmurs are of such low intensity as to be just at the threshold of hearing. Some

---

*Ertel PY, Lawrence M. Brown RK, Stern AM: Stethoscope Acoustics I. The doctor and his stethoscope. II. Transmission and filtration patterns. Circulation 34:889–909, 1966.

are almost completely high frequency, so that a stethoscope attenuating the high frequencies would make a murmur such as that due to aortic insufficiency completely inaudible.

MICROPHONE

As only a small portion of heart sounds are within the audible range, the use of electronics in heart-sound detection has been advocated. Unfortunately, physicians have not widely accepted the use of electronic stethoscopes. Graphic recording of heart sounds (phonocardiography) has achieved greater acceptance. This technique has been put to other uses, such as carotid phonoangiography.

Microphones used for the detection of heart sounds may be crystal, using the piezoelectric effect, or dynamic, based on Faraday's principle. At low frequencies, the piezoelectric shows a greater sensitivity then the dynamic microphone. The dynamic microphone has a low-frequency response and as such cannot be used for pulse-wave recordings.

These microphones may be contact, where the microphone is directly applied to the skin, or air-coupled, where there is an air-filled tube between the transducer and a cup on the skin. Air-coupled microphones are useful in recording carotid or the jugular venous pulse and apex cardiograms.

By carefully selecting diaphragm size and microphone bell, one can accomplish mechanical filtering by the same technique as that discussed above for the stethoscope, where the skin functions as a diaphragm, the more pressure being applied the more taut the skin becomes, and the greater the sensitivity to higher frequencies.

A frequency response of 25 to 2000 Hz is required to reproduce heart sounds and murmurs and a frequency response of 0.1 to 100 Hz is required for pulse waves. The readout can be either an oscilloscope or a high-frequency stripchart recorder.

CHAPTER 4

TECHNIQUES FOR MEASURING BLOOD PRESSURE AND BLOOD FLOW

BLOOD PRESSURE MEASUREMENTS
- Ankle Systolic Pressure
- Lower and Upper Extremity Segmental Systolic Pressure
- Systolic Blood Pressure in the Digits
- Skin Blood Pressure
- Ophthalmic Artery Pressure
- Peripheral Venous Pressure
- Direct Measurement of Arterial Blood Pressure
BLOOD FLOW MEASUREMENTS
- Doppler Ultrasonic Flowmetry
- Plethysmography
- Electromagnetic Flowmetry
- Temperature Gradients

The detection and treatment of vascular disease depends upon precise, quantitative test procedures that provide for an accurate anatomic and physiologic assessment of the vasculature. Such test procedures are valuable adjuncts to the complete history and physical examination. A vascular testing program should provide for the determinants of the presence, the degree of severity, and the location of the disease. The objective data should provide for an appropriate decision for a radiographic examination and subsequently for a decision for surgical intervention.

Criteria for an objective testing program include: (1) safe and relatively comfortable test procedures, (2) tests that can be repeated as often as required, (3) results that are reproducible, (4) test procedures that should be and are being done more by competent technicians, and (5) data that provide for objective assessment. Thus, a good test program provides for baseline data to be used for immediate decision making and for subsequent follow-up evaluations.

BLOOD PRESSURE MEASUREMENTS

Pressures in the arterial system are pulsatile and are affected by the forces, frequency, and magnitude of the cardiac contraction, the elasticity of the large and medium-sized arteries, and the state of the arterioles. Blood pressure can be measured by both direct and indirect methods. Conventional indirect methods utilize Korotkoff sounds or the return of palpable pulses. These methods are used most effectively to measure pressure in the upper and lower extremities in the absence of significant arterial occlusion. A systematic noninvasive measurement of blood pressure in several segments of the upper and lower limbs and of the fingers and toes requires special procedures but provides considerable information regarding the status of the circulation.

Indirect methods of measuring blood pressure require the use of an occlusion cuff or cuffs and a pulse sensor. When the cuff and the sensor are separated, the pressure is measured at the cuff location, not at the sensor location. Blood pressures are measured in millimeters of mercury (mm Hg). Pressure readings that reach a maximum of 100 to 150 mm Hg are recorded as systolic pressures, whereas pressures that reach a maximum of 70 to 90 mm Hg are designated diastolic pressures. Resting systolic pressures above 160 mm Hg and diastolic pressures above 90 mm Hg are generally considered abnormal. Factors such as exercise, emotional disturbances, trauma, and shock can have a profound effect on blood pressure.

Bilateral arm pressures (systolic and diastolic) should be done as part of a thorough physical examination. Detection of hypertension is important. Systolic pressure differences greater than 20 mm Hg between arms is suggestive of arterial occlusive disease in the arms or vessels leading to the arms, and blood pressure abnormalities in the lower extremities have special significance in the diagnosis of vascular disease.

BASIC SPHYGMOMANOMETRIC TECHNIQUES FOR MEASURING BRACHIAL SYSTOLIC AND DIASTOLIC PRESSURE

Instruments
1. Stethoscope
2. Compression cuff(s)
3. Sphygmomanometer(s)—mercury and/or aneroid
4. Rubber hand bulb with pressure valves

Procedures

1. Select the appropriate-sized compression cuff. Remember that the standard adult cuff will produce inaccurate readings in obese adults and small individuals.

2. Check the manometer periodically to determine the position of the mercury meniscus, which should be at zero when no pressure is applied. Check the aneroid manometer at intervals against a mercury manometer by connecting both instruments to the same pressure source.

3. Have the patient assume a comfortable sitting or supine position with the arm at approximately heart level. In either position the arm is abducted, slightly flexed, and supported by a relatively smooth firm surface. Generally there is little difference between resting blood pressure readings when sitting or lying down. If the individual complains of faintness or dizziness on standing, blood pressures should be taken in all three positions: standing, sitting, and lying.

4. The appropriate-sized deflated compression cuff is applied evenly and snugly around the upper arm. The lower edge of the cuff should be one inch above the bend in the arm or the point at which the bell of the stethoscope is to be positioned. The cuff is centered over the brachial artery in the front middle part of the arm. Remember that too high a reading will be obtained if the cuff is not centered over the artery, or if the cuff is applied too loosely, allowing the cuff to bulge (Fig. 4-1 a and b).

5. Palpate the radial artery and note the rate and rhythm (Fig. 4-2a). Inflate the compression cuff rapidly to approximately 30 mm Hg above the pressure at which the radial pulse disappears (Fig. 4-2b). Do not overinflate the cuff since this can be painful for the patient and can also produce falsely high readings.

6. Deflate the cuff at a rate of 2 to 3 mm Hg per heartbeat. Note the pressure at which the radial artery pulse returns and record this pressure as systolic arterial blood pressure.

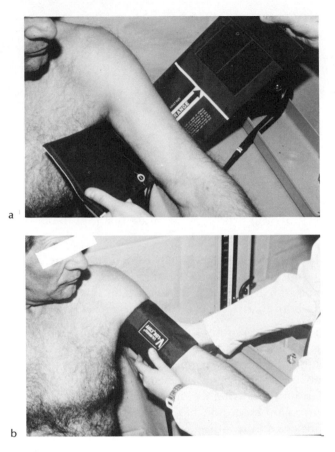

FIGURE 4-1a,b.   Application of pneumatic cuff.

7. Palpate the brachial artery on the inner aspect of the arm below the edge of the compression cuff (Fig 4-3a). If no pulsation is felt, palpate around the area at one to two o'clock. Place the bell of the stethoscope lightly but snugly over the palpable artery, producing an airtight seal (Fig. 4-3b). Inflate the compression cuff rapidly to 20 to 30 mm Hg above the systolic pressure previously recorded while palpating the radial artery (Fig. 4-3c).

8. Deflate the cuff at the rate of 2 to 3 mm Hg per heartbeat while observing the meniscus of the mercury column. Listen for characteristic changes in the Korotkoff sounds. The levels of pressure at which the quality of the sounds changes determine the systolic and diastolic pressures.

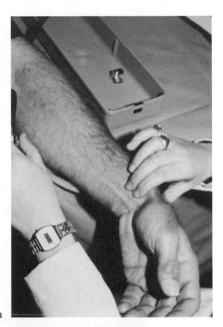

FIGURE 4-2a,b.   Palpation of radial artery.

a

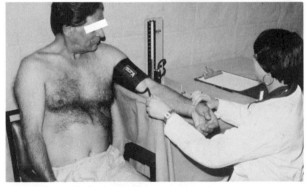

b

9. Systolic pressure is that pressure level at which the first Korotkoff sounds are heard. The sound is characterized by a beginning faint, clear rhythmic "tap" or "thump" of gradually increasing intensity. As pressure in the cuff is decreased the sound changes progress through a phase of "blowing" or swishing and then to a softer sound "thud." At the pressure within the cuff indicated by the level of the mercury column when the sound is suddenly muffled, the first diastolic pressure is recorded, and when the pressure in the cuff is at the level when the sound disappears, the second diastolic pressure is recorded, e.g., blood pressure = 125/90/ 80 mm Hg.

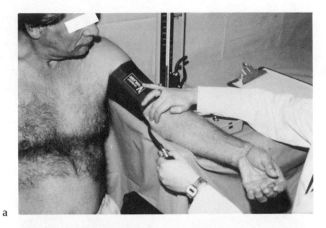

a

b

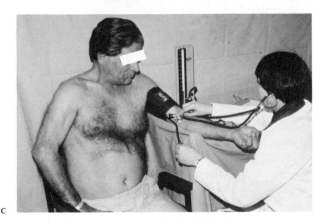

c

FIGURE 4-3a-c.   Palpation of brachial artery.

10. To obtain as accurate a reading as possible it is important to avoid all possible sources of error, such as the following. (a) Incorrect positioning of the extremity (the artery in which blood pressure is measured must be at the level of the heart). (b) Incorrect deflation of the compression cuff (at rates slower than 2 mm Hg per heartbeat, venous congestion may develop and the diastolic pressure reading will be too high). (c) Incorrect recording of the first blood pressure (because of possible arterial spasm and/or anxiety and apprehension first reading can be too high). Deflate the cuff completely, wait for venous return, repeat the measurements. (d) Incorrect position of the mercury column. (e) Disappearing sounds—the "gap." (To avoid recording incorrect low systolic readings remember to first record blood pressure by palpating radial artery). (f) Incorrect application of the cuff (bulging and ballooning of the cuff will produce readings that are too high). (g) Defective equipment such as the air release valve, porous rubber tubing, dirty mercury and glass tube, or an inaccurate aneroid manometer.

Figure 4-4 shows an example of a form that should be filled out for all patients undergoing a test for arm blood pressure.

ANKLE SYSTOLIC PRESSURE

Systolic arterial pressure can be determined at the ankle using a standard sphygmomanometer and the Doppler velocity meter. This technique is similar to conventional recording of blood pressure with the exception of the pick-up sensor. The Doppler probe is used instead of the stethoscope.

Instruments and Materials
1. Doppler velocity meter and probe(s)
2. Arm compression cuff(s)
3. Acoustic gel
4. Mercury and/or aneroid manometer

Procedure
1. Place an appropriate-sized arm cuff around the arm and palpate the brachial artery.

2. Apply ample acoustic gel over the artery. Position the Doppler probe over the palpated artery and listen for the arterial velocity signal (Fig. 4-5a). Keep the probe in this location.

3. Inflate the cuff until the signal disappears.

ARM BLOOD PRESSURE

Date: *6/15/78*

Name: *John/Jane Doe*   Telephone No.: *222-888-6666*

Address: *50 Clearview Blvd., Faraway, New York 12000*

Social Security Number: *001-01-0001*

Date of Birth: *1/20/20*   Height: *180* cm   Weight: *70* kg

Medications: (1)   (2)

(3)   (4)   None:

Time of Day: *13:00*   Time of Last Medication: *8:30*   Room Temp. *22 C*

Instruments:

Mercury Manometer   *X*   Aneroid Manometer   *No*

Arm Cuff Size   *12 cm x 23 cm*

Supine _____   Sitting _____   Standing _____

	Right Arm	*Left Arm*
Radial Artery		
Pulse rate (per minute)	*70*	*70*
Rhythm	*Regular*	*Regular*
Systolic Pressure (mm Hg)	*120*	*120*
Brachial Artery		
Systolic Pressure (mm Hg)	*120*	*120*
Diastolic Pressure 1.	*90*	*90*
Diastolic Pressure 2.	*80*	*80*

Comments: _____

_____ Technician: _____

FIGURE 4-4.   Example of an arm blood pressure form.

4. Slowly deflate the cuff and note the pressure at which the arterial signal returns. The velocity signal will not disappear during complete deflation of the cuff; therefore, diastolic pressure will not be determined.

5. Systolic blood pressure should be determined for both the right and left arms.

6. The same arm compression cuff is now placed around the ankle above the malleolus and will be inflated in the same manner as for arm systolic pressures (Fig. 4-5b, c, and d).

7. Palpate the dorsalis pedis and posterior tibial arteries. Select the strongest pulse. Note the sites at which the arteries are palpated. Apply ample acoustic gel over the artery.

8. Inflate the cuff to a pressure that occludes the artery. Deflate the cuff 2 to 3 mm Hg per heartbeat and note the pressure at which the velocity flow signal returns. Deflate the cuff completely.

9. Record all data on appropriate data sheets.

10. Points to remember: (a) The pneumatic bladder of the compression cuff must completely encircle the limb. Both the length and the width of the bladder affect the pressure. (b) Large extremities require wider and longer cuffs. Choice of manometer and Doppler probe depends upon ease of use and preference. (c) The mercury strain gauge or photosensor can be used instead of the Doppler probe. They are placed over the great toe, and a pulse wave instead of an audible signal is obtained. These sensors are discussed under Mercury Strain Gauge Plethysmography and Photoplethysmography.

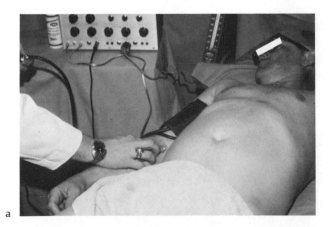

a

FIGURE 4-5a.   Procedure for determination of ankle systolic pressure using Doppler ultrasound.

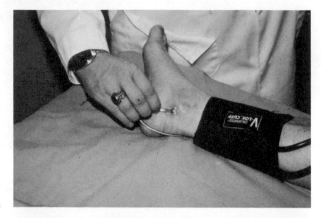

b

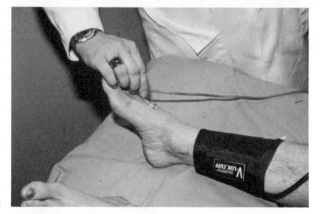

c

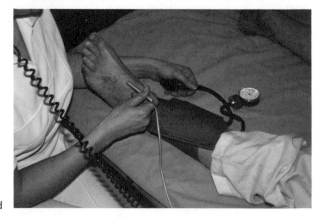

d

FIGURE 4-5b-d. Continued.

LOWER AND UPPER EXTREMITY SEGMENTAL SYSTOLIC PRESSURE

By applying an occluding cuff at various levels of the extremities and positioning a flow sensor over a peripheral artery, pressure profiles for each extremity are obtained. Any one of a variety of flow sensors can be used, for example, Doppler ultrasonic velocity detector, mercury in silastic strain gauge, and photosensor.

Instruments and Materials
1. A series of different-sized compression cuffs
2. Manometer—aneroid and/or mercury
3. Doppler instrument with earphones and probes
4. Acoustic gel
5. Pocket calculator
6. Measuring tape

Procedure
1. The patient assumes a supine position. All constricting clothing is removed or loosened and the skin surface areas over which pulses are palpable are made accessible.

2. Place compression cuff(s) on upper arms. Apply acoustic gel to the probe and over the palpable areas. Determine upper arm pressures at the brachial and radial arteries bilaterally.

3. Palpate the three vessels (posterior tibial, anterior tibial, and dorsalis pedis) at the ankle. Apply ample acoustic gel to the probe and select the artery with the strongest signal. This artery is to be used for systolic measurements at the four sites.

4. An appropriate cuff is positioned around the upper thigh and manometer attached. Doppler probe is positioned over the selected artery at the ankle. The thigh cuff is inflated until the audible signal disappears. The cuff is deflated slowly and the pressure at which the arterial signal returns is noted. In the same way, determine sequentially the pressures at the lower thigh (above knee), at the calf (below knee), and at the ankle (Fig. 4-6a, b, and c). Repeat these measurements on the other extremity. An alternate method is to position the four cuffs (high thigh, low thigh, calf, and ankle), sequentially determine the pressures at each site, and then proceed to the other limb.

5. Calculate

$$\frac{\text{ankle systolic pressure}}{\text{arm systolic pressure}} = \text{index}$$

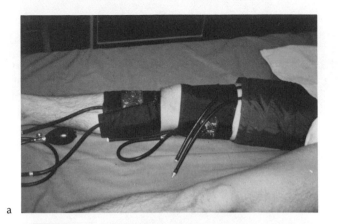

a

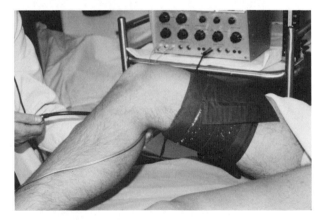

b

FIGURE 4-6a-c.   Doppler ultrasound procedure for measuring long extremity segmental systolic pressure and popliteal pressure.

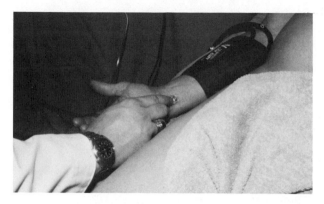

FIGURE 4-7.   Upper extremity sequential examination.

and note the pressure gradients segment to segment in same limb and compare measurements with opposite limb.

A similar segmental exam can be applied to the upper extremity. In this case the index is forearm–upper arm index and a normal index is equal to or greater than 1.0 (Fig. 4-7).

1. The patient assumes a supine position and all constricting clothing is loosened or removed and skin surface areas over which pulses are palpable are made accessible.

2. Place compression cuff(s) on upper and lower arm segments. Apply acoustic gel to the probe and over the palpable areas. Pressures are determined at the brachial, radial, and ulnar arteries bilaterally.

3. The probe is positioned over the appropriate vessel and the cuff is inflated while listening to the pulse sounds, which diminish as the pressure is increased. When the pulse is no longer audible the cuff pressure is increased approximately 20 to 30 mm Hg higher.

4. The cuff pressure is released at a slow, even pace while listening for the first audible pulse sound. This is the systolic pressure measurement for the particular area at which the cuff is placed.

SYSTOLIC BLOOD PRESSURE
IN THE DIGITS

In the evaluation of vascular disease, measurements should be made bilaterally at several locations along an extremity including the most distal areas, the digits. Assessment of the digital arterial supply can provide

---

PRETEST DATA

Date: _____   Time of Day: _____

Name: _____   SS#: _____ Tel. # _____

Date of Birth: _____   Ht.: _____cm Wt.: _____kg

Present Complaints:

Previous Vascular Procedures:

Associated Conditions:

Current Medications:

Time of Last Medication _____   Room Temperature _____

FIGURE 4-8.   Pretest data form to be used in vascular testing.

information with respect to the blood supply, especially if lesions are present and/or surgery is contemplated. The digits reflect the status of the circulation and respond to adverse external situations as well as the internal metabolic state. Figure 4-8 shows a pretest data form, which should be filled out for all patients undergoing vascular testing.

Instruments and Materials
1. Digital cuffs constructed of a velcro cuff and bladder attached to appropriate manometer and pressure bulb
2. Tape measure
3. Sensing device: Doppler probe; photosensor, silastic mercury strain gauge
4. Recorder for documenting pulsatile waveforms

Procedure (Fig. 4-9)
1. Patient is tested in the supine position at a comfortable room temperature (21 to 24C) avoiding any conditions that might produce vasospasm or increased vessel tone. In this position, the toes should be positioned slightly higher than heart level.

2. The circumference of each toe is determined at the base and the appropriate cuff applied with the proximal edge of the cuff not more than 1 cm from the base of the digit. Pressures will be overestimated if the cuff is too narrow and underestimated if the cuff is too wide.

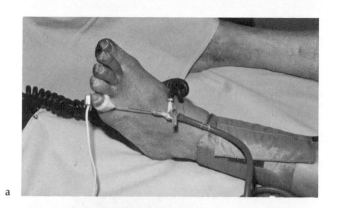

a

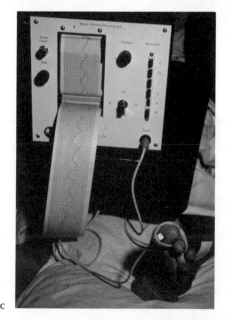

b

c

FIGURE 4-9a-c.   Technique for determining digital systolic pressure.

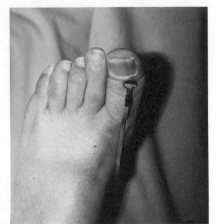

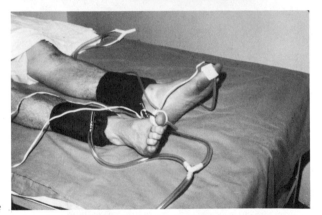

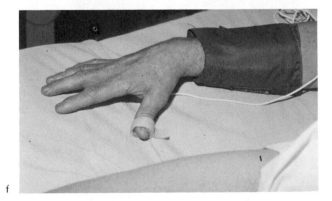

FIGURE 4-9d-f. Continued.

3. The sensing device is applied at the tip of the digit.

4. Very low or unmeasurable toe pressures in some patients can indicate little or no flow in the toes with the patient in the supine position. In some patients with no symptoms toe pressure may be slightly lower than those at the ankle or brachial artery. In patients with hypertension but no vascular disease higher systolic toe pressures can be observed. Abnormal toe pressures do reflect disease in the smaller distal vessels.

5. When recording digital pressures make note of the patient's physical condition and complaints, so that a total picture of the patient's status may be obtained.

SKIN BLOOD PRESSURE

By placing a photoelectric sensor beneath a compression cuff, pressures are detected in the cuff at which blood flow in skin directly under the cuff begins. This particular test is applicable to areas where a compression cuff can be applied. It has application in limb areas susceptible to lesions.

Instruments and Materials
1. Photoelectric probe
2. Recorder
3. Appropriate compression cuffs and manometers

Procedure
1. The photoelectric probe is taped to the skin surface and the compression cuff is placed so that the center of the bladder covers the probe. A second sensor may be placed distal to the occluding cuff.

2. Compression cuff is inflated to suprasystolic pressure. As suprasystolic pressure is reached the skin blanches and photo pulsewaves disappear.

3. Arm blood pressure is also recorded via the auscultatory method so that systolic and diastolic pressures are recorded.

4. Pressure in the cuff is released steadily at a rate of 2 to 3 mm Hg/sec. With release of the cuff pressure, the skin color returns at a well-defined pressure level, indicating systolic skin pressure. A pressure curve can be recorded as well as the pulsatile waveforms. Pressure in the deep vessels is determined by the appearance of waveforms in the sensor distal to the compression cuff. The pressure at which the photo waveforms reappear indicates the skin blood pressure. A drop in pressure from deep vessels to skin vessels may be anticipated.

Penile Blood Pressure

1. Brachial systolic blood pressure is measured in the usual manner and recorded.

2. The patient is then placed in the supine position.

3. A small (9 × 3 cm) pneumatic cuff is wrapped around the base of the penis and connected to the standard pressure transducer.

4. Distal to the cuff a photoplethysmographic (PPG) sensor is secured with a velcro band. The area is then covered to exclude extraneous light.

5. At zero cuff pressure the gain control of the PPG is advanced until a suitable waveform is obtained. These are recorded at a chart speed of 25 mm/sec.

6. The cuff is then inflated until the arterial signal disappears, then slowly deflated until flow returns. This test is recorded at 5 mm/sec on the two-channel stripchart.

7. The measurement is repeated several times until reproducible values are obtained. Recorder and PPG settings are noted.

8. Waveforms are analyzed and the penile systolic pressure is divided by the brachial systolic pressure to yield a penile-brachial index (PBI).

OPHTHALMIC ARTERY PRESSURE

Since the ophthalmic artery is the first major branch of the internal carotid artery, the indirect measurement of the ophthalmic systolic blood pressure is considered important in the assessment of cerebral vascular hemodynamics. Ophthalmodynamometry represents one of the earliest means for measuring this pressure. This technique utilizes a spring-loaded dynamometer that is placed directly on the eyeball while the examiner observes the retinal artery through an ophthalmoscope. The applied pressure is increased gradually until pulsations are observed in the retinal artery. The amount of pressure applied to the dynamometer in order to produce the pulsations is noted and compared with that observed for the other eye. When the internal carotid artery is occluded a pressure gradient can be observed between eyes. This technique is operator-dependent; frequently a gradient cannot be demonstrated in the presence of stenosis.

The introduction of the technique oculopneumoplethysmography for the determination of ophthalmic artery pressure has all but displaced the technique of ophthalmodynamometry.

With this technique, small suction cups are applied to each eye and a negative pressure of −300 mm Hg applied. This suction is equivalent to

+110 mm Hg ophthalmic artery pressure. Thus, with this current technique pressures greater than 110 mm Hg are not specified.

The patient usually assumes a supine position and the sclerae are anesthetized with appropriate ophthalmic solution. Each eye cup is placed on its respective sclera lateral to the cornea and held in place with suction. The patient's bilateral arm blood pressures are recorded. Any history of ocular injury or operation during the previous six months contraindicates this type of testing. Also excluded from this type of testing are patients with spontaneous retinal detachment or allergy to local anesthetics or epoxy materials, or patients with glaucoma and lens implantation.

The total instrument for this type of measurement will provide for the appropriate stripchart recording for vacuum level as well as pressure recordings for each eye. To date for observations made with this technique, normal ophthalmic artery blood pressures have been given a range of 60 to 95 percent of brachial blood pressure. The most valuable data obtained is that related to the bilateral eye measurements and their differences.

PERIPHERAL VENOUS PRESSURE

Venous function in the lower extremities can be assessed objectively by use of percutaneous pressure measurements in the saphenous and posterior tibial veins at the ankle during rest and during exercise. Venous pressure measurements can determine the presence of an obstruction to venous outflow from deep vessels proximal to the level at which the pressures are measured. The exact nature of the obstruction may not be delineated; however, characteristic pressure measurements can be determined for different degrees of venous dysfunction.

Instruments and Materials
1. Intravenous catheters and sterile heparinized saline
2. Pressure transducers
3. Four-channel recorder—two channels for pressure, one channel for EKG, and one channel for muscle potentials.

Procedure
1. Catheters are placed in the superficial long saphenous vein in front of the medial malleolus and posterior tibial vein (a deep intramuscular vein) via a cutdown. The catheter tips are placed 15 cm above the ankle and attached to the pressure transducers, which are adjusted to the level of the catheter tips.

2. Appropriate connections are then made to the recorder.

3. A standard exercise should be used, e.g., walking in place, or walking on a treadmill at a given speed and incline.

Observations

1. *Asymptomatic normal individual*

   a. *Quiet standing position.* Pressure in the saphenous vein and posterior tibial vein equals the hydrostatic pressure of a column of blood reaching to the heart level. This pressure is approximately 80 mm Hg for an individual 180 cm in height.

   b. *Walking in place.* With a few short steps the pressure in the veins falls to a level of approximately 30 to 40 mm Hg. The individual stops walking and stands quietly. Pressure returns to the resting value within 10 to 30 seconds. This is termed the pressure recovery time. During the exercise, the pressure in the intramuscular veins will exceed the pressure in the superficial veins. Blood does not return to the superficial vessels since functional perforating veins prevent retrograde flow. During relaxation of the muscles, the pressure in the deep veins drops below that in the superficial veins (approximately 10 mm Hg drop) and blood flows into the deep veins. As the individual remains motionless the pressures return to initial levels.

2. *Venous dysfunction*

   a. *Quiet standing position.* Pressure in the veins at the ankle equals the hydrostatic pressure of a column of blood reaching to the heart level (approximately 80 mm Hg).

   b. *Walking in place.* The pressure may increase slightly or may remain at the resting level. This is termed ambulatory venous hypertension. If there is a fall in pressure on walking, it will be much less than that observed in normal limbs and the recovery time is very short. The extent of pressure changes in venous dysfunction is dependent upon the degree and site of involvement. At the beginning of exercise, in a postthrombotic limb, there is little or no reduction in pressure, and during the exercise, the pressure continues to build up and may exceed the resting pressure by as much as 20 mm Hg. In this situation, the patient complains of a bursting type of pain in the limb. This will occur when walking, climbing stairs, and walking up an incline.

DIRECT MEASUREMENT OF ARTERIAL BLOOD PRESSURE

Direct measurement of arterial blood pressure requires arterial puncture, which is done by percutaneous insertion or by surgical cutdown for cannulation and/or catheterization of a vessel. For percutaneous insertion a needle or catheter is inserted in a vessel close to the point of entry of the skin. When a site distal to the point of entry is to be used, a long catheter is introduced through a superficial vessel and can be threaded to distal major vessels and to the heart. This technique can be used during injection of radiopaque dyes for x-ray, injection of colored dyes for indicator-dilution studies, and administration of drugs directly into the heart and specified vessels.

Two transducer systems are available for direct measurement of arterial blood pressure. In one instance the vasculature is coupled to an external transducer system through a liquid-filled catheter, and in the second, the pressure transducer is incorporated in the tip of a catheter that is inserted in the vessel itself.

For percutaneous insertions, a local anesthetic can be injected near the site of entry, the vessel is palpated, and then occluded by external pressure. A hollow needle with a guide and catheter is inserted at a slight angle to the vessel. The catheter may be left in place and the needle and guide withdrawn, or the in-dwelling needle may be used. Whichever device is secured in place at the site of entry, it is attached to a fluid-filled system leading directly to the extravascular transducer. In this instance the fluid-filled system consists of the catheter attached to a three-way stopcock and then to the dome of the transducer system, which is filled with sterile saline heparin solution. The system can be flushed periodically by means of the stopcock to avoid clotting at the tip.

The transducer is mounted near the patient at the same level as the site of pressure measurement in order to avoid errors due to hydrostatic pressure. To complete the systems, appropriate signal conditioning and recording or display instruments are selected.

Catheterization usually implies the use of a long tube inserted into a superficial vessel by means of a surgical cutdown. The catheter may then be threaded to the appropriate sensing site. In this system the transducer may be located in the tip of the catheter or the catheter may provide the channel through which the transducer is threaded. Again the catheter and transducer are coupled to the appropriate signal conditioning and display system(s).

During Surgery and Arteriography

During vascular surgery the direct measurement of arterial pressure proximal and distal to an occlusive lesion helps to determine the hemodynamic significance of the occlusion since the magnitude of a pressure gradient across a lesion is proportional to degree of occlusion. An important site for direct pressure measurement is the common femoral artery. All too frequently, when high-thigh pressure measurements are made utilizing the occlusion cuff method, an iliac artery stenosis can go undetected. This is most apt to occur when the thigh girth is large, in which case the measured pressure may exceed the brachial pressure by 30 to 40 mm Hg due to cuff artifact. An iliac stenosis that might cause a gradient of 15 to 20 mm Hg could thus go undetected. However, measurement of common femoral artery pressures and evaluation of pressure gradients across aortoiliac stenotic lesions at the time of angiography can be especially helpful in selection of the appropriate angiographic study.

The measurement of common femoral artery pressure at the time of surgery is also an aid in determining whether there is adequate pressure for perfusion of a distal reconstruction. Measurements immediately following the reconstruction can help to determine success or failure of the procedure. Disappearance of a prior gradient is an indication that the repair is adequate. No decrease or only a slight decrease in the gradient is an immediate indication for exploration of the reconstruction and/or an intraoperative arteriogram.

During carotid artery surgery, intraoperative pressure measurements of the retrograde pressure in the internal carotid artery will determine the need for an internal shunt during the procedure. Both the operating area and angiographic suites should be equipped with the appropriate instrumentation for routine direct measurement of arterial pressures.

BLOOD FLOW MEASUREMENTS

The primary role of the cardiovascular system is the movement of blood to and from the tissues. Measurement of this movement is of critical physiologic importance because adequate tissue perfusion, the primary determinant of tissue viability, is dependent upon adequate pulsatile blood flow. There is no ideal method that will accurately quantitatively describe all of the cardiovascular events in man. However, if the available flow-measuring devices or systems are utilized in the appropriate manner, the objective information with respect to the various components of blood flow (velocity, acceleration, pulsatility, volume, and elasticity of the vessels) can be obtained.

DOPPLER ULTRASONIC FLOWMETRY
(Using a Continuous-Wave System)

Blood Flow Velocity
Instruments and Materials
1. A Doppler instrument, probes, stethoscope earpieces, earphones or loudspeaker

2. Acoustic gel
3. Analog recorder
4. Audiofrequency analyzer
5. Tape recorder

Procedures. A systematic approach must be used. Careful note should be made of the conditions under which the measurements are made; a bilateral examination should be done as often as possible. The velocity signals will vary depending upon the artery or vein being examined, nature of the vascular bed (high or low resistance), cardiac function and rhythm, and position of the patient during the examination. Knowledge of the position of blood vessels and the landmarks for localizing them is essential. Certain tissue changes such as dense fibrosis, subcutaneous hemorrhage, excessive fat tissue, marked edema, and different bypass graft materials can interfere with sound transmission. Know the instruments and how they work. The examination is usually done with the patient resting comfortably in the supine position.

1. *Apply the transducer* (probe) to the surface of the skin (Fig. 4-10). Position the Doppler probe over the vessel to be examined at an angle of 45 to 60° to the skin surface. Within this range, the position of the probe can be adjusted until the signal of maximum intensity is obtained. The face of the transducer is coupled to the skin surface with acoustic gel. Avoid excessive pressure when applying the probe. The thin-walled veins are easily collapsed, especially when they lie just beneath the skin surface.

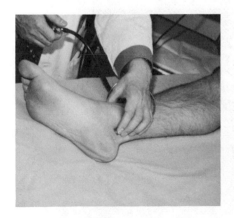
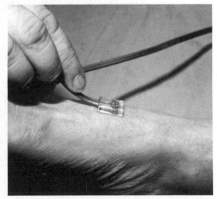

a   b

FIGURE 4-10a-b. Technique for recording Doppler ultrasonic waveforms.

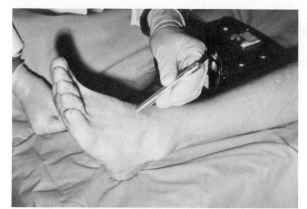

c

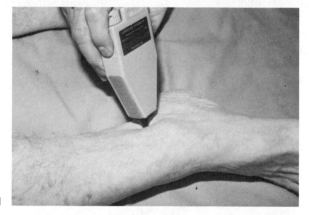

d

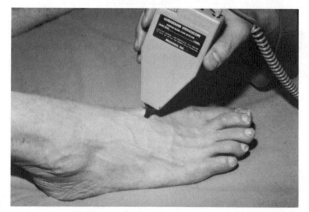

e

FIGURE 4-10c-e.   Continued.

2. *Examine the arteries*   (Figs. 4-11 and 4-12). Common, external, and internal carotid, vertebral, supraorbital, and superficial temporal in the head and neck; subclavian, axillary, brachial, radial, ulnar, palmar arch, and digital arteries in the upper extremities; external iliac, common femoral, superficial femoral, popliteal, anterior tibial, posterior tibial, dorsalis pedis, planter arch, and digital arteries in the lower extremities.

The *common carotid* is examined at the base of the neck. Flow in this vessel is into a low-resistance system via the internal carotid artery and during diastole flow does not return to zero. The common carotid is traced to its bifurcation into the external and internal carotid arteries. At the bifurcation an abrupt change in the frequency shift will be noted. Beyond this point it will be difficult to identify the internal carotid artery because of the many vessels in this area.

The *vertebral arteries* are difficult to examine since they lie deep in the neck. A directional velocity detector and a pencil probe should be used. The probe is positioned just above the clavicle and posterior to the sternal head of the sternocleidomastoid muscle. The carotid artery and jugular vein are identified; then using the probe tip, the artery and vein are displaced anteriorly and the probe tip is pressed into the neck toward the transverse processes of the cervical vertebrae. With experience the course of the vertebral artery can be examined.

When the innominate and/or subclavian arteries are occluded reversal of flow may be observed in the vertebral artery. If flow reversal is suspected, it can be further evaluated by placing a cuff around the upper arm and inflating it above brachial systolic pressure. The vertebral signal is located and recorded. After three minutes the arm cuff is deflated. The reverse flow velocity will be augmented until the hyperemia caused by the occluding cuff subsides. When subclavian steal is present, this flow reversal phenomenon will be observed in the vertebral artery and should be recorded.

To examine the supraorbital artery, use a directional velocity detector and pencil probe. The tip of the probe is positioned just below the supraorbital notch pointed slightly upward and adjusted until the best signal is obtained.

By placing the probe either above or below the clavicle and pointing in a medial direction the velocity waveform for the *subclavian artery* is detected. This is also a difficult artery to examine. The *axillary, brachial, radial*, and *ulnar* arteries are superficially positioned, making them easy to palpate and accessible for a Doppler examination. The sound patterns in the *palmar* and *digital arteries* are similar to these of the radial and ulnar arteries. Because of a large number of A-V shunts in the tips of the fingers the sound patterns express a high mean flow component.

All of the main arteries of the lower extremity can be examined

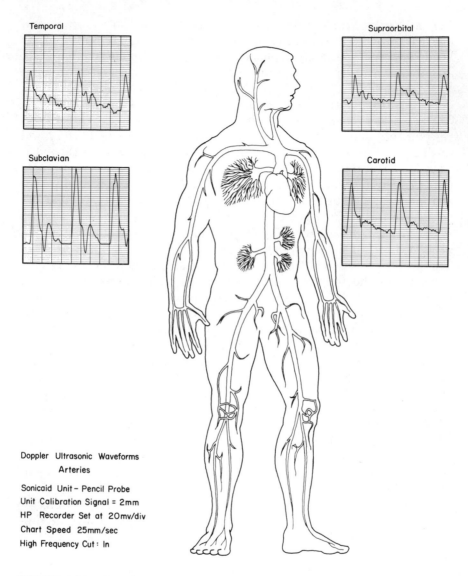

Temporal

Supraorbital

Subclavian

Carotid

Doppler Ultrasonic Waveforms
Arteries

Sonicaid Unit – Pencil Probe
Unit Calibration Signal = 2mm
HP   Recorder Set at 20mv/div
Chart Speed 25mm/sec
High Frequency Cut : In

FIGURE 4-11. Doppler ultrasonic waveforms obtained from the superficial temporal, supraorbital, carotid, and subclavian arteries.

throughout their course from the level of the *external iliac* artery down to and including the *digital arteries*. The arteries of the lower extremity are examined at sites closest to skin surface similar to points or sites at which the arteries are palpated.

3. *Examine the veins.* Internal jugular, axillary, brachial, external iliac,

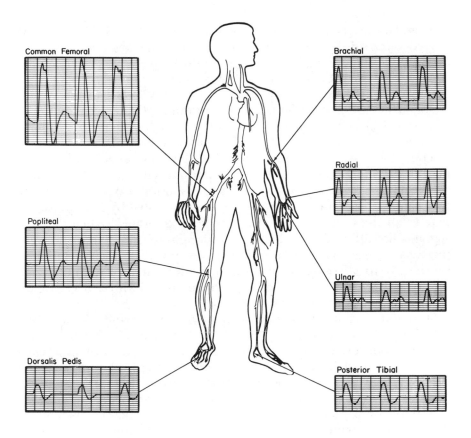

Doppler Ultrasonic Waveforms — Arteries
Sonicaid Unit — Pencil Probe.   Unit Calibration Signal = 2mm with Hewlett–Packard
recorder set at 20mv/div.   Chart speed 25mm/sec.   High frequency cut: in.

FIGURE 4-12.   Doppler ultrasonic waveforms obtained from the upper extremity at the brachial, radial, and ulnar arteries and from the lower extremity at the common femoral, popliteal, posterior tibial, and dorsalis pedis arteries.

common femoral, superficial femoral, popliteal, posterior tibial, greater and lesser saphenous, and perforating veins.

The major veins usually follow a straight course and are intimately related to the arteries. Collateral veins have a more circuitous course and are seldom associated with prominent arterial signals. In a systematic venous examination, the veins are located and identified by their anatomic relation to arteries of the same name.

To examine the veins, the patient assumes a supine position with the knees slightly flexed and the legs rotated externally at the hips. Once the concomitant artery of the vein to be examined is located, the probe is moved to the side of the artery in order to locate the low-pitched venous flow sounds. The probe is moved up and down the leg to determine the straight course of the major vein. A spontaneous flow signal should be obtained from all patent deep veins of the leg. When the signal is not spontaneous an obstruction is usually indicated. One exception is the posterior tibial vein. If the vein is patent, but the flow signal is not spontaneous, compression of the foot will result in a flow signal.

The velocity patterns of the veins of the lower extremity, with the patient in the supine position, reflect the periodic changes in the intraabdominal pressure occurring secondary to respiration. When the velocity flow signal varies with respiration and is interrupted by a deep breath, patency of the vein proximal to the probe is indicated. When the flow signal is not affected by a deep inspiration, an obstruction of the vein proximal to the probe may be indicated. The presence of an occlusion in the deep veins can cause the flow velocity patterns in the superficial veins of the same leg to be greatly increased as compared with flow velocity in comparable veins of the opposite leg.

During the examination, the examiner should determine whether the velocity flow signal can be augmented. In the normal, patent vein, compression of the extremity distal to the probe produces an increased velocity flow signal while compression proximal to the probe will stop the venous velocity flow signal. Release of the proximal compression is followed by an increased flow signal. The same procedures should be completed for comparable veins in the opposite leg. Valvular competence in the superficial femoral veins is determined by positioning the probe over the popliteal vein and forcibly squeezing the thigh. If the valves above the probe are incompetent, compression proximal to the probe causes blood to flow toward the probe. Release of the compression permits the blood to flow away from the probe.

To determine competency of the calf veins, the probe is positioned over the posterior tibial vein and the calf muscles are forcibly compressed. If the valves are incompetent the back-and-forth flow velocity signals will be detected with compression and release. The saphenous vein is examined by placing the probe at the distal site and then running the finger distally over the course of the vein. If the valves are incompetent the back-and-forth reflux sounds can be detected. Flow reversal in the femoral vein can be detected during quiet respiration when the patient is tilted to the head-up position.

4. *Process the flow velocity signals.* Listen to the frequency shift during the examination, record the frequency shift on magnetic tape and analyze with an audiofrequency analyzer to produce a sonogram, process the signal through a zero-crossing frequency to voltage converter, DC amplifier, and stripchart recorder.

5. *Listen to the signal.* Listening to the frequency shift is a simple procedure. However, to do this effectively, the examiner must be able to recognize normal velocity patterns and know how they are changed with disease of the vessels. The ability to recognize sound patterns is a skill that is best developed by examining normals and abnormals. Normal arterial signals are multiphasic with a prominent systolic component and one or more diastolic sounds. Distal to an arterial obstruction the sound is more monophasic with attenuation of the systolic component and an absence of the diastolic sounds. Distal to a significant stenosis, the velocity signal may be high-pitched or turbulent with a mixture of high and low frequencies and loss of multiphasic pulsatile flow velocity pattern. The venous signals are lower in pitch and are affected by changes in the respiratory cycle.

Recording the Doppler Velocity Waveform (Zero-Crossing Technique)

The audible signals are converted to an electrical signal with a frequency voltage (DC) converter. Both the directional and nondirectional continuous-wave Doppler instruments use this technique to obtain waveforms from accessible arteries and veins. Waveforms recorded from normal arteries coincide with the heart sounds with the first deflection denoting forward flow during systole, negative deflection denoting reverse flow during early diastole, and a third deflection representing return to forward flow, which occurs in late diastole and is secondary to elastic recoil of the arterial wall. Flow waveforms recorded distal to an occlusion are monophasic with marked attenuation of the systolic component. Waveforms recorded immediately distal to a stenosis display a high-frequency component during systole but no reverse flow. Depending upon the vasomotor tone of the distal arterial tree reverse flow may be present or absent.

Audiospectral Analysis of the Doppler Signal— Ultrasonic Sonography

The Doppler signals from specific locations are recorded on tape using a high-fidelity system. The tape is then played through a sound spectrum analyzer providing a graphic recording (sonogram) with the frequency plotted on the ordinate and time on the abscissa. The frequency is proportional to blood cell velocity. The amplitude of the Doppler signal at any frequency is proportional to the number of blood cells moving at a given velocity and is expressed in different gray scales. The darker the contour, the greater the sound intensity. This system is considered to be capable of defining flow velocity aberrations associated with minor stenoses.

To obtain venous waveforms a directional instrument is used. The types and patterns recorded depend upon the vein examined and the position of the subject during the examination. When recording from the central venous circulation, *internal jugular vein,* an EKG should be recorded at the same time. This is a complex velocity waveform related to jugular venous pressure and the electrocardiogram. With the patient in the supine position waveforms recorded from veins in the extremities reflect velocity changes occurring with respiration.

PLETHYSMOGRAPHY

Plethysmography (volume measurement) is a technique that permits the observation of changes in the size of a part as it is modified by the blood circulating through it. The term is derived from the Greek *plethysmos,* increase, and *graphine,* to write. The plethysmograph is the instrument used to determine and register variations in the (1) size of an organ, part, or limb, and (2) amount of blood present or passing through it.

Venous Occlusion Plethysmography
(Measurement of Arterial Blood Flow)
This technique is based on the principle of measurement of the volume increase of an organ during temporary arrest of venous return. With venous occlusion, the change in tissue volume distal to the occlusion cuff is recorded. During the first few seconds of venous occlusion, the volume change is proportional to the arterial inflow. The arterial inflow will remain *relatively* constant over a range of subdiastolic pressures. Thus, a number of pressure levels are tested before selection of the appropriate occlusion pressure.

Instruments
1. Volume-sensing instrument to be placed around the part or segment to be assessed
2. Pneumatic cuffs, one positioned proximal to the sensing instrument and one (optional) positioned at the ankle
3. Appropriate recording device(s)

Three types of plethysmographs are used to measure volume change. The water-filled plethysmograph measures volume change directly since the part to be assessed is positioned in a rigid water-filled container.

Thus a change in volume of the enclosed structure will displace a quantity of enclosed fluid, which is measured by a suitable device. The air-filled plethysmograph is similar to the water-filled device, completely encasing the structure to be assessed, or more conveniently, an air-filled cuff can be placed around the structure. In this arrangement, an increase in volume of the structure within the cylinder or cuff will compress the contained air and cause an increase in air pressure, which can be recorded via an appropriate transducer.

The easiest and simplest instrument to use clinically is the mercury strain gauge, which detects a change in volume via a change in circumference of the structure around which the guage is positioned. The device is calibrated to determine volume change. This device is especially good for the hand, foot, individual digits, and limb segments.

Blood flow measured by means of a plethysmograph is expressed as the volume of blood flow per unit volume of tissue (within the plethysmograph) per unit of time.

Mercury Strain Gauge Plethysmography

Instruments
1. Mercury strain gauge plethysmograph
2. Series of mercury strain gauges for digits and leg segments
3. Analog recorder (single or multichannel)

Procedure
1. Patient is placed in a comfortable supine position.

2. The silastic tube(s) is placed around terminal digit from which pulse waveforms are recorded. The gauge is placed around the terminal digit so that the nonexpansible portion is positioned at the base of the nail.

3. The amplitude and shape of the waveform determines the status or quality of circulation to the digit.

The mercury strain gauge is used for digit volume changes and systolic blood pressure measurements in the extemities.

Measurement of Calf Blood Flow Using the Mercury Strain Gauge
1. Patient is placed in comfortable position.

2. The appropriate mercury strain gauge is positioned around the calf.

3. A pneumatic cuff is positioned just above the knee. This cuff is connected to a device that ensures rapid controlled inflation of the pneumatic cuff and can be inflated for either venous occlusion or complete occlusion of the circulation.

4. A pneumatic cuff may also be positioned distally at the ankle and inflated above systolic blood pressure, thus excluding foot blood flow during the study. This is an optional procedure.

Electrical Impedance Plethysmography

The technique of electrical impedance plethysmography is based on the concept that a fluid-filled region of the body offers impedance to flow of electric current. Thus, a change in volume of the region should show a change in the impedance. It is well known that as the volume of blood in the limbs varies with each cardiac cycle so do the physical and electrical characteristics of the limb. Electrical conductivity is modified by the change in limb volume. As the fluid volume and geometric configuration of the limb body segment or part change with each cardiac cycle, so will the response to an externally induced electrical current applied to the limb, segment, or part.

Instruments
1. Impedance instrument (Fig. 4-13)
2. Electrode bands and conducting gel
3. Recorder stripchart, tape, oscilloscope
4. Online computer

Procedure.   The procedures described for this technique are general. With slight modifications, depending upon the objectives of the test, they can be adapted for any tetrapolar impedance device.

1. Preparation of the patient for lower extremity bilateral impedance measurements: The patient should wear short trunks and his legs and

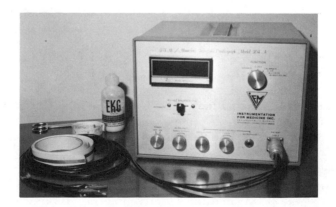

FIGURE 4-13.   The impedance plethysmograph.

feet should be bare. He assumes a supine position on the examination table.

2. The thickest portion of the calf is located and a small "pencil" mark is made 5 cm above and 5 cm below this point. Repeat for the other leg. Another two points are made 5 cm above upper edge of kneecap and 15 cm above kneecap. Similar procedures for thigh.

3. The circumference of the limbs at each location is determined. A total of six electrode strips will be made for each leg (three thigh and three calf). The electrode tapes of appropriate length are cut from a tape roll and placed on a flat surface with protective backing removed from the corner of each strip and strips anchored to flat surface and protective backing removed. Conductive cream is applied in thin strips to each silver electrode strip leaving about 1 to 1.5″ at either end free of cream. The silver electrode strips are placed around the thighs and calves at previously marked positions, conductive cream in contact with the skin surface. As the ends of the strips are brought together the ends are aligned. The high-thigh and above-ankle electrodes are the forcing electrodes, and the others pick-up electrodes.

4. Leads from the impedance device are clipped in place (Fig. 4-14), one leg at a time, red lead at the most distal electrode strip (just above ankle) and second lead at the most proximal electrode on high-thigh region. These remain in position throughout the test. The black clipper leads are variable leads and are placed in the following sequence:

a. To measure impedance and to obtain pulsatile waveform in the calf region, leads are clipped to electrode strips in calf region.

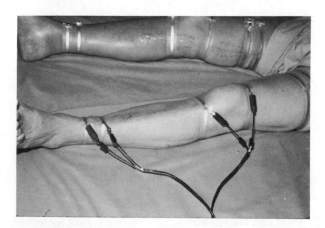

FIGURE 4-14.   Placement of electrodes in peripheral impedance study of lower extremity.

b. To measure impedance in popliteal region, leads are placed on strip below knee and above knee.

c. To measure impedance in the thigh region, leads are placed on electrode strips encompassing the thigh region.

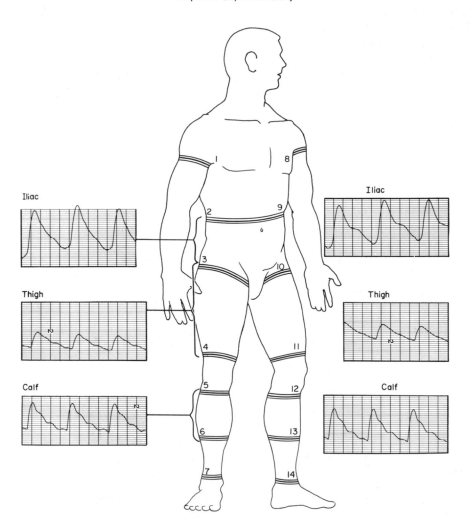

FIGURE 4-15.   Peripheral arterial impedance study showing waveforms obtained in evaluating the iliac, thigh, and calf regions.

5. The procedure is repeated for the opposite leg. Typical arterial impedance waveforms are shown in Figure 4-15.

6. A similar procedure can be used on the arm (Fig. 4-16).

Photoplethysmography

Supraorbital photoplethysmography refers to recording abnormal flow dynamics in frontal and supraorbital arteries (terminal branches of the ophthalmic artery). It is used to detect significant obstruction of the extracranial internal carotid artery.

Instruments
1. Photoplethysmograph (transducer with power source and stripchart recorder) (Fig. 4-17).
2. Two-channel or other appropriate recorder.

The *transducer* contains an infrared light-emitting diode and an adjacent phototransistor which detects backscattered light. It functions on the reflectance principle of photoplethysmography; a phototransistor sensitive to variations in infrared light is reflected back from tissue microcirculation. The infrared portion of the light spectrum has the advantage of not being significantly influenced by the degree of hemoglobin

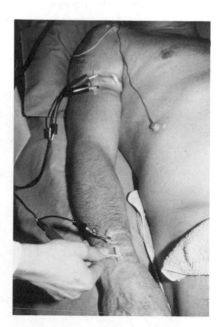

FIGURE 4-16.   Placement of electrodes in peripheral impedance study of upper extremity.

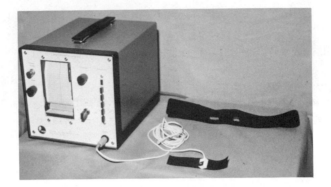

FIGURE 4-17.   Photoplethysmograph.

saturation of the blood. A low-power source in the recorder activates the light-emitting diode and has no heating effect on the transducer. Output of the phototransistor pulse pickup is connected to a high-gain amplifier with appropriate filtering to provide stable tracing on recorder with a low-frequency cutoff of 0.53 Hz.

Procedure

1. Patient assumes supine position.

2. Place photoplethysmograph transducer on forehead above eyebrow over medial aspect of each eye (region of forehead supplied by frontal and supraorbital arteries—terminal branches of ophthalmic artery) (Fig. 4-18a).

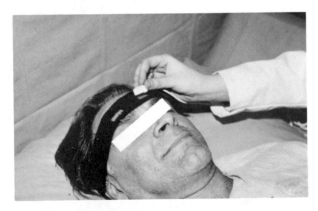

FIGURE 4-18a.   Technique for carrying out a supraorbital photoplethysmographic examination for the detection of extracranial cerebrovascular occlusive disease.

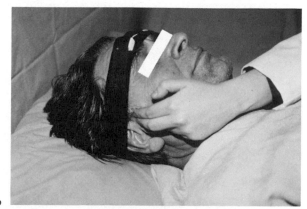

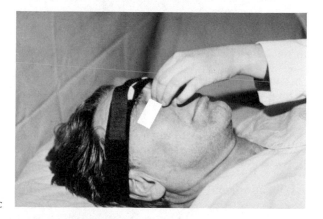

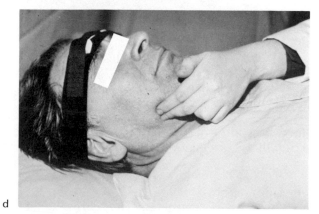

FIGURE 4-18b-d.   Continued.

3. Transducers held in place via headband to avoid any pressure that might attenuate trace.

4. Transducers connected via their power source to the recorder.

5. Pulsatile tracings from each supraorbital area are recorded simultaneously on two-channel recorder.

6. Adjust gain of amplifier channel so that amplitude of pulsations are approximately equal in magnitude and at least 20 mm in height.

7. A paper speed of 5 mm/sec is suitable.

8. Activate recorder with foot switch during examination.

9. Supraorbital PPG examination: Record simultaneous pulsations during series of sequential bilateral maneuvers to compress major branches of each external carotid artery and then in tandem each common carotid artery.

10. Activate recorder via foot switch.

11. Carry out simultaneously three-second compression maneuvers of each superficial temporal artery (Fig. 4-18b), angular artery (Fig. 4-18c), and facial artery (Fig. 4-18d).

12. Each common carotid artery is transiently compressed (less than three seconds) low in neck to avoid stimulating carotid sinus or dislodging emboli from a diseased carotid bifurcation.

13. If there is an abnormal response during bilateral compression of the branches' external carotid artery, compress each branch in tandem in order to determine source of abnormal collateral circulation.

Interpretation

1. *Normal supraorbital tracing* (Fig. 4-19) (PPG) compression of temporal and facial branches of external carotid artery show no significant attenuation. Transient compression of *ipsilateral common carotid artery* results in diminished waveform or tracing.

2. Significant obstruction ⩾50% stenosis or occlusion of internal carotid artery equals significant attenuation of supraorbital pulsation.

Oculoplethysmography

The instrumentation for extracranial cerebrovascular examination uses a ± millisecond pulse delay measurement system that detects and eliminates the effect of noise and artifact and provides a digital display

Supraorbital

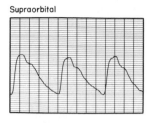

Finger

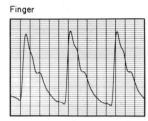

Toe

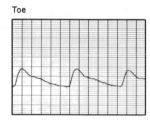

Bionic Unit
Unit Sensitivity : X4
Hewlett—Packard Recorder Set at 20mv/div

FIGURE 4-19. Photoplethysmographic waveforms obtained from the supraorbital artery and the fingers and toes.

of relative eye and ear pulse delays. Digital display is an average of eight noise-free, blink-free pulses and is simultaneously displayed as relative pulse delay ear to ear for external carotid artery, eye to eye for internal carotid artery, and eye to ear for bilateral evaluation of internal and external carotid arteries.

Instruments
1. Oculoplethysmograph (Fig. 4-20)
2. Topical ophthalmic anesthesia

Procedure
1. Calibrate the oculoplethysmograph as per directions.

2. Screen patient for potential contraindications (although reported to be safe for use in cases of previous eye surgery or eye pathology, we prefer not to use the technique on such patients).

3. The patient should be in a supine position. The machine is ready. Apply one to two drops topical ophthalmic anesthesia to each eye (Fig. 4-21a).

4. Rotate eye cup apparatus to a position over the patient's forehead and rub ear lobes to stimulate circulation.

5. Ear clips are attached to the right and left ear lobes and eye cups placed over right and left eyes (Figs. 4-21b, c).

6. Pay particular attention to attaching ear clips and eye cups labeled "right" to right side and "left" to left side. Ensure that vacuum applied to maintain position of eye cups is appropriate and check using "suction

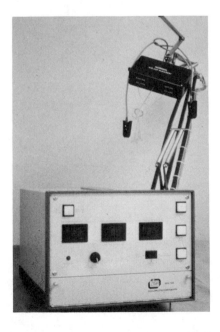

FIGURE 4-20. Oculoplethysmograph.

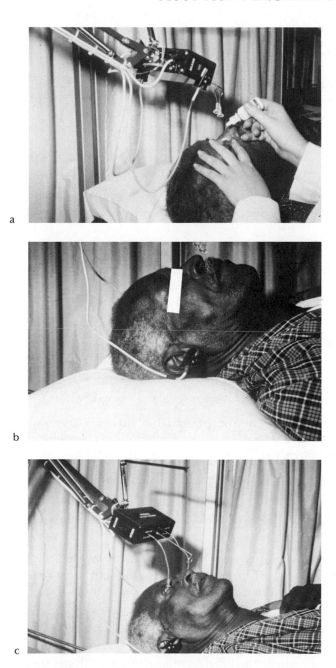

FIGURE 4-21a-c.   The technique of oculoplethysmography, which utilizes pulse arrival delay in detecting extracranial cerebrovascular occlusive disease.

check" switch. If vacuum is inadequate or if eye cup–cornea contact is lost, release vacuum and reapply eye cups.

7. Once the ear clips and eye cups are adequately placed, instruct patient to relax, hold eyes open, and try not to blink. The instrument is set in pulse measurement mode. If excessive blinking prohibits measurement, the noise-blink sensitivity is adjusted downward.

8. Once the eye-to-eye digital display is stabilized (eight blink-free cardiac cycles), institute the auto average mode, which holds the digital display average to eight blink-free and noise-free measurements.

9. Reset and repeat blink-free and noise-free measurements and display average. Recording three average displays is usually adequate for a test.

10. At completion of the examination instruct the patient not to rub eyes for approximately 2 hours, until the effect of the topical anesthesia has dissipated.

Fluid Oculoplethysmograph. The technique of fluid-filled oculoplethysmography is used for the detection of extracranial cerebrovascular occlusive disease (Figs. 4-22a–c).

Procedure

1. Calibrate the oculoplethysmograph as per directions.

2. Screen the patient for potential contraindications (although reported to be safe for use in cases of previous eye surgery or eye pathology, we prefer not to use the technique on such patients).

3. Patient is seated, ear lobes are massaged, and left and right ear clips are attached to respective ears.

4. One or two drops of topical ophthalmic anesthesia are placed in each eye.

5. Have the patient position himself comfortably, place his feet flat on the floor in front of him, and place his chin and forehead in the headstand during the ear pulse and eye pulse measurements.

6. To measure ear pulse, be sure the USE/CAL switch is in the USE position; the gain switch is on "1"; power switch is ON. Turn the function switch on the OPG electronics to the EAR position. Adjust the pulse amplitudes to where the beams swing three-fourths of the width of the screen. Push the recorder drive and record five or more ear pulses.

7. To place the eye cups in the normal position, put the stopcock for

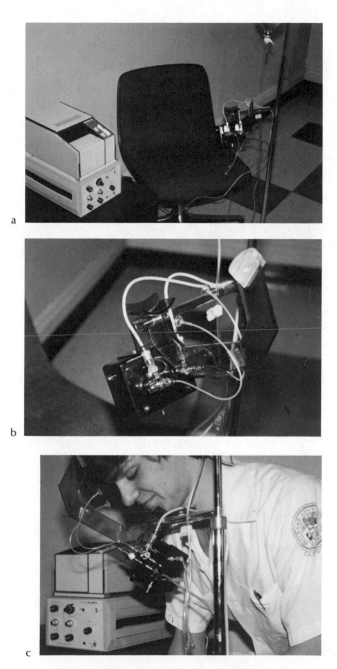

FIGURE 4-22a-c.   The technique of fluid-filled oculoplethysmography, used for the detection of extracranial cerebrovascular occlusive disease.

fluid-filled eye cup being applied in the "up" position, and turn on intermittent suction. Firmly grasp the patient's upper and lower lid just below the lashes. Ask the patient to look down, preferably at an object on the floor in front of his feet. Place the fluid-filled eye cup on the eye. Place the bottom edge of the eye cup in contact with the eye just below the cornea. Rotate the cup stem up to place the fluid-filled cup in full contact with the eye over the cornea, and hold in place for two or three "clicks" of the intermittent suction. Remove your hand and visually inspect for placement and for air bubbles in the eye cup.

8. Place the function selection switch in the PRESS (pressure) position. To equalize suction, bring the suction switch on the manifold forward (continuous) for approximately two or three seconds, and return it to middle (off) position. Look in the recording window and observe two light beams at the top left-hand corner. They must be within the top (left) 2 cm of the window. Beams must also be within 0.5 cm of each other.
Push recorder drive and record a sample strip; run at least two or three inches of paper (10 cm/sec).

9. To record eye pulses turn the function switch on the OPG electronics to EYE. Reset button: Push the reset button as required to bring the light beams to their calibrated position. Gain adjustment: If after one or two seconds, the light beams or pulses are going beyond the borders of the window, it may be necessary to place the gain to "½" and thus make the eye pulses "½" in size. Try to use gain of "1" as much as possible. To record, push DRIVE ON and record at least five or six "clean" waveforms as viewed in the viewing window during recording.
With this "normal" placement, the left eye will be recorded as the light trace on the recording. The right ear, right eye, and differential traces will appear as the darker traces on the recording.

10. To remove the eye cups, gently hold the eye cup by its stem. Tell the patient to open his eye, and that he will feel a "rush of water." Bring the stopcock forward and the eye cup will release from the eye.

11. Apply the eye cups in cross placement. It is desirable in most studies to obtain a diagnostically confirming strip by reapplying the eye cups to opposite eyes and repeating the ocular pulse portion of the study.

ELECTROMAGNETIC FLOWMETRY

Intraoperative
As reconstructive arterial surgery developed, the vascular surgeon became aware of the need to know more about blood flow measurement.

This was most apparent during the vascular procedure(s). Electromagnetic flowmetry was found to be most suited for this purpose. (See Procedure below.) It requires a precise setup and the services of a well-trained biomedical technologist. With careful planning and structuring, a small portable laboratory can be established for the purpose of making physiologic measurements during surgery.

Electromagnetic flowmetry provides the vascular surgeon with a quantitative method of simultaneously measuring *mean* and *pulsatile blood flow* in situ and an instantaneous evaluation of preoperative flow rates and postoperative changes before the patient is released to the recovery room. Each vascular procedure can be evaluated in this manner.

Since the electromagnetic flow probe is applied to intact blood vessels, the need for a vascular incision is eliminated. This technique is far better than reliance on the feel of the pulse as an indicator of flow, since a vessel can pulsate even when there is no blood flowing through it and the immediate assessment of the technical results of the surgical procedure is of considerable practical value. The instantaneous values obtained with this technique are utilized to define pulsatile flow waveforms, the characteristics of which provide information regarding the quantity of flow through the vessel(s) observed.

Instruments
1. Calibrated flow probes of varying diameters (clean, free of debris and deposits, gas-sterilized)
2. Multichannel recorder (direct writing and/or oscilloscope), tape recorder

Use of intraoperative electromagnetic flowmetry is not without some sources of error. (1) The blood flow velocity profile can be distorted and inaccuracies produced depending on the location of the flow probe. The best results are obtained if the probe is placed on a straight relatively uniform section of a vessel, which should be located several centimeters from a junction or sharp bend. Measurements should not be made in the area of a plaque(s). Several readings should be made at each site and averaged, to reduce the magnitude of any error. It is likely that an area free of plaque(s) or curvature(s) can be found; caution should be observed in interpretation of all readings. (2) Probe fit is critical and good electrical contact with the vessel wall is essential. To make good contact, use a probe 5 to 20 percent smaller in diameter than the vessel to which the probe will be applied. This will produce only a small reduction in luminal diameter, and little effect on pressure gradient or flow characteristics is anticipated. (3) During use the probe should not be allowed to dry and should be surrounded by body fluids at all times. (4) Determine the patient's hematocrit before the test. An increased hematocrit can lead to a decreased flow signal, while a decreased hematocrit can lead to an increased signal. A large error should not be expected over a range of 35 to 50 percent hematocrit if the conditions for probe calibration and use at operation are similar. (5) The structure of the vessel wall can influence the measurements. Thickened vessels with extensive plaques change the values. Careful note should be made of the position of the probe and the condition of the vessel. (6) Calibration of the flowmeter probe is critical; this should be the responsibility of the technician in charge of instrumentation. To make the flow measurement, a stable zero baseline is established. This is done either electronically or mechanically determined by the flowmeter system utilized.

Procedure.   The general procedure is to have available a supply of calibrated probes of varying diameters (gas-sterilized), clean and free of debris or deposits. Dissect a length of vessel approximately three times the width of the probe and with a silk tie or caliper, determine the circumference or diameter of the vessel. After this measurement, select probe with a slightly smaller diameter (5 to 20 percent). Disconnect electric equipment, especially electrocautery, to eliminate electrical interference. Position the probe and momentarily occlude this vessel distally to adjust zero. Allow seconds to several minutes for resultant hyperemia to subside and then record pulsatile and mean flow. With branched vessels or end-to-side grafts with two or more outflow tracts, attempt to occlude each outflow tract or branch in turn, giving some idea of flow distribution. When feasible do an in vivo calibration. Upon removal of probes rinse, wash, and prepare for resterilization.

Practical Potential—Uses During Reconstructive Surgery
1. Detect operative accidents
2. Assess capacity of the run-off bed distal to the reconstruction
3. Predict success or failure of reconstruction
4. Assess hemodynamics of pulsatile flow
5. Analyze waveform
6. Evaluate use of an intraoperative vasodilator.

Use of the Electromagnetic Flowmeter (Carolina Medical Model 301) During Surgery (Fig. 4-23.)

Procedure

Probe Table
1. Set up a small table with the probe switch box. The entire table is covered with a sterile drape
2. Three sterile beakers are half-filled' with saline and set on the sterile drape.

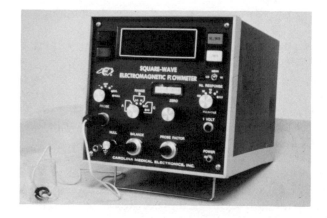

FIGURE 4-23. Instrumentation for standard intraoperative electromagnetic flowmetry.

Electromagnetic Flowmeter
1. The pulsatile flow and mean flow outputs are connected to the DC 8802A preamplifier inputs.
2. The #3 input from the FM recording adapter Vetter Model FM 3 is connected to the left DC 8802A preamplifier output for pulsatile flow and the Vetter #2 input is connected to the right DC 8802A preamplifier output for mean flow.
3. The monitor scope with stripchart recorder (Hewlett-Packard), electromagnetic flowmeter, tape recorder (Pioneer Stereo Tape Recorder Model Rt 701), and the Vetter units are turned ON and warmed up for 20 minutes.
4. The controls of the electromagnetic flowmeter are set:

probe	off
multiplier	10
time constant	30 ms
output zero	dial to zero
balance	When using the probe switch box, the EMF balance control is set to 500 and locked.
balance control	All balancing is then done with the probe switch balance controls.
probe factor	This control is set specifically for each probe used.

Stripchart Recorder
1. The 8802A DC preamplifiers are nulled (screw control) in the off position.
2. Each preamplifier is then calibrated to a deflection of 25 mm with the calibration switch and locked.
3. The attenuator controls are initially set to 50.

4. The ground wire must be attached from the patient to the recorder frame.

5. Pertinent patient data, the surgical procedure, and the date are written on the stripchart.

Vetter Unit
1. The control is set to playback position.
2. The dial pointer is set to zero (center) using the left stereo volume control with the recorder in "pause" position.

Magnetic Tape Recorder
1. Recorder is set to "record" position with pause control engaged.
2. Pertinent patient data, surgical procedure, and the date are then voice recorded on right stereo channel.
3. The recorder is left in the record position with the pause control engaged.

Blood Flow Recording
1. Measure the silk suture. Record the name of the artery and circumference.
2. The EMF probe is selected based on the circumference measurement. Open the outer wrapper and pass the probe to the surgeon.
3. The plug end of the probe is inserted into the switch box receptacle #1 and the surgeon places the other end into sterile saline solution.
4. The EMF probe is then balanced by shifting the probe control between plus and off, with correction made on the switch box balance #1 control until little movement is observed on the chart by this shifting. The probe factor is placed on the EMF probe factor dial and locked.
5. The probe is then positioned around the vessel and the probe control is switched to plus.
6. The waveforms are observed. When stable, the stripchart recorder is started at 5 mm/sec, and this is followed in sequence by magnetic recording of flow.
7. The stripchart recorder is then switched to 25 mm/sec and this is followed by the recording of at least ten waveforms at 125 mm/sec.
8. Following the acquisition of pulsatile waveforms and mean blood flow in the preceding step, the recorder is switched to 5 mm/sec and the surgeon occludes the vessel.
9. The blood flow dial is observed and subsequent zero occlusion numbers are obtained with the difference multiplied by 100 and recorded as mean flow.
10. The stripchart recorder and magnetic recorder are stopped. Probe control is returned to off. Data regarding the vessel studied, balance

control setting, and time constant (t.c.) setting are recorded on the data sheet.

11. Each time a new probe is used all procedures from step 2 on are repeated.

12. Follow-up flow observations are done by balancing per step 4 and utilizing the correct probe factor for the probe to be used.

13. At the end of the procedure, the EMF probes are scrubbed with soap, keeping the solution away from the contact plug end. The probes are then returned to the charge nurse, who prepares them by sterilization by gas.

Figure 4-24 shows standard electromagnetic flowmetry pulsatile waveforms obtained from various arteries. A flow chart of the mechanical connections is shown in Figure 4-25. Figure 4-26 shows an intraoperative data sheet for flow and pressure measurements and Figure 4-27 is a sample sheet for reports to the patient's chart.

ELECTROMAGNETIC FLOWMETRY

Noninvasive
The use of the noninvasive electromagnetic flowmeter is based on the principle that the movement of an electrical conductor through a magnetic field produces a voltage across the conductor that is proportional to the number of magnetic lines of force cut per unit time. As blood is a moving conductive fluid, the application of an external magnet induces a voltage across the segment that is detectable using skin electrodes and can be calibrated in terms of flow.

Instruments (Fig. 4-28a–c)
1. Noninvasive electromagnetic flowmeter
2. Alcohol
3. Sandpaper
4. Electrodes
5. Contact gel

Procedure
1. With the patient in a supine position, leg is flexed upward; the midcalf and thigh are measured in centimeters.

2. At the thickest point or midpoint of the calf and thigh, the area for placement of the electrodes is marked both medially and laterally to form an imaginary horizontal line between the two points.

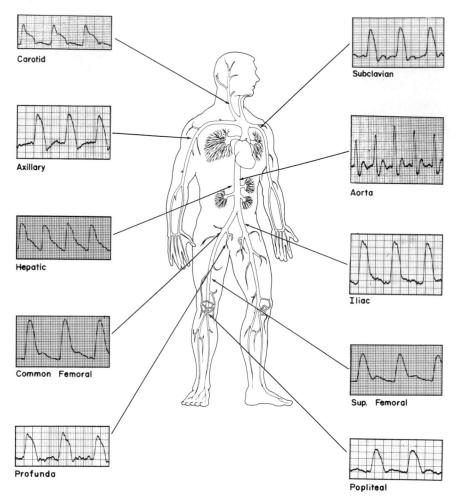

FIGURE 4-24. Intraoperative arterial pulsatile waveforms using standard electromagnetic flowmetry.

3. At the marks, an area of approximately one square inch is shaved. Removal of hair is essential to obtaining good electrical contact.

4. The shaved area is wiped with an alcohol pad and a piece of fine sandpaper is used to gently stimulate the area. Use caution so as to minimize trauma to the skin.

5. A small amount of contact gel is gently rubbed into the skin and wiped off.

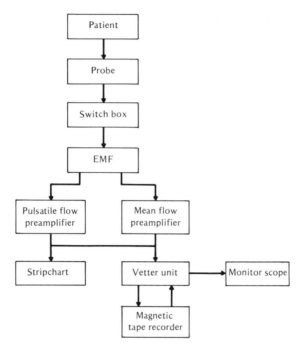

FIGURE 4-25.   Flow chart of mechanical connections.

6. The area for electrode attachment is then tested to ensure good electrical contact. If good contact has not been achieved, the preparation procedure should be repeated.

7. When good electrical contact has been achieved, the electrodes can be attached to the patient and coupled to the computer (Fig. 4-29). EKG electrodes are additionally attached to the patient.

The computer of the noninvasive electromagnetic flowmeter has five main modes of operation: (1) In the *enter data* mode, specific patient data (ID number, limb segment circumference) can be entered. (2) In the *scope* mode, the screen displays the trigger channel, flow channel, and BA channel in real time. (3) In the *options* mode, the operator is asked a series of questions as to the acquisition of the data (see below). (4) The *pause* mode is used when the operator needs to interrupt the data acquisition but does not wish to lose data or process the data previously acquired during the run. (5) The *start* mode is for the acquisition of data.

1. The computer is turned on and following a few seconds of warm-up, "Enter ID#" is displayed. A number of nine digits maximum can be

OPERATING ROOM HEMODYNAMIC MEASUREMENTS

Blood Flow Measurements	Cir.	Probe	Factor	Mult.	T.C.	Gain	Flow
Vessel:							
Vessel:							
Vessel:							
Vessel:							
Vessel:							

Blood Pressure Measurements	B/P	Pulse	Mean		B/P	Pulse	Mean

Patient: _____   Date: _____

SS#: _____   DOB: _____

Operation Performed: _____

FIGURE 4-26.   Example of an intraoperative data sheet for flow and pressure measurements.

entered. If a mistake is made, the "clear" button is pressed, which recycles the computer, and the correct number can be entered.

2. Once the ID number has been entered, the "enter" button is pressed and the computer advances to the next question:

"Circ A":   Enter the limb circumference in centimeters for Channel A.
"Fact A":   Enter the geometrical coefficient for Channel A; 100 for thighs and 74 for calves.
"Circ B":   Enter the limb circumference for Channel B.
"Fact B":   Enter the geometrical coefficient for Channel B.
"Sweeps":   Enter the number of sweeps to be taken for the acquisition of data (from 0 to 2048).
"Field":   Enter the field strength of the magnet in guess (1000).

Name:_____   SS#: _____

Date:_____   DOB:_____

Operation:_____

Blood Flow (ml/min.)			Blood Pressure (mm Hg.)					
	Before	After	Before			After		
			Syst.	Dias.	Pulse	Syst.	Dias.	Pulse
Iliac								
C. Femoral								
S. Femoral								
Profunda								
Popliteal								
Tibial								

FIGURE 4-27.   Example of a sample sheet for reports to the patient's chart.

3. Set the gain. This determines the size of the recorded signal. Gains of 1, 2, and 4 are available. Press the proper digit followed by "enter" to set the gain on one channel. Pressing the "channel select" displays the alternate channel so the gain can be set. The gain can be changed any number of times but only in the enter mode. One now enters the options mode.

4. The options mode asks a series of four questions that are answered either yes or no, pressing one for yes and zero for no.

  a. "Bypass Auto BAR?": Answering no automatically removes the BA; if yes, the BA is not automatically removed.

  b. "Remove local EKG?": This should be answered yes for measurements above the knee to remove local EKG effects that can affect data. For measurements below the knee, a no answer can be made.

  c. "Bypass Channel B?": This should be answered yes if only one limb is being evaluated at one level.

  d. "Beep on QRS?": Answering yes will cause a beep on each valid trigger received, which is useful for monitoring on the initital setting of the trigger level in the scope mode.

  At this point the computer automatically switches to the scope mode for the aquisition of data.

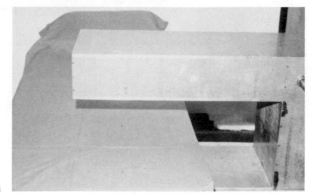

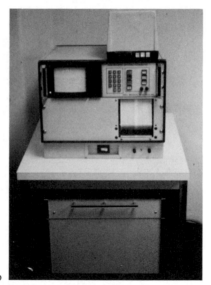

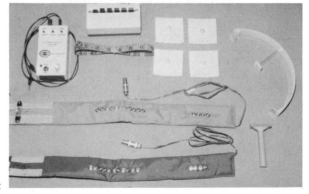

FIGURE 4-28a-c. The instrumentation for noninvasive electromagnetic electromagnetic flowmetry: (a) magnet; (b) computer; (c) electrodes.

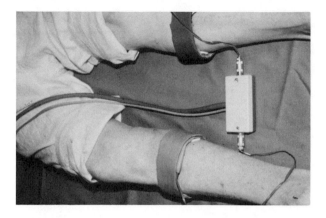

FIGURE 4-29.   Electrodes in place and patient attached to computer.

5. Pressing the "start" button initiates data acquisition. The screen will display data from Channel A or B and BA signals are not shown.

6. As data are acquired, four numbers and a letter are shown at the top of the screen. In the upper left corner, the pass number is displayed as 0 to 4.

a. Pass 0: Eight sweeps are taken and averaged to obtain the average R-R interval.

Pass 1 and 2 are done only when local EKG is to be removed as in measurements above the knee. They should be done with the magnet removed.

b. Pass 1: Eight additional sweeps are taken and R-R intervals of ac-mode. Acceptable data are averaged and the waveform is processed and stored in the reference area of the computer to be subtracted from data

c. Pass 2: As many sweeps are taken as entered in the enter data mode. Acceptable data is averaged and the waveform is processed and stored in the reference area of the computer to be subtracted from data acquired during pass 4.

d. Pass 3: Eight sweeps are taken as in pass 1 only with the magnet in place (Fig. 4-30). The pass 3 noise window is used to discriminate data in pass 4.

e. Pass 4: This is the same as pass 2 except with the magnet in place. The acquired data are stored apart from pass 2. The two sets of data are subtracted and the final output is displayed.

Following the pass number in the upper left corner is the letter A or B for which channel is displayed, followed by the number of sweeps rejected by the noise window, followed by the number of R-R interval

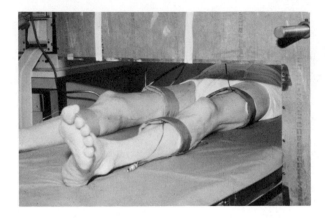

FIGURE 4-30.   Patient with magnet in place ready for testing.

rejections. The final digits in the upper right corner signifies the number or sweeps to go for completion.

7. A number of options are available during the acquisition of the data.

a. "Abort": If the run must be terminated, pressing this button during pass 2 or 4 will stop data collection and initiate processing of the data already obtained.

b. "Pause": Pressing this button will suspend data collection but will not initiate processing.

c. "Continue": Pressing this button will resume the acquisition of data from the point where "Pause" was initiated.

d. "S": Pressing this button will return the computer to the scope mode.

e. "Channel Select": Pressing this button will permit monitoring of the alternate channel. If one is viewing Channel A, this button will display Channel B and if viewing Channel B, this button will display Channel A.

8. After averaging one may set the zero line and the onset of systole to complete the data processing.

9. The final flow waveform is displayed as is "Number of Copies: 1" with a flashing underline under the number. The number of prints required (from 0 to 99) is entered on the keyboard and "enter" is pressed and the wave is printed (Fig. 4-31).

On the printed wave, the first wave is the actual averaged and corrected wave with a spike before and after that represents 8 ml. The wave that follows is a normalized wave that allows comparison of waves of

Noninvasive Electromagnetic Flowmeter

Normal Pulsatile Waveform and Averaged Blood Flow.

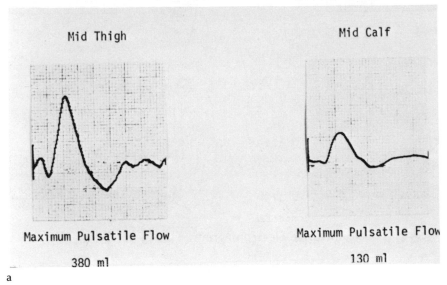

a

FIGURE 4-31a.   Pulsatile waveforms in noninvasive electromagnetic flowmetry.

widely disparate amplitude and qualitative examination of the waveform shape of the small flow waves seen in the presence of disease.

Printed above the curve is the patient ID number and 12 parameters.

The numbers to the right of the slash are for the top trace or Channel A and the numbers to the left of the slash are for the bottom trace or Channel B. The parameters are as follows:

a. R = heart rate (average); the reciprocal of the average period is multiplied by 60 sec/min to obtain beats/min.

b. S = onset of systole. This point is set by the operator and is called the zero line.

c. C = duration of systole taken as the interval between the onset of systole and the first successive zero crossing.

d. M = time to reach maximum flow taken as the length of time from the triggering to the maximum positive peak.

e. N = time to reach minimum flow taken as the length of time from the triggering to the most negative excursion.

f. P = systolic pressure indicator (ml/sec/sec) taken as the peak flow rate value divided by the time interval from triggering to peak.

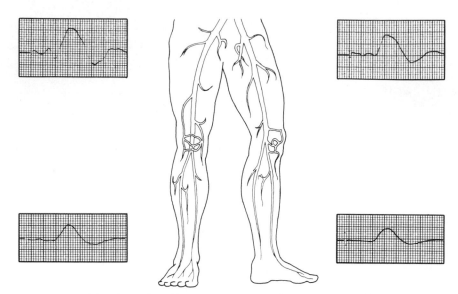

Noninvasive Electromagnetic Flowmeter Study

J. E.V.   Age 46 Male

	Rt.(59)	Thigh	L.(57)
Cal. 3mm			
Peak Flow Rate			
Q ml/sec	31.76		26.36
Stroke			
U. Vol.	4.96		3.98
Stroke Vol. x			
F. Heart Rate	331.21		265.33
Peak Pulsative			
(Q x 60)	1905.6		1581.6
Heart Rate 67			

	Rt.(40)	Calf	L.(39.5)
Cal. 6mm			
Q.	8.95		7.9
U.	1.11		1.11
F.	74.51		74.24
Peak Pulsative	537.		474.

b

FIGURE 4-31b.   Continued.

g. A = ascending slope (ml/sec/sec) taken as the peak flow rate value divided by the interval between the onset of systole and peak flow rate.

h. D = descending slope (ml/sec/sec) taken as the peak flow rate value divided by the interval between the peak flow rate and the first successive zero crossing. If no zero crossing follows the peak, then 600 msec after triggering or minimum accepted period (whichever is smaller) is used as the time interval.

i. E = elasticity constant, which is taken as the difference between the flow rate maximum and minimum divided by the absolute value of the minimum.

j. G = peak flow rate (ml/sec) and is the maximum blood flow rate.

k. V = stroke volume (ml) as the positive area under the systolic portion of the wave.

l. F = mean flow (ml/min) taken as the stroke volume multiplied by the average heart rate.

With minor modifications, the noninvasive electromagnetic flowmeter may be used to evaluate blood flow in the brachial and posterior tibial arteries.

TEMPERATURE GRADIENTS

The evaluation of skin temperature can provide an indication of the magnitude of blood flow to that particular region, as blood flow is influenced by temperature and vice versa. In the presence of adequate blood flow, skin temperature is normal, while decreases in blood flow lead to decreases in skin temperature. The opposite also holds true.

The blood flow is also influenced to a great extent by the ambient room temperature. For example, it has been found that at 15 C, blood flow to the foot is approximately 0.2 ml/100 ml/min. If the ambient room temperature is increased to 44 C, the blood flow to the foot increases to about 16.5 ml/100 ml/min. The nutritional blood flow to a region is less sensitive to temperature fluctuations than is skin blood flow, due to the preponderance of arteriovenous anastomoses in the skin.

There are several methods available for determining the presence of temperature gradients (see Thermometry in Chapter 3). When using thermometry, thermistor probes can be placed over any region of the body and the skin temperature simply read off the meter. When using liquid crystals, they may be sprayed on to monitor temperature variations over a large area (particularly applicable in breast cancer, as are thermograms) or liquid crystal tape may simply be applied over any particular area. In either instance, the color of the liquid crystal is simply interpreted as the skin temperature. Either of these two techniques can

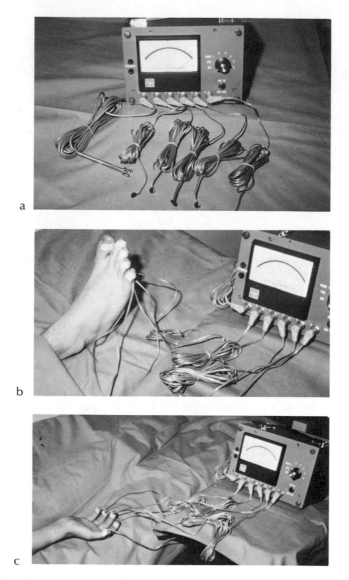

FIGURE 4-32a-c.   Technique for determining the presence of temperature gradients.

be applied in various instances: in evaluating the vascularity of gangrenous lesions or ulcerations, as an aid in determining the most distal level
of amputation possible consistent with wound healing, in monitoring toe
temperatures for an indication of bypass graft patency and for the early
detection of shock, for preoperative and postoperative studies in evaluat-

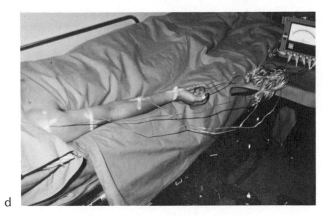

d

FIGURE 4-32d. Continued.

ing the success of bypass procedures or sympathectomy. The illustrations included here demonstrate some of these applications (Fig. 4-32).

An area where temperature is an important diagnostic tool is in the evaluation for Raynaud's disease and phenomenon. At identical temperatures, one can note a precipitous drop in digital temperature upon exposure in the patient with Raynaud's, as compared with a normal individual. Frequently the patient's digits may appear perfectly normal even though they feel cold. At a room temperature of 20 C, the normal temperature of the volar surface of the index finger is about 30 C, while in the patient with Raynaud's disease the temperature is 22 to 24 C.

CHAPTER 5

OBJECTIVE ASSESSMENT OF THE VASCULAR SYSTEM

EXTRACRANIAL CEREBROVASCULAR SYSTEM

Stroke ranks third overall among the leading causes of death and second in deaths due to cardiovascular disease in the United States. It has been estimated that there are approximately 160 new strokes annually per

155

100,000 population. A factor just as serious as mortality is the fact that those who survive are often disabled, which places a burden on patients' families and on society as a whole.

Perhaps the most significant factor in the development of extracranial cerebrovascular occlusive disease leading to stroke is advancing age. As the longevity of today's population increases, one can anticipate an increasing incidence in the occurrence of stroke. The incidence of stroke has been reported to be 0.3 percent for the 55-to-64-year age group. This incidence increases to 0.6 percent for the 65-to-74-year age group and and to 1.8 percent for the greater-than-75-year age group—a five-fold increase over the incidence of stroke in the 55-to-64-year age group. Interestingly, the incidence of stroke in males is 1.5 times greater than in females. This report of the population of Rochester, Minnesota,[1] shows a high (38%) initial mortality rate following initial stroke. Of those patients that survived the inital stroke, only 29% had a complete recovery; 71 percent had a neurologic deficit of which 4 percent required total nursing care, 18 percent were disabled but capable of self-care, and 10 percent were aphasic. In the patients that survived, there was a 10% chance of a recurrence of stroke during the first year and a 20% chance of recurrence during the first five years. Another study[2] shows an equally high initial mortality rate of 40 percent. The overall recurrence of symptoms in this study was 38 percent, with 26 percent developing recurring stroke, 20 percent developing transient ischemic attacks, and 2 percent developing both (for definition of transient ischemic attack and a discussion of symptoms, see "Clinical Manifestations" in this section). There was a very high initial mortality rate (62%) following recurrence of stroke. The data from these two studies shows stroke to produce a significant degree of morbidity and mortality that greatly increases in the patient who survives the initial infarction and subsequently has a recurrence of stroke.

Although there are references to what we today call stroke in the early writings of the Greeks (e.g., Hippocrates and Aretaeus), it was not until the seventeenth century that Wepfer recognized the relation of interrupted cerebral blood flow to the production of apoplexy (cerebral infarction). The earliest report linking stroke with extracranial cerebrovascular occlusive disease is attributed to Gowers in 1875, in describing a patient with right hemiplegia and blindness of the left eye. This was noted by Hunt in 1914. It was not until 1937 when Moniz demonstrated the use of arteriography of the carotid artery in diagnosing occlusive disease that work in the area of extracranial cerebrovascular occlusive disease was undertaken. In 1954 Eastcott, Pickering, and Rob reported the first successful surgical procedure on an extracranial carotid artery.

Since then, carotid endarterectomy has become one of the most common and successful surgical procedures carried out on the vascular system.

Once cerebral infarction is initiated, it is not possible to limit its extent or reverse the process. The only effective treatment is prevention. The noninvasive tests that will be discussed here are of significant value in providing for the early detection of hemodynamically significant oc-clusive disease of the extracranial cerebral circulation, allowing prompt institution of treatment that can frequently prevent the occurrence of a devastating frank stroke.

ANATOMY OF THE EXTRACRANIAL ARTERIAL CIRCULATION

The anatomical region that applies to the topic of extracranial cere-brovascular occlusive disease is that area of arteries that lies between and includes the arch of the aorta and the circle of Willis.

As the aorta arises from the left ventricle, it arches to the left and descends to transport blood to the region of the body below the heart. Arising from the arch of the aorta, there are three branches that supply blood to the upper extremity, neck, and head. The first branch is the innominate or brachiocephalic artery, the second is the left common carotid artery, and the third is the left subclavian artery.

As the innominate artery arises from the aortic arch, it proceeds supe-riorly and posteriorly to the point of the sternoclavicular junction, where it divides, giving rise to the right common carotid artery and the right subclavian artery, which arches laterally and posteriorly, traveling be-hind the scalenus anticus muscle to the right arm.

The left common carotid artery, arising from the aortic arch directly, runs parallel to the right common carotid artery. At the midcervical region (the upper border of the thyroid cartilage), the right and left common carotid arteries bifurcate into the right and left internal and external carotid arteries; the point of bifurcation may vary considerably.

The left subclavian artery as it arises directly from the aortic arch proceeds superiorly to the base of the neck where it arches laterally to pass behind the left scalenus anticus muscle to the left arm. As they pass behind the scalenus anticus muscles, the right and left subclavian arteries give rise to the right and left vertebral, internal mammary, thyrocervical, costocervical, and transverse cervical arteries. The vertebral artery is the branch that has significance in the normal cerebral circulation, but if it is occluded, the other branches of the subclavian arteries are important as collateral channels.

Blood is supplied to the face, scalp, oronasopharynx, skull, and meninges via the external carotid arteries. The external carotid arteries and their branches are of minor importance in the normal cerebral circulation. However, as with the cervical branches of the subclavian artery in the presence of vertebral artery stenosis, they take on importance as collateral pathways in the presence of internal carotid artery disease. The branches of the external carotid that are important in noninvasive diagnostic techniques are the superficial temporal artery and the facial or external maxillary artery. The facial artery courses upward and forward to the medial angles of the eye, where it is referred to as the angular artery.

The internal carotid arteries are most important in the cerebral circulation and can be divided into four segments: cervical, petrous, cavernous, and cerebral. The cervical segment has no branches and the fine branches arising from the petrous and cavernous portions are relatively minor. The first major branch of the cerebral segment is the ophthalmic artery, which enters the orbit from behind. The cerebral segment of the internal carotid continues and terminates in the anterior and middle cerebral arteries and the posterior communicating artery.

The vertebral arteries arising from the subclavian arteries are only free for a short distance prior to entering and passing through the foramina of the transverse processes of the upper six cervical vertebrae. They enter the cranium via the foramen magnum and unite to form the basilar artery. From its cervical portion, the vertebral arteries give rise to muscular and spinal branches which are clinically important as collateral channels. From its cranial portion, the vertebrals give rise to meningeal, posterior and anterior spinal, posterior inferior cerebellar, and medullary arteries. As the basilar artery proceeds along the underside of the brain stem it has a number of branches; it terminates in the posterior cerebral arteries which, in addition to a number of other areas, supply the visual portion of the cerebral cortex.

The posterior cerebral arteries form the posterior portion of the circle of Willis. Clinically, the circle of Willis is most significant as its arrangement allows blood from the posterior circulation to support the anterior circulation and vice versa if there is disease present. This arrangement is frequently incomplete, as a number of variations in structure can occur and interrupt the circle of blood flow. The anterior portion of the circle of Willis is formed by the anterior communicating artery joining the anterior cerebral arteries. The posterior portion is formed by the posterior communicating arteries that arise from the point of termination of the basilar artery and the origin of the posterior cerebral arteries. Laterally, the internal carotid arteries and middle cerebral arteries additionally supply inflow to the circle.

CLINICAL MANIFESTATIONS

The clinical manifestations of extracranial cerebrovascular occlusive disease range from fleeting episodes of neurologic dysfunction of less than 24 hours in duration to the permanent incapacitating neurologic deficit resulting from a major cerebral infarction. The actual symptoms with which a particular patient presents depend on the artery involved and thus provide a means of classification of symptoms into those signifying disease involvement of the carotid system (hemispheric symptoms or anterior ischemia) or of the vertebrobasilar system (nonhemispheric symptoms or posterior ischemia).

The most characteristic clinical manifestation and most definite of warnings is the transient ischemic attack. A transient ischemic attack (TIA) is an episode of temporary and focal cerebral dysfunction of vascular origin. A TIA is characteristically rapid in onset with symptoms reaching maximal effect in less than five minutes, frequently in less than one minute. The typical TIA is variable in duration, ranging from as brief a period of time as 2 to 15 minutes to as long as 24 hours. If the neurologic dysfunction persists for a period of time longer than 24 hours, the patient has had an actual cerebral infarction, although it is sometimes referred to as a TIA with incomplete recovery. The resolution of a TIA is rapid, frequently requiring only a few minutes; prolonged attacks take longer to be resolved.

Symptoms characteristic of a TIA involving the carotid system, hemispheric symptoms of anterior ischemia, include one or any combination of the following:

1. Motor defect. Generally a decrease or absence of function usually involving both upper and lower extremities unilaterally and manifested as weakness, paralysis, or clumsiness.
2. Sensory defect. Unilateral and generally manifested as numbness or paresthesia (a spontaneous sensation such as burning, pricking, numbness) involving the upper or lower extremities or the face.
3. Aphasia. A minor or major disturbance in speech and/or language with the possibility of impairment in reading, writing, or the capability of doing calculations.
4. Amaurosis fugax. Before the onset of the TIA, the patient's vision is normal, and following the attack, total or partial vision is transiently lost in one eye. The symptom is quite characteristic and the patient usually describes the occurrence as a window shade being slowly drawn across the field of vision.
5. Homonymous hemianopia. A loss of vision in the corresponding right or left lateral halves of the eyes.

Symptoms characteristic of a TIA involving the vertebrobasilar system, nonhemispheric symptoms of posterior ischemia, may include any one or a combination of the following:

1. Motor defect. Similar to motor defects seen in carotid system TIAs; however, with weakness, paralysis, or clumsiness of all four extremities with possible quadriplegia. The defect sometimes alternates between left and right sides in separate attacks.
2. Sensory defect. As with a TIA involving the carotid system; however, numbness or paresthesia occurs in any combination of or all four extremities or both sides of the face or mouth. The sensory defect is frequently bilateral and may alternate sides in separate attacks.
3. Homonymous hemianopia. A loss of vision in the corresponding right or left lateral halves of the eyes.
4. Bilateral homonymous hemianopia. Complete or partial loss of vision in both homonymous fields or altitudinal field defect.
5. Unilateral or bilateral loss of hearing.
6. Ataxia (loss of muscular coordination), disequilibrium, unsteadiness, or imbalance not associated with vertigo.

The symptoms of vertigo (dizziness, either with or without vomiting), diplopia (double vision), dysphagia (difficulty in swallowing), or dysarthria (difficulty in articulation) should not be considered as symptomatic of a TIA when they are manifested singly; however, if they occur in combination with one another or in combination with motor, sensory, or vision defects, they may be considered symptomatic of TIA. Vertigo can often be precipitated or aggravated by positional changes of the head or neck. "Drop attacks" may be considered symptomatic of a TIA; however, syncope (fainting), which is not a characteristic of a TIA, is commonly taken as a drop attack. A drop attack should be carefully characterized as a transient paraparesis (a slight degree of paralysis affecting the lower extremities) in which a normal individual suddenly feels his legs giving way and falls helplessly to the ground.

Symptoms mimicking those characteristics of vertebrobasilar insufficiency are frequently seen secondary to subclavian steal syndrome. In this syndrome, the origin of the subclavian artery is compromised and, in response to upper extremity muscular activity, blood flow in the branches of the first portion of the subclavian artery is reversed to supply blood to the exercising muscles. As the vertebral artery is a major branch of the subclavian artery, it functions as a major collateral pathway in the presence of a stenotic origin of the subclavian artery. Thus, blood flow in the ipsilateral vertebral artery is compromised by the subclavian artery stenosis and shunts blood from the basilar artery to supply the exercising upper extremity. The complex of symptoms is characteristically brought on by exercise of the upper extremity and typically consists of vertigo and/or presyncope. Frequently, a patient may have angiographic evidence of subclavian steal but not manifest symptoms, or manifest symptoms related to posture but independent of exercise.

The patient with a completed stroke is easily identifiable. Where the carotid system is involved in a complete stroke, the patient may present with minor weakness or catastrophic hemiplegia and aphasia. There may be complete unilateral loss of motor function or loss of only five-finger manipulation capability. Neurologic dysfunction that involves the dominant cerebral hemisphere will produce an associated express dysphasia varying in degree. Immediately following the stroke, the persisting neurologic deficit, motor and/or sensory defect, is at its maximum. This is followed by a gradual recovery of function that may be due to a reduction of acute edema, the formation of collateral channels, or compensation by adjacent regions of the cerebral cortex.

Patients presenting with a progressive stroke do not follow the above pattern. Such patients present with a modest neurologic deficit that progressively worsens.

A completed stroke involving the vertebrobasilar system is frequently fatal, as the vital functions of the brain stem are interrupted. Minor stroke involving the vertebrobasilar system does occur, although much less frequently than stroke involving the carotid system. Minor stroke in the vertebrobasilar system may leave the patient with paralysis of extraocular function, loss of hearing, persistent vertigo, ataxia, or bilateral asymmetric paralysis.

PATHOLOGY AND MECHANISM OF SYMPTOMS

Atherosclerosis is the primary pathologic factor in extracranial cerebrovascular occlusive disease and 90% of all instances are due to this factor. The remaining 10 percent of cases of cerebrovascular dysfunction are due to a variety of pathologies: fibromuscular dysplasia, kinking of the artery, extrinsic compression, traumatic occlusion or intimal dissection of the internal carotid artery, inflammatory angiopathies (e.g., Takayasu-Onishi arteritis), and migraine.

The plaque of atherosclerosis is an intimal disposition of a nodule of fat, primarily cholesterol, associated with an inflammatory response giving rise to fibroblastic proliferation. The plaque is grossly whitish in appearance, protruding into the arterial lumen. Calcification of the plaque may subsequently occur and, as the plaque becomes enlarged, it may rupture through the intima, leading to embolization. Rupture of the plaque may leave an ulcerated area that is ideal for formation of thrombus or platelet aggregation, giving rise to secondary emboli. Hemorrhage may occur, extending the lesion to a point where it may cause acute occlusion.

Plaque formation is most likely to occur at the point of arterial bifurcation. In extracranial cerebrovascular occlusive disease, the most common point of plaque formation is therefore at the bifurcation of common carotid arteries into the internal and external carotid arteries. Less frequent points of plaque formation are at the base of the great vessels as they arise from the aortic arch, at the origin of the vertebral arteries from the subclavian ateries, and intracranially at the origin of the anterior cerebral and posterior cerebral arteries and other branches of the basilar artery.

Elongation of the cervical portion of the carotid system may be congenital or acquired and is seen in approximately 15 to 20 percent of carotid angiograms. Such elongation may lead to redundancy with subsequent kinking, causing a compromise of cerebral blood flow.

Extrinsic compression that compromises cerebral blood flow is most frequently noted at the vertebral arteries, where hyperostosis or bone spur formation in the foramina of the cervical vertebral transverse processes can encroach upon the vertebral artery, causing obstruction of flow. Movement of the head will accentuate the obstruction. A desmoplastic response to radiation therapy may further obstruct vertebral artery flow.

Infrequently, extracranial obstruction of cerebral blood flow may be secondary to inflammatory angiopathies. An example is Takayasu-Onishi arteritis, an inflammatory disease affecting the major branches of the aortic arch. It occurs predominantly in females (about 90 percent) and in Asia. It is characterized by weak or absent pulses in the arm (sometimes referred to as "pulseless disease") and low brachial blood pressure.

The mechanism through which atherosclerotic involvement of the extracranial arterial circulation produces the symptoms that are characteristic of transient ischemic attacks is important to the clinician in determining the appropriate diagnostic and therapeutic modalities to be used. The mechanism of transient ischemic attacks has been variously attributed to mechanical obstruction to flow, embolization from ulcerated plaques, cerebroangiospasm, kinking or compression of arteries, polycythemia, anemia, and shunting of blood. The most probable mechanism is either mechanical obstruction to flow or embolization from ulcerated plaques.

In the mechanical theory, a transient ischemic attack is likened to a form of cerebral intermittent claudication. Although this theory has had support in the past, there is evidence showing it not to be the case. Studies have shown total cerebral blood flow to be equal before and after carotid endarterectomy. Also, the presence of a constant stenosis makes it difficult to envision it causing intermittent attacks of ischemia, as there is no significant variation in cerebral blood flow requirements.

Studies demonstrating the disappearance of TIAs following endarterectomy before the atherosclerotic plaque is a sufficient size to reduce blood flow, and TIAs disappearing following total arterial occlusion, lend support to the embolization theory. Although it would seem likely that embolization should lead to random neurologic dysfunction rather than the repetitive pattern characteristic of TIAs, the work of Milliken[3] has shown that due to laminar flow properties, particles released from the same point in the carotid artery are consistently carried to the same terminal branch.

Transient ischemic attacks with dizziness, vertigo, ataxia, or syncope (nonlateralizing) are due to a reduction of blood flow to the brain stem. Postural changes frequently bring on such symptoms, lending support to the theory of their flow-related mechanism.

With subclavian steal syndrome, shunting of blood is the obvious mechanism for symptoms, as the vertebral artery functions as a collateral vessel and shunts blood away from the brain stem.

The completed stroke corresponds to a definite area of infarcted cerebral tissue, which may be due to embolic occlusion or thrombosis of a critical end vessel, or an acute absence of blood flow by a proximal occlusion with inadequate collateral flow through the circle of Willis. The size, composition, and final disposition of the embolus play a role in whether a TIA or a stroke will ensue.

The mechanism for a progressing stroke has several theories: a series of emboli from a single lesion, a series of thromboemboli breaking off a totally occluding internal carotid artery thrombus, or expansion of the original area of infarction due to local edema. Each theory would account for a progressive increase in the degree of neurologic dysfunction occurring over a period of time.

EVALUATION OF THE PATIENT

History and Physical Examination

An accurate patient history is essential to a clinician's evaluation. The history of the sequence of episodes of neurologic dysfunction is basic to the evaluation and diagnosis of extracranial cerebrovascular occlusive disease. It should be carefully noted whether the patient's symptoms are hemispheric or nonhemispheric and thus whether they involve the carotid or vertebrobasilar system (see "Clinical Manifestations"). The duration of any form of neurologic deficit differentiates a transient ischemic attack from an actual cerebral infarction. Distinguishing between actual extracranial cerebrovascular occlusive disease and seizure disorders is facilitated by questioning the patient as to the presence of an aura, a preceding headache, or motor activity.

The patient's family or close friends can frequently indicate whether there has been any deterioration in intellectual capacity, which the patient may be unable to determine.

High-risk factors such as hypertension, a family history of stroke, diabetes, and the presence of intermittent claudication, angina pectoris, or previous myocardial infarction should be carefully evaluated, as they increase the likelihood of extracranial cerebrovascular occlusive disease.

The details of a thorough physical examination have been treated previously (see Chapters 1 and 2). Particular care should be given to several aspects of the physical examination in evaluating the patient for the presence of extracranial cerebrovascular occlusive disease.

Bilateral arm blood pressures are of importance as a unilaterally reduced arm pressure is often the initial sign of occlusive disease involvement of the great vessel arising from the aortic arch. Hypertension also increases the probability of atherosclerotic involvement of the extracranial vasculature. Segmental blood pressure evaluation of the extremities should be carried out, as peripheral vascular occlusive disease in an additional high-risk factor.

The detection of a neck bruit on physical examination is most characteristic of the presence of extracranial cerebrovascular disease. A bruit is the sound produced by turbulent flow as the blood flows past an arterial lesion and can be simply detected using a stethoscope. An important fact to be remembered when listening for a bruit is that the sound produced by turbulent flow is propagated distally from the point of the lesion. Therefore, if there is a significant lesion at the carotid bifurcation, for example, the bruit will not be heard if one listens at a point proximal to the bifurcation. The technique for screening a patient for detection of a carotid bruit has been detailed previously. It is recommended that the clinician listen for carotid bruits at three locations: the base of the neck, the midcervical region, and the angle of the jaw. The patient should be requested to take several deep breaths and then to hold his breath as one listens for the presence of bruits at these three locations. Listening at the three locations aids the clinician in distinguishing between a carotid bruit and the propagated sound of an aortic systolic murmur. As the clinician moves the stethoscope distal to the carotid bifurcation, the sound produced by a murmur, when present, will change pitch. Listening for bruits bilaterally will facilitate differentiation between a murmur and a carotid bruit.

Another recommended location is bilaterally over the supraclavicular fossae for the detection of a bruit arising from the subclavian arteries.

It should be noted that the absence of a bruit is not conclusive proof of the absence of significant extracranial cerebrovascular occlusive disease; as many as 40 percent of patients with arteriographically documented carotid stenosis do not present with a detectable carotid bruit. The presence of a bruit, however, is strongly suggestive of the presence of carotid occlusive disease.

An additional aspect of the physical examination for extracranial cerebrovascular occlusive disease is the evaluation of the pulses in the cervical region. This is of importance in detecting stenosis of the great vessels as they arise from the aortic arch. There will be reduced pulsation in the cervical portion of these vessels in the presence of hemodynamically significant stenoses at their origin. The presence of a stenosis in the cervical portion of the carotids usually does not yield a reduction in the quality of the pulse. In evaluating the pulses of the cervical region, the clinician should use care in avoiding massage of the carotid bifurcation, which can precipitate a reflex bradycardia. Compression of the carotids has been infrequently used in an attempt to reproduce the patient's symptoms. This procedure should be avoided as it may cause dislodgement of an embolus, precipitating a cerebral infarction.

A complete neurologic examination should be a routine part of examining the patient for extracranial cerebrovascular occlusive disease. Such an examination will document the presence of a remaining neurologic deficit, thus differentiating a cerebral infarction from a transient ischemic attack. It may also suggest the possible presence of additional pathology, e.g., brain tumor. The neurologic examination establishes a baseline for comparison with posttherapy examination.

An ophthalmoscopic examination is useful in detecting cholesterol emboli in the retinal arteries, which is indicative of an embolus-producing lesion in the carotid system. The emboli are typically trapped at arteriolar bifurcations in the retina and do not completely obstruct blood flow. The embolus is characteristically seen as a bright yellow refractile particle. This examination is probably best carried out by a trained ophthalmologist.

The role of a clinical laboratory examination in the evaluation of patients for extracranial cerebrovascular occlusive disease is relatively minor. Polycythemia vera may infrequently produce symptoms characteristic of cerebrovascular disease and its presence can be detected by a complete blood count. Temporal arteritis can be ruled out by a normal erythrocyte sedimentation rate. Blood sugar and serum cholesterol studies are helpful in establishing the presence of the risk factors of diabetes mellitus and familial hypercholesterolemia, respectively.

Application of Noninvasive Techniques

Doppler Ultrasound. The use of Doppler ultrasound in the evaluation of the patient with extracranial cerebrovascular occlusive disease is based on the collateral pathway that exists between the branches of the internal and external carotid arteries.

The ophthalmic artery is the first major branch of the internal carotid artery. It enters the orbit, gives off branches to the retina, and continues toward the supraorbital ridge, where it bifurcates to give rise to the frontal artery, which is medial, and the supraorbital artery, which is lateral. Both branches have a collateral relationship with a branch of the external carotid artery: the superficial temporal artery (from the external carotid) with the supraorbital artery (from the internal carotid) and the angular artery (from the external carotid) with the frontal artery (from the internal carotid). In normal individuals, flow in the supraorbital artery is directed out of the orbit and is augmented or unaffected by ipsilateral superficial temporal artery compression. In the presence of hemodynamically significant stenosis or occlusion of the internal carotid artery, flow in the supraorbital artery may be reversed and may be attenuated or obliterated by ipsilateral superficial temporal artery compression.

The instrumentation required for this examination is a directional Doppler ultrasonic flowmeter. This may be attached to a stripchart recorder for recording waveforms or a simple audio output for listening to the Doppler sounds with direction of flow being read off the flowmeter. We routinely use the recording of waveforms for detecting flow direction and augmentation or attentuation of waveforms on compression. The Doppler output may also be recorded with an instrumentation tape recorder for future analysis. The technique of the Doppler ultrasound cerebrovascular examination is detailed in Chapter 4.

In normal individuals, flow in the supraorbital artery is directed out of the orbit toward the forehead. This is interpreted as forward flow and is seen on the stripchart recording as a velocity waveform above the zero velocity baseline (Fig. 5-1). The presence of hemodynamically significant stenosis (greater than 50 percent reduction in internal arterial diameter) or occlusion of the extracranial internal carotid artery is seen as reverse flow in the supraorbital artery (flow into the orbit) and a velocity waveform below the zero velocity baseline. In rare instances, there may be paradoxical forward flow in the supraorbital artery due to extracranial collateral circulation in the presence of a stenosed internal carotid artery.

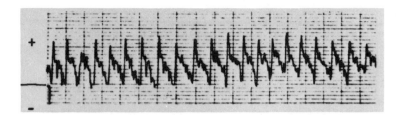

FIGURE 5-1.   Normal tracing of the supraorbital artery flow by Doppler ultrasound.

The various compression maneuvers distinguish between normal and paradoxical forward flow.

Forward supraorbital artery flow is either augmented or not affected by compression of the ipsilateral superficial temporal artery (Fig. 5-2). In the presence of hemodynamically significant internal carotid artery stenosis, supraorbital artery flow is reversed and ipsilateral superficial temporal artery compression attenuates or obliterates the waveform. Similar responses are seen with ipsilateral compression of the facial and angular arteries (Fig. 5-3). Sequential compression of all three branches of the external carotid artery should be carried out even in the presence of normal forward flow in the supraorbital artery to detect the presence of paradoxical forward flow. The extracranial collateral flow that provides for paradoxical forward supraorbital artery flow is probably supplied by the facial artery via the angular and nasal arteries. Frequently, contralateral sequential compression of the branches of the external carotid artery will obliterate reverse flow in the supraorbital artery where ipsilateral compression will not.

Common carotid cartery compression is used to rule out intracranial collateral circulation in the presence of normal supraorbital artery flow. The aforementioned hazards of carotid artery compression may be avoided by compression low in the neck away from the carotid sinus and bifurcation. This compression maneuver is not required in the presence of reverse supraorbital artery flow and may be omitted unless there is strong suspicion of intracranial collateral circulation. When the maneuver is necessary, the compression should be done only for one or two heartbeats. In the normal study, compression of the ipsilateral common carotid will attentuate, obliterate, or cause reverse supraorbital artery flow (Fig. 5-4). Such a response obviates the need for contralateral compression of the common carotid artery. In the presence of intracranial collateral flow due to significant carotid artery stenosis, supraorbital artery flow is unchanged or augmented by ipsilateral common carotid

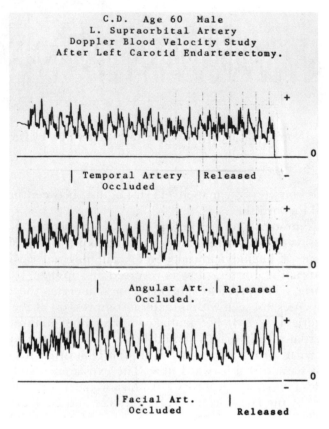

FIGURE 5-2.   A normal series of compression maneuvers in the Doppler cerebrovascular examination.

artery compression. If supraorbital artery flow is attenuated or obliterated by compression of the contralateral common carotid artery, there is intracranial collateral flow via the circle of Willis from the contralateral common carotid artery. The presence of collateral flow via the vertebrobasilar system in the presence of an obstructed internal carotid artery is detected by no change or an augmentation of supraorbital artery flow with ipsilateral and contralateral common carotid artery compression.

An algorithm outlining the steps and interpretation of the Doppler cerebrovascular examination is shown in Figure 5-5.

Photoplethysmography. The use of photoplethysmography in evaluating the extracranial cerebral circulation is based on the same anatomical relationships as is the use of Doppler ultrasound, i.e., the collateral relationships between the superficial temporal branch of the

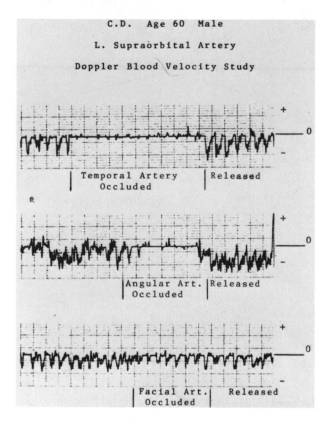

FIGURE 5-3. A series of compression maneuvers in the Doppler cerebrovascular examination indicating the presence of extracranial cerebrovascular occlusive disease.

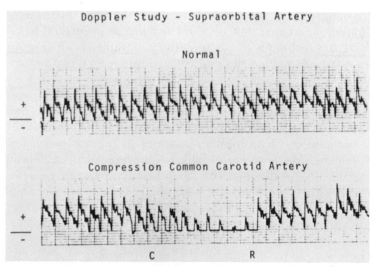

FIGURE 5-4. Compression of ipsilateral common carotid artery in a normal study.

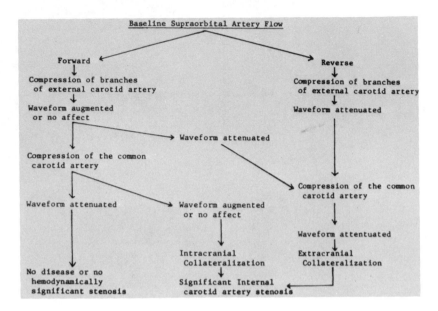

FIGURE 5-5.   An algorithim for the Doppler cerebrovascular examination.

external carotid artery and the supraorbital branch of the internal carotid artery and between the facial branch of the external carotid artery and the frontal branch of the internal carotid artery. The technique using the photoplethysmograph is basically the same as that used with Doppler ultrasound. The only instrumentation required is a photoplethysmograph. The technique for using the photoplethysmograph in evaluating the extracranial cerebral circulation is detailed in Chapter 4.

Using this technique of photoplethysmography, both supraorbital arteries may be examined simultaneously employing a two-channel photoplethysmograph with two probes. With the use of two probes over the supraorbital arteries, compression maneuvers are done ipsilaterally and contralaterally simultaneously for each branch of the external carotid and common carotid arteries. The baseline waveform should be adjusted with the gain of each amplifier channel so the waveform heights are approximately equal and of suitable height (greater than 20 millimeters). Using the dual technique, the photoplethysmograph recorder is best activated with a foot switch. If, with bilateral compression, an abnormal response is noted, each branch of the external carotid artery is then compressed sequentially to determine the source of the collateral circulation.

The photoplethysmographic tracing is normally not significantly attenuated by compression maneuvers carried out on the branches of the

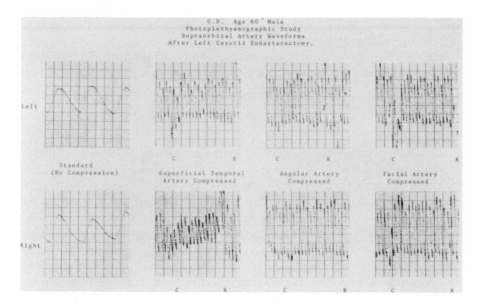

FIGURE 5-6. A normal supraorbital photoplethysmographic study (upper trace) showing no effect on compression of the branches of the external carotid artery.

external carotid artery and there is no diminution of the waveform only with transient ipsilateral compression of the common carotid artery. However, in the presence of a hemodynamically significant stenosis of the intenal carotid artery giving rise to extracranial collateral circulation, there is a significant attentuation of the supraorbital photoplethysmographic waveform on ipsilateral or contralateral compression of the branches of the external carotid artery. Studies have shown that an attenuation of more than 33 percent of the baseline waveform with ipsilateral compression is indicative of the presence of hemodynamically significant internal carotid artery stenosis. Attenuation of the baseline waveform of greater than 15 percent with contralateral compression is indicative of significant internal carotid artery stenosis (Fig. 5-6).

Common carotid artery compression is used for the documentation of the presence of intracranial collateral circulation. As mentioned above, a normal response to transient common carotid artery compression is a diminution of the supraorbital photoplethysmographic waveform only with ipsilateral compression. In the presence of intracranial collateralization, ipsilateral common carotid artery compression has a minimal or no effect on the supraorbital photoplethysmographic tracing. If the response to external carotid artery compression is normal and there is attenuation of the supraorbital photoplethysmograph waveform on contralateral compression, there is intracranial collateral circulation by way of the contralateral internal carotid artery. If neither ipsilateral or contralateral common carotid artery compression has an effect on the supraorbital photoplethysmographic waveform, collateral flow by way of the vertebrobasilar system is indicated. It should be noted that the supraorbital photoplethysmograph is not influenced by the presence of equally severe bilateral disease.

Oculoplethysmography. The use of the technique of oculoplethysmography in the noninvasive diagnosis of extracranial cerebrovascular occlusive disease is based upon the relative arrival time of the ocular pulse. The ocular pulse is a reflection of internal carotid artery flow via the transmission of the pulse pressure through the ophthalmic and retinal arteries to the intraocular fluid. The assumption is made that this transmission of pulse pressure is a reflection of the impedance to flow in the proximal portion of the internal carotid artery, as the ophthalmic artery is the first major branch of the internal carotid artery. It should be noted at this point that oculoplethysmography is a measure of total collateral flow as well as primary flow to the eye.

Evaluating the relative arrival time of the right and left ocular pulses provides an indication of the presence of hemodynamically significant right or left internal carotid artery stenosis. Additionally, an evaluation of the relative pulse arrival time at the ears provides an indication of the presence of right or left external carotid artery stenosis of hemodynamic significance. Plastic eye cups are attached to the eye by means of a low vacuum and the pulse wave is detected as a manifestation of a negative pressure exerted as the cornea is slightly pulled away from the cup, as the eye expands with the arrival of each arterial pulse. The relative delay in the pulse arrival time may be displayed digitally or may be ascertained through examination of the analog recording of the pulsatile waveform. Relative delay in the arrival of the pulse pressure wave at the ears can be detected using ear clips with a built-in photoplethysmograph that are clipped to the ear lobes. As with the eye cups, relative delay in the pulse arrival time may be displayed digitally or through an examination of the analog pulsatile waveform recording.

An oculoplethysmograph that provides a digital display of relative pulse arrival delay is perhaps most advantageous as waveform analysis is obviated. Such instrumentation, however, can be easily modified to also provide an analog output. The instrument uses an accurate (± 1 millisecond) pulse delay measurement system that detects and eliminates the effect of noise and artifact and provides a digital display of the relative eye and ear pulse delays. The digital display is the average of eight noise-free, blink-free pulses and is simultaneously displayed as relative pulse delay ear to ear for the external carotid artery, eye to eye for the internal carotid artery, and eye to ear for the bilateral evaluation of the internal and external carotid arteries. The procedure of oculoplethysmography is detailed in Chapter 4.

A technically valid examination should show a consistency in the pulse delay averages of ±3 ms for the eye-to-eye digital display and ±5 ms for the ear-to-ear and eye-to-ear digital display, and a confirmation of the pulse delay side. With cross-cup placement, the indicated side should read the opposite of the side obtained with normal cup placement, e.g., normal placement, L8, and with the cross-cup placement, R7.

The digital ear-to-ear pulse delay display evaluates the external carotid artery for the presence of hemodynamically significant stenosis. A digital display of 0 to 30 ms is within normal range; a display of a greater than 30 ms delay is indicative of hemodynamically significant stenosis of the external carotid artery on the indicated side (e.g., R35). The digital eye-to-eye pulse delay display evaluates the internal carotid artery for the presence of hemodynamically significant stenosis. The normal range of eye-to-eye pulse delay is 0 to 10 ms. A pulse delay display greater than 10 ms is indicative of the presence of hemodynamically significant stenosis of the internal carotid artery corresponding to the indicated side (e.g., L15). The evaluation of eye-to-ear pulse delay can be used to assess the presence of bilateral internal or external carotid artery stenosis. A 0 to 30 ms pulse delay for eye to ear is within normal range. The presence of hemodynamically significant bilateral stenosis of the internal carotid artery is indicated by a greater-than-30 ms "eye" delay (e.g., eye 36) and of the external carotid artery a greater-than-30 ms "ear" delay (e.g., ear 35). See Tables 5-1 and 5-2.

In the rare instance of symmetrical bilateral internal and external carotid artery stenosis, a false negative result would be obtained. A false positive result will be obtained in the presence of ophthalmic artery disease in the absence of internal carotid stenosis. Additionally, total internal carotid artery occlusion of long duration that has excellent collateralization can display an eye-to-eye pulse delay that is less than expected (a pulse delay display of 15 to 20 ms). In such instances, compression of the ipsilateral superficial temporal artery will demonstrate the actual presence of pulse delay greater than 20 ms.

Instead of a digital display, an analysis of the ocular pulse tracing can be done. The most widespread use is made of the fluid-filled oculoplethysmograph. The stripchart that is obtained traces the right ear pulse, the left and right eye pulses, and a left-right eye pulse differential. A brief visual inspection of the stripchart is made to reject isolated waveforms that may be artifact. The presence of any readily visible ear-eye pulse delays is noted.

TABLE 5-1.   NORMAL OCULOPLETHYSMOGRAPHIC
EXAMINATION OF 60-YEAR-OLD MALE.

Ear/Ear		Eye/Eye		Eye/Ear	
R		R		Eye	
L		L		Ear	
R	20	L	8	Ear	8
R	15	L	8	Ear	13
R	23	L	4	Ear	2
R	24	L	8	Ear	2
R	24	L	10	Ear	2
R	29	L	4	Eye	1
R	50	L	7	Eye	23

TABLE 5-2.   AN ABNORMAL OCULOPLETHYSMO-
GRAPHIC EXAMINATION OF 53-YEAR-OLD MALE,
SIGNIFYING THE PRESENCE OF SIGNIFICANT
EXTRACRANIAL CEREBROVASCULAR OCCLUSUVE
DISEASE.

Ear/Ear		Eye/Eye		Eye/Ear	
R		R		Eye	
L		L		Ear	
L	27	L	28	Ear	22
L	24	L	28	Ear	24
L	33	L	27	Ear	23
L	28	L	24	Ear	20
L	33	L	28	Ear	19
L	26	L	33	Ear	15
L	31	L	28	Ear	16

If the left-right eye pulse differential trace is flat, there is no eye pulse delay. A vertical line is drawn at the trough of the first ocular pulse denoting the beginning of the arterial phase and also at the second ocular pulse peak of each complex. Intersections of the vertical lines and the differential trace are identified and joined by straight lines. The drawn baseline following the differential but deviating from the horizontal is representative of the ocular pulse amplitude differences. The direction of the baseline deviation indicates the side of the delayed pulse (Figs. 5-7 and 5-8).

Carotid Phonoangiography.   Carotid phonoangiography is an audiovisual analysis of recordings made of cervical carotid bruits. The technique is similar to but more sensitive than the technique of standard

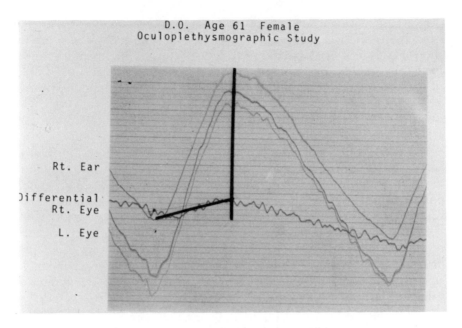

FIGURE 5-7.   Normal fluid-filled oculoplethysmographic examination.

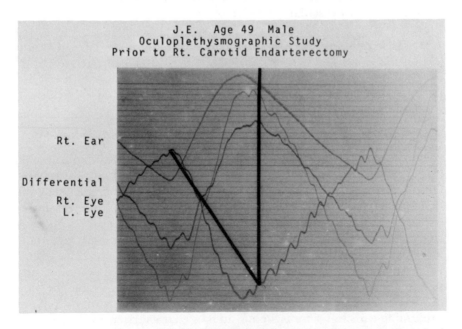

FIGURE 5-8.   An abnormal fluid-filled oculoplethysmographic examination signifying the presence of significant extracranial cerebrovascular occlusive disease.

clinical auscultation using a stethoscope for the detection of bruits arising from the cervical carotid arteries (see "History and Physical Examination" in this section). With the technique of carotid phonoangiography, a specially adapted microphone is placed over the cervical carotid arteries at three levels: low, middle, and high, and recordings of carotid bruits are made and analyzed to determine the degree of underlying stenosis. The reader is referred to Chapter 6, "Carotid Phonoangiography" for a more extensive discussion of phonoangiography.

The analysis of a carotid phonoangiogram is in terms of the relative amplitude and duration of the bruit waveform in relation to the first and second heart sounds. The low placement of the specially adapted microphone at the base of the neck functions in detecting bruits radiating superiorly from below the carotid bifurcation.

Carotid phonoangiography yields a relatively small incidence of false positive results emphasizing the significance of detecting cervical carotid bruits in determining the presence of extracranial cerebrovascular occlusive disease. Carotid phonoangiography is recognized to be limited in value for the detection of total occlusion of the cervical carotid artery, but it is more sensitive in detecting the presence of stenotic lesions of a lesser degree that are associated with minimal flow reduction. Additionally, carotid phonoangiography is more sensitive to symmetrical bilateral extracranial cerebrovascular occlusive disease.

Doppler Imaging.   A discussion of the application of ultrasound (echography and Doppler ultrasonic angiography) as it pertains to the evaluation of extracranial cerebrovascular occlusive disease as well as peripheral vascular occlusive disease is detailed in Chapter 6, "Ultrasonography."

Application of Arteriography

The detection of the presence of a stenotic lesion in the extracranial cerebrovascular circulation is often overshadowed by the need to determine the presence and topography of a nonstenotic plaque. A plaque that is rough or ulcerative is often the source of a clot, atherosclerotic debris, or platelet aggregates that can embolize. A lesion with these characteristics may be of a size sufficient to be stenotic, but it is frequently too small to yield a reduction in flow or cause turbulent flow yet still produce symptom-causing emboli. As such, the detection of a nonstenotic, symptomatic ulcerative plaque will not be possible by noninvasive techniques. Highly symptomatic patients, particularly patients presenting with transient ischemic attacks characterized by hemispheric symptoms (see "Clinical Manifestations"), should therefore undergo routine arteriography whether or not noninvasive techniques demonstrate the presence of an underlying ulcerative plaque responsible for the production of cerebral emboli.

Although radiocontrast arteriography remains the essential method for localizing the site of the stenotic lesion, for the detection of non-stenotic ulcerative plaques, and demonstrating total internal carotid artery occlusion, the noninvasive techniques outlined in this chapter have several advantages over arteriography in the assessment of extracranial cerebrovascular occlusive disease. Noninvasive techniques are particularly advantageous in the assessment of the hemodynamic significance of occlusive lesions (e.g., fibromuscular hyperplasia) or kinking, which do not have a single area of stenosis. Noninvasive techniques additionally facilitate the periodic evaluation of patients with asymptomatic carotid bruits or suspected extracranial cerebrovascular occlusive disease or screening patients considered to be at high risk for the development of extracranial cerebrovascular disease. These noninvasive techniques also provide an objective means of assessing the postoperative success in the reestablishment of cerebral blood flow. The application of these noninvasive techniques will increase the positive yield of carotid angiography. It should be noted that these noninvasive techiniques do not replace arteriography but should be considered complementary.

SUMMARY

The topic of extracranial cerebrovascular occlusive disease is the subject of some controversy due to a lack of objective data on its natural history. This has led some physicians to question the need for surgical intervention in such patients. The nonivasive diagnostic techniques that we have presented should do much in the way of alleviating this difficulty.

In addition to providing some clarification on the currently existing therapeutic controversies via a study of the natural history of extracranial cerebrovascular occlusive disease, these noninvasive diagnositic techniques are useful in the screening of the general population or patients with indefinite symptoms or symptoms not typical of the presence of disease: in the follow-up of patients who have undergone carotid endarterectomy for the early detection of re-stenosis; as a baseline for the evaluation of the immediate success of the procedure; and in evaluating patients prior to major surgery where perioperative episodes of hypotension may be expected.

The detection of the presence of a true carotid bruit is highly indicative of the presence of extracranial cerebrovascular occlusive disease. As a bruit is produced with a lesser degree of stenosis (approximately 35 percent) as compared with that required to precipitate a reduction in flow (approximately 75 percent), the presence of a bruit can detect the presence of disease at an earlier stage than possible with other non-invasive techniques that require a reduction in flow in order to detect the presence of disease. If a bruit is not detected, this is not an indication of the absence of significant extracranial cerebrovascular occlusive disease, because a bruit will disappear as a stenotic lesion approaches complete occlusion.

Oculoplethysmography has been reported as a highly reliable technique for the detection of significant occlusive disease. This is particularly true when there is unilateral involvement of the carotid system. A negative result with oculoplethysmography only rules out the presence of a lesion advanced enough to precipitate a reduction in flow. A negative result will also be reported in the presence of bilaterally equal occlusive disease as well as in the presence of an ulcerative plaque. The technique, however, is highly useful as a screening technique and in preoperative and postoperative patients.

The techniques of photoplethysmography and Doppler ultrasound flow detection are relatively simple examinations that are easily applicable to bedside or office use. The instrumentation is quite portable and relatively inexpensive. As with oculoplethysmography, these two techniques are readily applicable for screening and preoperative and postoperative studies.

In the highly symptomatic patient, a normal noninvasive study should not rule out the presence of extracranial cerebrovascular occlusive disease. Those patients with signs that are characteristic of transient ischemic attacks or patients who may benefit from surgical intervention should undergo carotid arteriography in the presence of a normal noninvasive study.

PERIPHERAL ARTERIAL SYSTEM

Recent estimates show that over 200,000 deaths annually may be attributed to atherothrombotic disease of the major arterial vessels. An additional 600,000 deaths annually are due to atherosclerotic coronary heart disease.

The patient with peripheral arterial disease may be seen by a physician of any number of specialties—family practitioner, internist, orthopedist, neurologist, etc. Such patients are usually, or should be, referred to a vascular surgeon for definitive diagnosis and therapy. In view of this fact, it is unfortunate that many vascular surgeons do not perform a complete physiologic evaluation of their patients. While a simple clinical examination may be adequate for the experienced vascular surgeon to make a diagnosis and possibly establish the location of the major blockage, the primary physician does not have the necessary experience. In this case a quick, simple, and noninvasive testing technique would be especially valuable. The techniques that follow range from simple, inexpensive means of determining ankle pressure, particularly applicable to office use, to sophisticated instrumentation for evaluating blood flow.

ARTERIAL PRESSURES

The measurement of arterial systolic pressures is a simple and inexpensive technique that can be repeatedly carried out by noninvasive means. Systolic pressure measurement provides a sensitive and objecive quantitative index of the presence and severity of atherosclerotic occlusive disease and complements the information that is obtained through physical examination. The equipment required is a penumatic cuff and a flow sensor, which may be Doppler ultrasound, strain gauge, or photoplethysmograph. The pneumatic cuff is simply placed around the anatomical area to be evaluated and the flow sensor is placed distally (e.g., the Doppler probe is positioned over a distal peripheral artery; the strain gauge is placed around the forearm, calf, finger, or toe; the photoplethysmograph is placed on the finger or toe). The pneumatic cuff is inflated to where the arterial signal is obliterated and then gradually deflated. The pressure at which the arterial flow signal returns is taken as the systolic pressure. Using Doppler ultrasound, this point is easily detected at the return of the audio output; with strain gauge or photoplethysmography, it is detected by the return of the arterial blood flow waveform.

Ankle Pressures

The measurement of a patient's ankle pressure provides a means for a rapid and reliable assessment of a patient's circulatory status in the lower extremity. The presence of atherosclerotic occlusive disease is readily detected and the technique is readily applicable to follow-up studies and assessing the immediate success of an arterial reconstruction in the recovery room. Ankle pressures may play an additional role in predicting the possible beneficial effect of lumbar sympathectomy, the healing of ischemic ulceration or gangrene, and in selecting the lowest level of amputation possible consistent with wound healing.

The basic technique consists of placing a pneumatic cuff just proximal to the ankle, with the Doppler probe placed either over the posterior tibial artery or dorsalis pedis artery, which is an extension of the anterior tibial artery at the dorsum of the foot. The difference between the ankle pressure measurements at the posterior tibial and dorsalis pedis arteries normally range from no difference to approximately 10 mm Hg. If there is a difference greater than 15 mm Hg in the two ankle pressure measurements, the artery with the lowest pressure is probably stenosed or occluded. In rare instances, a patient may present with stenosis or occlusion of the posterior and anterior tibial arteries and yet have "normal" ankle pressures due to the presence of a large and disease-free peroneal artery.

In terms of absolute pressure, normal ankle systolic pressure is typically 0 to 20 mm Hg greater than brachial systolic pressure. This increase in ankle pressure above the brachial pressure is due to the augmentation of the systolic pressure as the pressure pulse is propagated distally, a decrease in the diastolic pressure, and an increased pulse pressure due to the presence of reflected pressure waves, and the increasing stiffness of the arterial wall. In the presence of atherosclerotic occlusive disease, the ankle systolic pressure is reduced below brachial systolic pressure due to the flow of blood through a stenosed artery or, in the presence of arterial occlusion, blood flowing through collateral vessels of a much smaller diameter, which offer a greater resistance to flow and a consequent drop in systolic pressure.

Using the absolute ankle systolic pressure, it is possible to classify patients into one of three categories: normal patients, patients with intermittent claudication, or patients with rest pain, gangrene, or ulceration. Patients with absolute ankle systolic pressures greater than 50 to 60 mm Hg rarely present with rest pain, gangrene, or ulceration unless there is concomitant disease involvement of the pedal or digital arteries. Patients who present with rest pain, gangrene, or ulceration typically have ankle systolic pressures below 40 to 50 mm Hg.

The absolute ankle systolic pressure should not be overemphazied as it can frequently be misleading. For example, of two patients with identical ankle pressures of 115 mm Hg, one may present with intermittent claudication and one may not. If one compares the ankle systolic pressure with the brachial systolic pressure to obtain an ankle/brachial systolic pressure ratio or ischemic index, one obtains a more reliable indication of the presence and severity of the disease process. In normal patients, the ischemic index is usually greater than 1.0, indicative of a normally higher ankle pressure as compared with brachial pressure. The lower limit of normal individuals for the ischemic index can be taken as approximately 0.97. With increasing age, the lower limit of normality for the ischemic index may increase due to stiffening of the arterial wall; an ischemic index of 0.97 in an elderly patient does not rule out the presence of mild atherosclerotic occlusive disease. In the presence of disease, the ischemic index is less than 1.0, indicating an ankle pressure of 115 mm Hg with a brachial pressure of 110 mm Hg would probably not have intermittent claudication as his ischemic index would be greater than 1.0. However, if another patient had an ankle systolic pressure of 115 mm Hg with a brachial pressure of 150 mm Hg, he could possibly have intermittent claudication as his ischemic index is much less than 1.0. In the presence of disease that is confined to the popliteal artery or other arteries below the knee, the ischemic index values would be comparatively high but below normal. With diffuse or multilevel disease, the ischemic index values would be relatively low. Similarly, the presence of gangrene, rest pain, or ulceration yields very low ischemic indices while with mild intermittent claudication, high ischemic indices may be seen. Complete arterial occlusion yields ischemic indices markedly lower as compared with the presence of mild disease involvement, which seems to emphasize the greater importance of arterial diameters rather than the extent of occlusion or collateralization.

Ankle as well as segmental pressures that are obtained at rest often do not accurately reflect the true status of the patient's circulatory reserve. A relatively accurate evaluation of the circulatory reserve can be obtained through an examination of the pressure or flow response to hyperemia. This can be observed following a period of exercise testing or with the reactive hyperemia test.

In the normal subject, a period of moderate exercise on a treadmill (2 mph at a grade of 12 percent) will produce little or no drop in ankle pressure (Fig. 5-9). The ankle pressure may actually increase in response to exercise. Following a period of strenuous exercise, the ankle pressure in the normal subject may decrease a few millimeters of mercury but characteristically exhibits a rapid return to baseline. In a patient with arterial occlusive disease, even a period of moderate exercise will be enough to precipitate a fall in ankle pressure. The extent of the decrease in the ankle pressure and the period of time required to return to baseline are a function of the extent of the disease process. The more extensive the disease process, the greater the drop in ankle pressure and the longer the time required to return to baseline. It is not unusual in some patients for ankle pressure not to return to baseline even 20 to 30 minutes following exercise (Fig. 5-10). In patients who are incapable of walking on a treadmill, simple foot flex exercise can precipitate a similar response in the presence of disease. In some patients, the reactive hyperemia test may also be used.

With the reactive hyperemia test, a pneumatic cuff placed proximally on the thigh is inflated to suprasystolic pressure to produce a transient period of total limb ischemia (usually lasting 3 minutes before release of

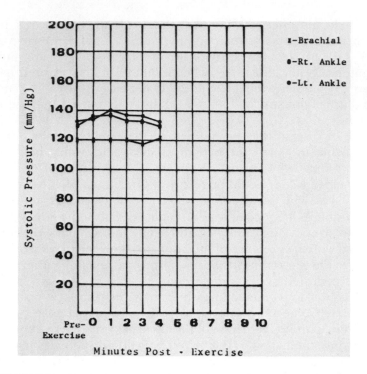

FIGURE 5-9.   Normal response of arterial pressure to a period of exercise.

the cuff). Following release of the thigh cuff, the peripheral arteriolar bed becomes dilated, providing a large increase in blood flow, which normally exhibits a rapid return to baseline. In the normal, there may be a slight decrease in ankle pressure following release of the proximal occluding cuff but the pressure should return to baseline in approximately 30 seconds. In the presence of disease, a similar response as with exercise testing is noted—a greater pressure drop and a prolonged period of time to return to baseline. The more extensive the disease process, the greater the pressure drop and the longer the time to return to baseline. The reactive hyperemia test is probably easier than exercise testing as a treadmill is not required. This is particularly advantageous in the evaluation of amputees or the elderly. Additionally, the reactive hyperemia test is amenable to use of mercury strain gauge or photoplethysmography.

Segmental Pressures

The localization and partial quantification of the presence of arterial obstruction can be obtained using segmental limb pressures. In a similar

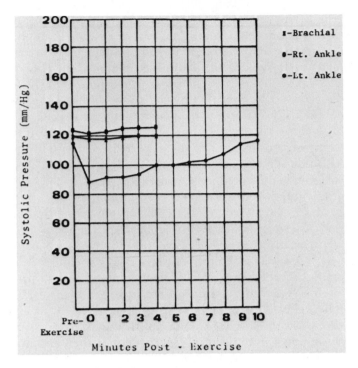

FIGURE 5-10.   Abnormal response of arterial pressure to a period of exercise.

fashion as outlined above for the measurement of ankle systolic pressures, the pressure gradient down the leg can be assessed using segmental pressure measurements with pneumatic cuff placement at the high thigh, above the knee, at the calf, and at the ankle.

Pressures at the high-thigh and above-the-knee segments are particularly important in distinguishing between aortoiliac, femoropopliteal, or combined disease. Due to the use of a relatively small pneumatic cuff as compared with the size of the thigh, normal thigh pressures should be 30 mm Hg or greater than brachial systolic pressure. The absolute thigh systolic pressure will vary with the size of the patient, being higher in the patients with large thighs and lower in patients with smaller thighs.

The presence of significant aortoiliac occlusive disease is indicated by a thigh pressure that is less than brachial pressure or less than approximately 30 mm Hg greater than the brachial pressure. It should be remembered that a patient with a smaller thigh diameter will have thigh pressures that approach brachial pressure and thus may not be indicative of the presence of disease. In such instances, comparison with the contralateral thigh pressure may be of value. The presence of a bilateral difference in thigh pressure of 20 mm Hg or greater is indicative of the presence of disease on the side with the lower pressure. A thigh/brachial index that is greater than 1.20 indicates the probable absence of significant aortoiliac occlusive disease. An index greater than approximately 0.80 but less than 1.20 indicates the presence of stenosis of the aortoiliac region with indices below approximately 0.80 indicating the probability of complete occlusion. If on physical examination an excellent femoral pulse is palpated and the patient has a low high-thigh pressure, there is probable complete obstruction of the superficial femoral artery with a stenotic profunda femoris artery.

As one examines the pressure down the leg, there should not be a pressure gradient between any two levels of more than 20 to 30 mm Hg. Pressure gradients greater than 20 to 30 mm Hg are indicative of significant atherosclerotic occlusive disease between the two segments. In the presence of complete arterial obsruction the pressure gradient between the two segments is typically 40 mm Hg or greater.

As mentioned above, comparison of segmental pressures with the contralateral limb is frequently helpful. A pressure gradient of 20 mm Hg or greater between left and right segments is indicative of significant occlusive disease at the level of the limb with the lower pressure.

At times, one may note distal pressures higher than proximal pressures. This may be attributed to calcification of the arterial wall interfering with compression of the arterial wall by the pneumatic cuff. Such is frequently the case in diabetic patients, where the ankle pressure or other segmental pressures may exceed 300 mm Hg.

In the measurement of the systolic pressure in the calf segment, a systolic pressure of 10 to 20 mm Hg greater than brachial pressure should be expected. A patient with a large drop in pressure from the calf to the ankle would be expected to have significant disease in the run-off vessels.

By comparing segmental pressures down the leg and with the contralateral limb, one should, in most cases, be able to determine the location of the obstructive process as well as obtain some idea of the functional significance of the disease process. In the presence of multilevel disease, one may not be able to determine which obstruction is the most functionally significant. This is particularly the case in the presence of combined aortoiliac-femoropopliteal occlusive disease. An extremely low thigh pressure may be reflected in low distal pressures, making diagnosis of combined occlusive disease difficult (Figs. 5-11 to 5-15).

Digital Pressures
For the detection of small vessel disease, the techniques of photoplethysmography and mercury strain-gauge plethysmography are particu-

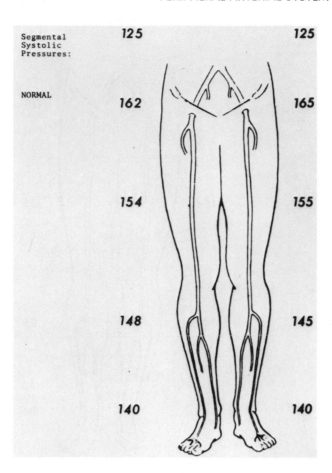

Segmental
Systolic
Pressures:

NORMAL

125   125

162   165

154   155

148   145

140   140

FIGURE 5-11.   Normal segmental pressure profile showing no significant pressure gradient vertically or horizontally.

larly advantageous. With placement of standard pneumatic cuffs at the ankle or metatarsal areas, or a specially adapted cuff around the digit with the photoplethysmograph probe on the ventral surface of the toes, the return of the pulsatile photoplethysmographic waveform as the cuff is deflated indicates the ankle, metatarsal, or digital pressure. The test can be repeated for each of the digits to evaluate each digit's blood supply. This technique may be particularly beneficial when applied to the patient with gangrenous involvement of the toes when amputation is necessary. If the patient has good metatarsal pressures, amputation of only the involved digit is frequently sufficient to salvage the patient's foot. With more extensive gangrenous involvement of the toes, a good

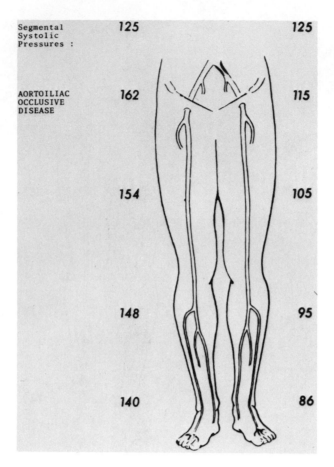

FIGURE 5-12.   Pressure profile indicative of aortoiliac occlusive disease as shown on the right side of the figure.

metatarsal pressure would indicate a good prognosis for transmetatarsal amputation.

The technique of photoplethysmography is also useful in detecting microembolization from an atheromatous plaque or aneurysm. In such patients, Doppler systolic segmental limb pressures may in fact be normal down to the ankle; however, the photoplethysmograph would show a decreased metatarsal pressure due to peripheral embolization (Table 5-3, p. 190.)

In assessing finger pressures, systolic pressure should be equal to or slightly greater than brachial pressure depending upon the age of the

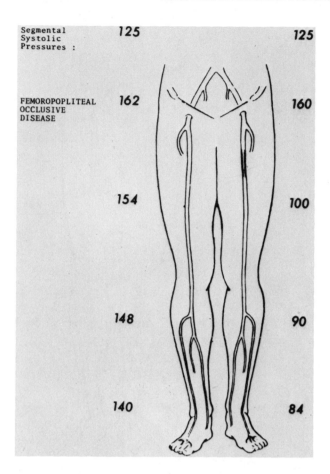

Segmental
Systolic
Pressures :

FEMOROPOPLITEAL
OCCLUSIVE
DISEASE

FIGURE 5-13.   Pressure profile characteristic of femoropopliteal occlusive disease—a large pressure gradient between high-thigh and above-knee segments.

patient: equal in older patients, and greater finger pressures as compared with brachial pressure in young patients. In general, a 15 mm Hg or greater pressure difference between fingers, a wrist-to-finger gradient of 30 mm Hg or greater, or an absolute finger systolic pressure less than 70 mm Hg should be considered to be abnormal. Abnormal finger pressures are noted in the presence of occlusive disease involving the digital arteries, the common digital artery, the palmar arch, the radial or ulnar arteries, the brachial or subclavian arteries. Involvement of only one digital artery or only the radial or ulnar artery may not be sufficient to cause a significant pressure gradient. Additionally, measurements of

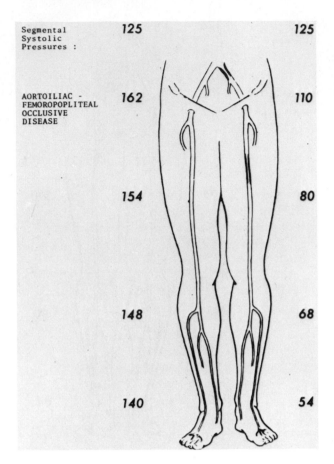

FIGURE 5-14. Pressure profile characteristic of combined aortoiliac-femoropopliteal occlusive disease.

finger pressures may be beneficial in distinguishing between Raynaud's disease (cold sensitivity due to vasospasm) or Raynaud's phenomenon (arterial obstruction due to collagen vascular disease, arteritis, etc.). At room temperature in the absence of an occlusive lesion, finger pressures will be normal. If sensitivity to cold or other ischemic manifestations are secondary to arterial obstruction, finger pressures will be low at room temperature and may be decreased further if the digit is warmed.

In assessing toe pressures, the pressure at the toes is usually slightly less as compared with brachial pressure and ankle pressure. A toe/brachial systolic pressure index below 0.7 should be considered to

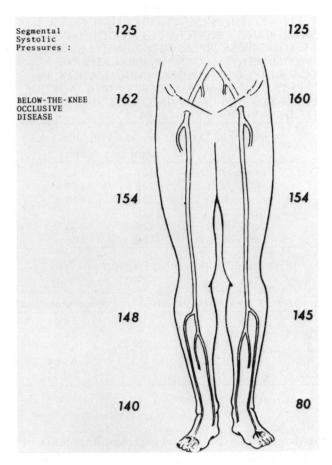

Segmental
Systolic
Pressures :   125   125

BELOW-THE-KNEE   162   160
OCCLUSIVE
DISEASE

154   154

148   145

140   80

FIGURE 5-15.   Pressure profile characteristic of occlusive disease present below the knee.

be abnormal. Measurement of toe pressure is usually done at the base of the toe and thus will not detect the presence of disease at the tip of the toe. As each digit is supplied by two main lateral arteries, occlusion of only one of the main lateral arteries will not be detected (Figs. 5-16 and 5-17).

Penile Pressures

The presence of impotence may be secondary to neurogenic, hormonal, psychogenic, or arterial factors and is an area of increasing interest. The new operative technique of epigastricocavernous anastomosis

TABLE 5-3.   THE PRESENCE OF DIGITAL PRESSURES, SIGNIFICANTLY REDUCED BELOW DOPPLER ANKLE SYSTOLIC PRESSURE, AS DETERMINED USING PHOTOPLETHYSMOGRAPHY, INDICATES THE POSSIBILITY OF PERIPHERAL EMBOLIZATION. IN THIS PATIENT A SACCULAR ABDOMINAL AORTIC ANEURYSM WAS DETERMINED TO BE THE SOURCE OF THE PERIPHERAL EMBOLIZATION.

Segmental Doppler Systolic Pressures		
	Right	Left
Brachial	122	112
High Thigh	128	114
Above Knee	128	118
Calf	126	90
Post. Tibial	124	100
Dors. Pedis	116	106

Photoplethysmographic Pressures At Toes		
Toe	Right	Left
	Ankle/Metatarsal	Ankle/Metatarsal
1.	72/55	75/64
2.	74/20	74/69
3.	55/80	46/55
4.	105/25	83/64
5.	104/54	80/37

has made the detection of the arterial origin of impotence of value. The occurrence of impotence following aortoiliac reconstructive procedures has also contributed to this increasing interest.

In the normal potent male the pressure gradient between the penile and brachial systolic pressures is typically less than 40 mm Hg and the penile-brachial index is usually greater than 0.75. These pressure values in the presence of acceptable pulsatile waveforms are suggestive of the presence of adequate penile blood flow. In the patient with a penile-brachial systolic pressure gradient of more than 60 mm Hg, a penile-brachial index less than 0.60, and poor pulsatile waveforms, there is a strong possibility that impotence, when present, is of vascular origin (Figs. 5-18 and 5-19). There is considerable overlap in these pressure values, and the age of the patient has considerable influence on the type of waveforms obtained. As there are numerous exceptions to the above criteria, it is currently difficult to determine which patients would be expected to benefit from penile revascularization.

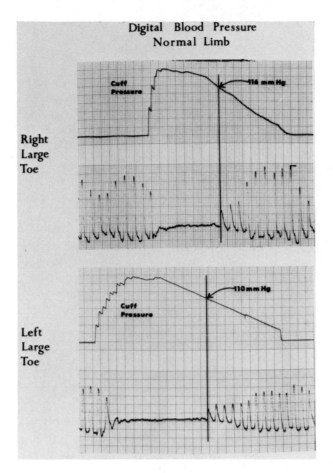

FIGURE 5-16.   Normal digital pressure as determined with the photoplethysmograph.

VELOCITY WAVEFORM

By using a directional Doppler instrument with the angle of the probe adjusted to obtain a maximal velocity waveform tracing, velocity waveforms may be obtained from any peripheral artery (Fig. 5-20).

In the absence of disease, the normal arterial velocity waveform is multiphasic, usually composed of one systolic and a variable number of diastolic components. The waveforms obtained are representative of the average forward and reverse flow velocities at a given time. As such, when the waveform traces below the zero line, the average reverse flow

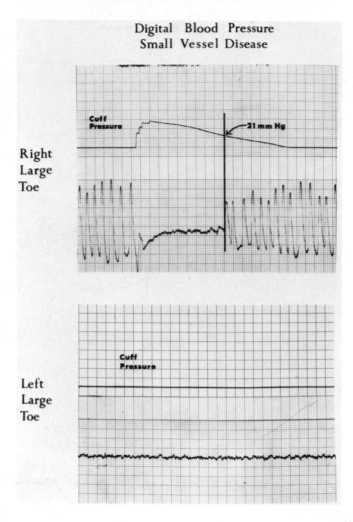

FIGURE 5-17.   Abnormal digital pressures as determined with the photoplethysmograph. The lower trace shows an absence of pulsatile blood flow on photoplethysmography.

at that particular time is greater than the average forward flow. In the normal, the initial large positive deflection (indicative of a high net forward flow) is the systolic component and is characteristic of a large inflow of blood. The second component is a negative deflection, indicative of a net reversal of flow. This is followed by another positive deflection, indicative of diastolic forward flow. The flow reversal noted in the normal arterial velocity waveform is the result of the generally higher re-

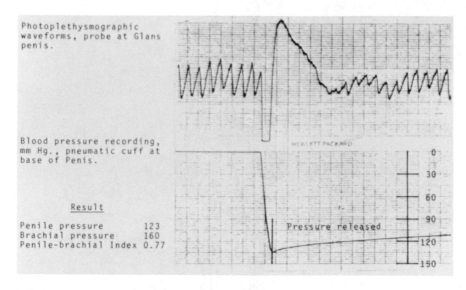

FIGURE 5-18.   Normal penile pressure study.

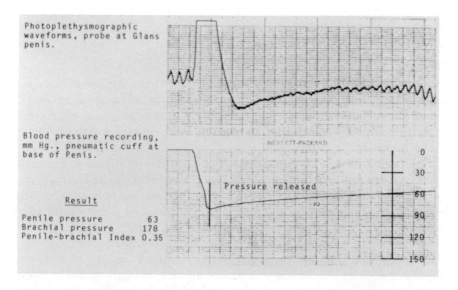

FIGURE 5-19.   Abnormal penile pressure study.

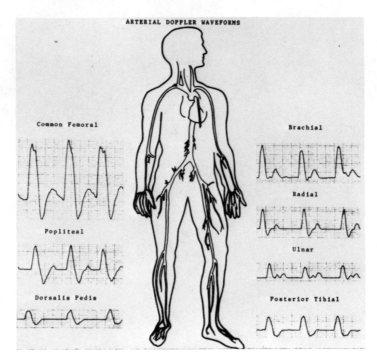

FIGURE 5-20.   Normal Doppler velocity waveforms demonstrating a normal multiphasic pattern, a prominent reverse flow component, rapid acceleration and deceleration, and a sharp peak.

sistance found in the peripheral vascular bed. If the higher peripheral vascular resistance is decreased, as by the administration of vasodilators, the net reversal of flow is eliminated. In addition to being characteristically multiphasic, the Doppler velocity waveform cycles with each beat of the heart, i.e., it is pulsatile.

The qualitative evaluation of the velocity waveform, the recognition of the waveform pattern, is most widely used. The primary deviations from the norm looked for are the absence of reverse flow component, a rounding of the velocity waveform peak, and a prolonged acceleration (upslope) or deceleration (downslope) of the waveform.

In comparing abnormal velocity waveforms obtained proximal and distal to an occlusion and proximal, distal, and over an area of stenosis, the abnormalities in the waveform are similar enough to make their qualitative differentiation somewhat difficult. In most cases, the simple qualitative differentiation of normal from abnormal is all that is required.

The arterial velocity waveform may also be quantitated. From the obtained tracing of the velocity waveform, one can directly measure the pulse rise time and decay time, and peak forward and reverse velocity. Mean velocity may also be obtained electronically. The pulse rise time is measured as the time from the onset of the initial component to the waveform peak and the pulse delay time is taken as the time from the peak to the waveforms' return to baseline. From these parameters, acceleration (peak forward velocity divided by pulse rise time), deceleration (peak forward velocity divided by the pulse decay time) as well as various ratios (e.g., acceleration/deceleration and peak velocity/mean velocity) can be calculated. Although this method of quantification does not allow determination of the level of disease involvement, it can differentiate single level from multilevel involvement.

PULSATILE WAVEFORMS

Arterial Impedance Plethysmography

The technique of arterial impedance plethysmography is concerned with the detection of blood volume changes in the limb. Basically, a constant, high-frequency current is forced between two circumferential electrodes positioned on a limb. Resultant voltages are measured between two inner electrodes and impedance waveforms are generated. The changes in impedance are due to segmental volume fluctuations and can be recorded and quantified using waveform analysis techniques.

The shape of the waveform is influenced by a number of physiologic parameters that includes the magnitude of ventricular contraction, vessel and tissue elasticity, and proximal and distal resistance. Arterial impedance plethysmographic waveforms can be obtained from the thigh-to-ankle, above-the-knee, popliteal, and below-the-knee segments. In normals, the impedance waveform is characterized by a steep systolic rise (rapid acceleration), a narrow peak, and a dicrotic notch on the diastolic downslope (deceleration) (Figs. 5-21 and 5-22). In the presence of occlusive disease distal to the segment being examined, there is a prolongation of the pulsatile waveform acceleration and a rounded peak. Proximal to an obstruction, the acceleration may be relatively normal; however, the peak will be rounded and the deceleration of the curve prolonged (Fig. 5-23). As with systolic pressure measurements, a period of exercise or temporary total ischemia can often bring about changes in the impedance waveform, indicating occlusive disease that is not apparent in the resting state (Figs. 5-24 through 5-26).

Noninvasive Electromagnetic Flowmetry

The noninvasive electromagnetic flowmeter provides a direct measure of pulsatile blood flow by means of Faraday's law of electromagnetic

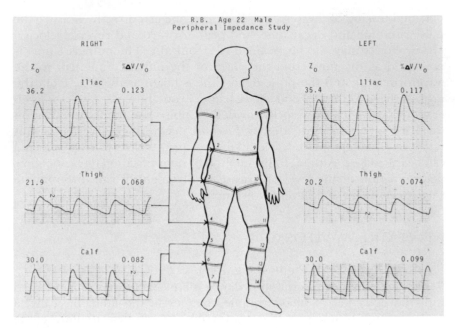

FIGURE 5-21. A normal peripheral arterial impedance study. Z_0 is the base impedance and the value % $\Delta V/V_0$ is a measurement of the lateral expansion of the segment being evaluated and is sensitive to the pulsatile component of pressure and the arteries' compliance.

induction. A magnetic field is generated by a large permanent magnet exterior to the body. Blood, a moving conductive fluid, generates an electrical potential perpendicular to both the magnetic field and the direction of flow. Skin electrodes detect the voltages, which are proportional to the quantity of flowing blood. The data are processed to distinguish between the blood flow signal and background noise due to ECG and myoelectric potentials. These measurements of peak pulsatile flow are made over a cross section of an extremity with the enclosed arteries contributing to the resultant signal. The blood flow waveform is printed on a stripchart with the peak height corresponding to peak pulsatile blood flow. A normal thigh flow with the noninvasive electromagnetic flowmeter is approximately 130 ml/min or greater; the waveform has a relatively sharp acceleration and deceleration (Figs. 5-27 through 5-29). The presence of occlusive disease prolongs the acceleration in the presence of proximal disease and the deceleration in the presence of distal disease (Fig. 5-30). Patients with symptoms characteristic of intermittent claudication have been found to have thigh peak pulsatile flow values in

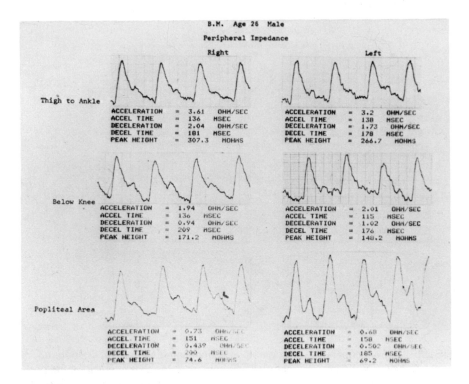

FIGURE 5-22. Normal peripheral arterial impedance study showing computer analysis.

the range of 150 to 200 ml/min and calf peak pulsatile flow values in the range of 50 to 100 ml/min. Patients with rest pain or severe ischemia have thigh peak pulsatile flow values below 150 ml/min and calf peak pulsatile flow values below 50 ml/min.

The noninvasive electromagnetic flowmeter has been found to be particularly useful in diabetic patients where severely calcified arteries yield highly exaggerated pressures when there is in fact vastly reduced arterial blood flow (Fig. 5-31). We have often found the noninvasive electromagnetic flowmeter to be capable of detecting the presence of occlusive disease that is not apparent by arteriography (Chapter 9, "Multiple Segment Involvement").

Photoplethysmography

The technique of photoplethysmography has been presented previously as a most useful technique in the evaluation of the extracranial cerebrovascular system (under "Evaluation of the Patient" in this chap-

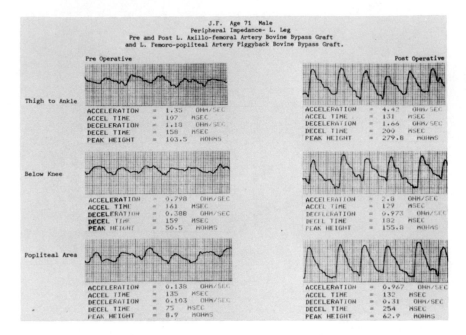

FIGURE 5-23.   Preoperative-postoperative comparison of peripheral arterial impedance. Tracings on the left, preoperative, show waveforms characteristic of the presence of disease. Tracings on the right show marked improvement in waveform
characteristics following operation.

ter), in the determination of digital pressures for the determination of
small vessel disease and peripheral embolization, and the determination
of penile pressures for the detection of arterial insufficiency as a cause of
impotence (under "Arterial Pressures").

The sensing probe of the photoplethysmograph contains a tiny light
source and photosensitive cell. The photosensitive cell responds to the
light reflected from the arterial blood in the vascular bed over which the
probe is placed. The amount of detected pulsating light is directly proportional to the amount of pulsating blood.

In the presence of ulcerations or other wounds, photoplethysmography can be used in the assessment of wound-healing potentials. The
presence of good, pulsatile photoplethysmographic waveforms around
the wound is indicative of good tissue perfusion and wound healing with
conservative management. In the absence of pulsatile photoplethysmographic waveforms, there is poor tissue perfusion and poor wound healing potential, suggesting the need for surgical intervention to obtain
primary healing (Figs. 5-32 through 5-35).

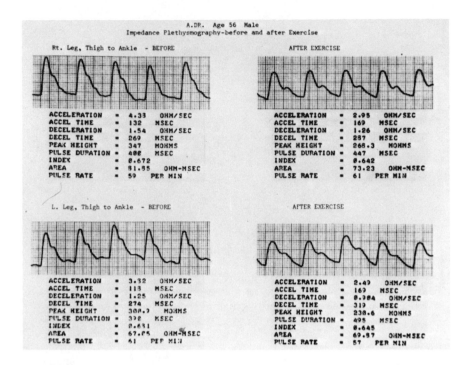

FIGURE 5-24.   Tracings on left, prior to exercise, appear relatively normal. The tracings on the right show changes in the waveform characteristic of underlying disease following a brief period of exercise.

The photoplethysmograph is also capable of quantitating skin perfusion pressure—a useful measurement in the determination of amputation level. The sensing probe of the photoplethysmograph is affixed to the diaphram of a pressure transducer and the apparatus is simply applied to the desired area with manual pressure (Fig. 5-36). As the manual pressure is increased, there is an obliteration of the photowaveform, which returns as the pressure is reduced. The pressure at which the photowaveform returns is taken as the skin perfusion pressure. A skin perfusion pressure of 40 mm Hg or greater can reasonably be expected to yield wound healing (Fig. 5-37).

TEMPERATURE PROFILE

The skin surface temperature can be used as an indication of cutaneous blood flow when it is related to internal or forehead temperatures

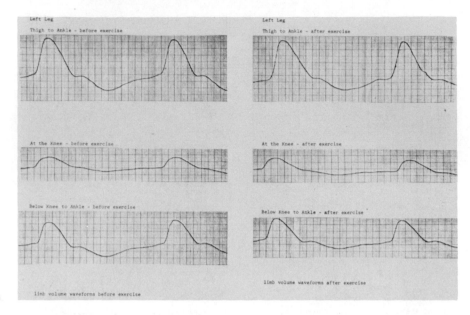

FIGURE 5-25. This patient shows a normal exercise response for the left lower extremity. The quality of the waveform is maintained following exercise.

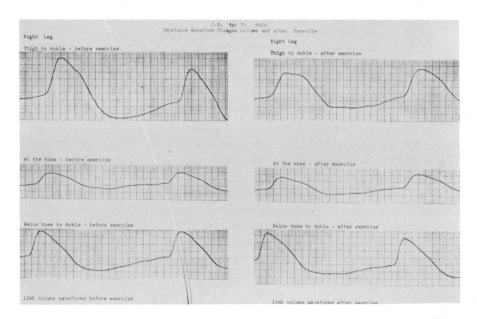

FIGURE 5-26. The same patient (as in Figure 5-25) shows an abnormal exercise response on the right lower extremity. The quality of the waveform is lost following exercise.

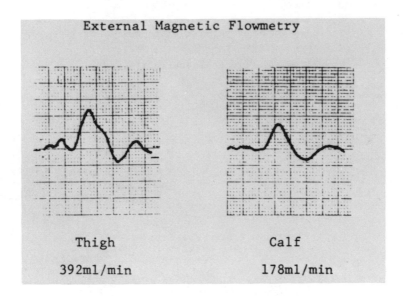

FIGURE 5-27.   Normal pulsatile waveforms and flow values obtained by non-invasive electromagnetic flowmetry for the thigh and calf segments.

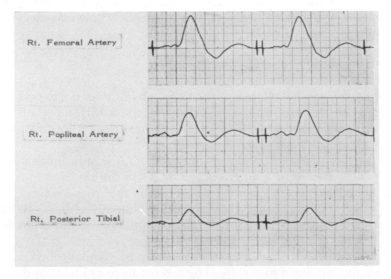

FIGURE 5-28.   Noninvasive electromagnetic flowmetry study in the normal at the femoral, popliteal, and posterior tibial regions demonstrating the basic similarity of waveform shape.

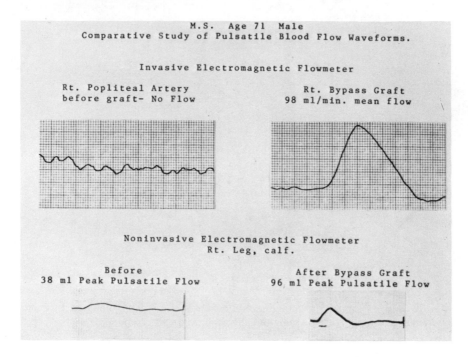

FIGURE 5-29. Comparison of noninvasive with standard intraoperative electromagnetic flowmetry showing a close agreement in terms of flow values and waveform shape.

and the environmental temperature. Although one does not expect identical temperatures at symmetrical skin surfaces, a difference of more than one degree centigrade between two symmetrical points during repeated tests is evidence of an abnormality.

Measurement of finger and toe temperatures is significant in peripheral vascular disease as temperature changes in the digits are an indication of changes in the vasomotor tone of the superficial vessels. Prior to a surface area breaking down, there is frequently a three- to four-degree contrast between the inflamed area and an adjacent uninvolved area.

In the normal, there is an ascending gradient of vascular tonus extending from the hip down to the toe. The temperature gradient of the skin is the reverse of the gradient of vascular tonus. In the presence of vascular disease, the temperature gradient from the thigh to the toe may be as great as nine degrees centigrade in the severely ischemic extremity.

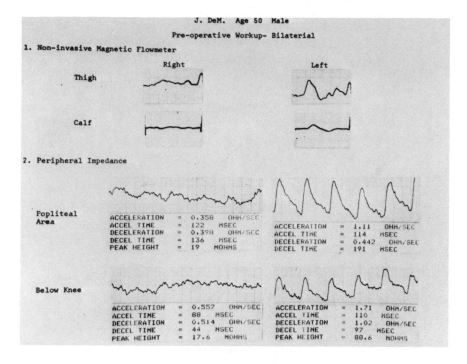

FIGURE 5-30.   Preoperative-postoperative compression of noninvasive electromagnetic flowmetry and peripheral arterial impedance. Preoperatively, waveforms obtained were erratic and nonpulsatile. Following femoropopliteal bypass (modified human umbilical vein) obtained waveforms show excellent pulsatility.

ARTERIOGRAPHY, ECHOGRAPHY, RADIONUCLIDE ARTERIOGRAPHY

These three topics are considered in detail in Chapter 6 and only brief mention shall be made here.

The use of arteriography should be limited in use to establish a precise delineation of the disease process and provide anatomic information that may be required for the physician to make a therapeutic decision as to the management of a particular patient. The noninvasive techniques that have been presented provide more than adequate information for the establishment of the diagnosis.

Echography, also known as pulse echo ultrasonography, is most extensively used in the examination of abdominal aortic aneurysms. In this

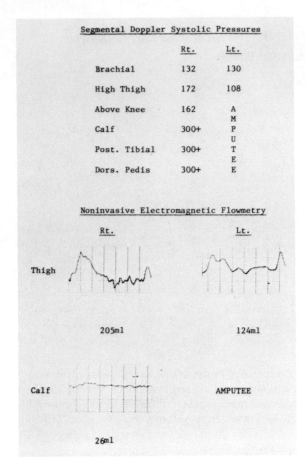

Segmental Doppler Systolic Pressures		
	Rt.	Lt.
Brachial	132	130
High Thigh	172	108
Above Knee	162	A
		M
Calf	300+	P
		U
Post. Tibial	300+	T
		E
Dors. Pedis	300+	E

Noninvasive Electromagnetic Flowmetry

Rt.   Lt.

Thigh

205ml   124ml

Calf   AMPUTEE

26ml

FIGURE 5-31. In patients with severely calcified arteries noninvasive electromagnetic flowmetry is capable of supplying accurate information as to blood flow. This patient had vastly reduced pulsatile flow in the presence of ankle systolic pressure of +300 mm Hg.

regard, it is a particularly advantageous technique as compared with arteriography, in that echography can be used serially to follow the development of the aneurysm in high-risk or elderly patients.

Radionuclide arteriography can be applied in the evaluation of arterial perfusion of the tissues at rest and also to monitor changes in tissue perfusion following physiological or pharmacological stimuli. The use of radionuclides can also be applied to visualizing the arterial lumen.

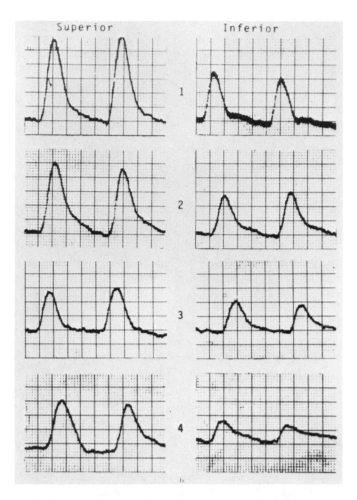

FIGURE 5-32. Photoplethysmographic study superior and inferior to an ulcer showing excellent pulsatile waveforms indicative of a good healing potential.

SUMMARY

The determination of the ankle pressure and the calculation of an ischemic index is the quickest and simplest method of establishing the presence of atherosclerotic occlusive disease. If this technique is taken a step further, one can obtain segmental limb pressures for establishing the most proximal level of disease, the presence of distal disease, and the

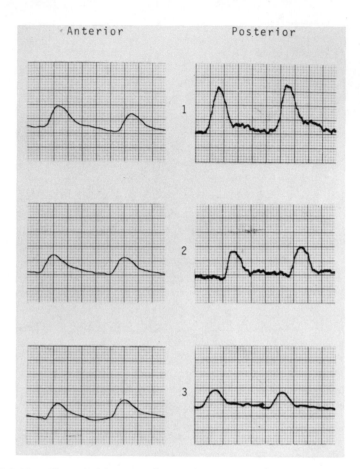

FIGURE 5-33.   Photoplethysmographic study anterior and posterior to an ulcer showing excellent pulsatile waveforms indicative of a good healing potential.

status of the run-off vessels. If the patient's pressure profile is normal, in all likelihood there is an absence of arterial disease. Taking the test a step further, determination of the digit pressures can rule out the presence of small vessel disease. These tests are relatively inexpensive, simple, and can be done rather quickly, making them particularly applicable for office use. Further testing is probably best carried out in a centrally based vascular laboratory.

The determination of a patient's circulatory response to exercise or transient ischemia is important as it can frequently detect the presence of underlying disease that is not readily apparent in the resting state. Reac-

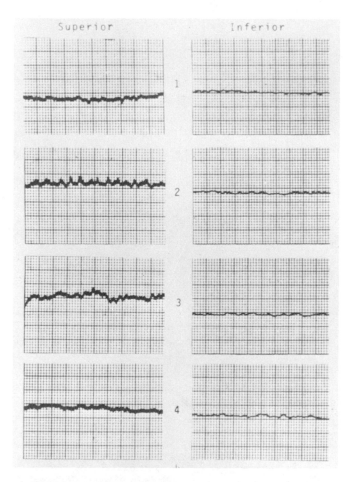

FIGURE 5-34. Photoplethysmographic study superior and inferior to an ulcer showing an absence of pulsatile flow, indicating a poor healing potential.

tive hyperemia testing or foot flex exercise can be adequately done in the physician's office. Exercise testing with a treadmill is the realm of the vascular laboratory.

The other techniques mentioned previously, noninvasive electromagnetic flowmetry and various plethysmographic techniques exclusive of the phototechnique are realistically applicable only in the vascular laboratory. This should not lessen their importance as they often provide information that is not available by other techniques, as in a diabetic patient with systolic pressures of 300+ mm Hg in the presence of greatly reduced blood flow.

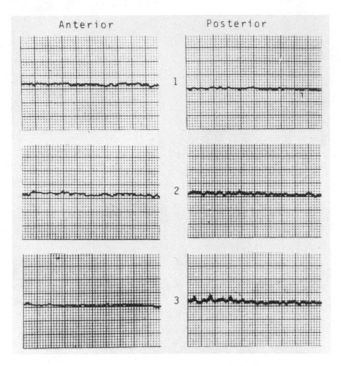

FIGURE 5-35.   Photoplethysmographic study anterior and posterior to an ulcer showing an absence of pulsatile flow, indicating a poor healing potential.

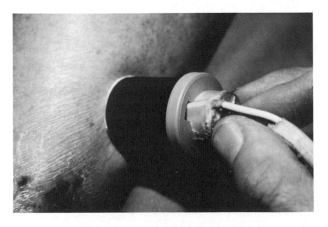

FIGURE 5-36.   In evaluating skin perfusion pressure, the photoplethysmograph probe-pressure transducer apparatus is simply applied to the desired area.

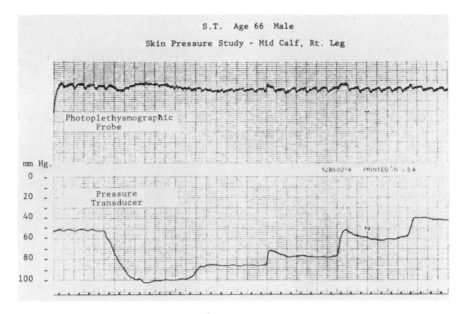

S.T.   Age 66   Male

Skin Pressure Study - Mid Calf, Rt. Leg

Photoplethysmographic
Probe

mm Hg.

0

20   Pressure
          Transducer

40

60

80

100

FIGURE 5-37.   The skin perfusion pressure is determined as that pressure at which the photoplethysmographic waveform returns.

PERIPHERAL VENOUS SYSTEM

The topic of venous disorders is usually treated lightly by the clinician as most of the patients presenting with venous disease may not be considered to be in danger of losing life or limb. Such an attitude is indeed unfortunate as venous disorders are responsible for significant morbidity and their successful management requires a great deal of care.

Reports of the incidence of venous disease vary greatly due to differences in selection of patients, the method of examination, and the interpretation of results. Surveys of clinicians note an incidence of 60 percent while governmental health surveys place it at 2 percent. The age of the patients appears to be a most influential factor. The incidence of varicose veins has been reported to be four times more prevalent in 60-year-olds than in 20-year-olds, and chronic venous insufficiency has been found to be seven times more prevalent in 60-year-olds. Sex is another important factor; varicose veins are seen twice as frequently in females.

The diagnosis of such venous disorders as superficial thrombophlebitis, phlegmasia cerulea, and phlegmasia alba dolens is typically easy to make on clinical examination alone. In the case of deep venous thrombosis, however, clinical diagnosis may be notably inaccurate. An apparently healthy limb may have a deep venous thrombosis, or phlebography may show a limb with all the signs of deep venous thrombosis to have a normal venous system. Many well-documented reports demonstrate the incidence of massive pulmonary embolism leading to deaths, without any clinical signs or symptoms of thrombophlebitis. Some reports of a clinically certain diagnosis of deep venous thrombosis show only 55% accuracy for clinical diagnosis.

One must conclude from such reports that classical clinical signs and symptoms of deep vein thrombosis (pain, swelling, tenderness, skin temperature changes, Homan's sign, Lowenberg's sign, etc.) are unreliable in detecting or ruling out deep venous thrombosis. The need for noninvasive diagnositc techniques is readily apparent.

VENOUS PRESSURE MEASUREMENTS

Venous pressure measurements may be made either centrally or peripherally. The central venous pressure (in reality, right atrial pressure) is primarily of value in the assessment of cardiac function in the critical care setting. The measurement of peripheral venous pressure can be used for the detection of venous pressure gradients, venous obstruction, or dysfunction of the muscular-venous pumps. Although the measurement of peripheral venous pressure provides useful information in relation to venous pathology, the technique is most frequently applied in clinical research.

An important prerequisite for the accurate measurement of peripheral venous pressure is the determination of a reference point, as small variations in venous pressure are of greater diagnostic significance than similar minor changes in arterial pressure. In order to obtain an absolute venous pressure, the manometer must be level with the tip of the intravenous cannula. In the relaxed, upright patient, lower limb venous pressure is equal to that of a column of blood extending to the phlebostatic axis. The phlebostatic axis is defined as the intersection of a horizontal plane through the fourth chondrosternal junction with a vertical plane in the mid-axillary line. A more meaningful expression of the peripheral venous pressure is its difference from the central venous pressure. With the manometers at the same level, the difference in the two venous pressures represents the hydraulic pressure gradient between the catheter tips. If the central venous pressure is not measured, one may assume it to be normal for the purposes of calculations.

The mean peripheral venous pressure is normally reduced during exercise well below the normal hydrostatic level for both the superficial and deep venous system. The level of blood flow to muscle and skin determines the amount of reduction. This normal reduction in mean peripheral venous pressure seems to increase the perfusion pressure of the exercising muscles and allow a redistribution of the blood volume. A reduction in mean peripheral venous pressure is even seen during the relatively minor movement of muscle required during quiet standing. This reduction in the subcutaneous venous pressure is sufficient to reduce the rate of subcutaneous fluid accumulation.

Incompetence of the subcutaneous vein valves is seen in the presence of primary varicose veins, particularly in the great saphenous system. Depending upon the diameter of the dilated veins, the fall in the subcutaneous venous pressure during exercise is greater or lesser. This is brought about if the size of the valveless vein leading to the central venous reservoir is in excess of the pumping capacity of the leg. The use of tourniquet occlusion of the great saphenous vein can lead to a normal exercise response and can be used to predict the operative success in managing such patients.

In measuring the peripheral venous pressure in a patient following an episode of deep venous thrombosis, there may be an increase in the deep venous pressure rather than a decrease during exercise. A similar response may also be seen in the subcutaneous venous pressure. Such an increase in the peripheral venous pressure is due to a narrowing of the lumen of the major deep veins, causing an obstruction to the venous outflow. More often, there may be damage to the valves of the deep and perforating veins, which places the two systems in free communication with each other. The subcutaneous venous pressure does not fall upon exercise, particularly in the presence of obstruction to the venous outflow.

Such pressure measurements may be useful in the diagnosis of venous pathology, in the planning of surgical management, and also as an index of operative success. One can quantify the level of venous function by comparing the rate with which pressure drops and the level it drops to during exercise and the time for its return to baseline.

DOPPLER ULTRASOUND

The use of Doppler ultrasound in assessing the venous system is based upon the fact that an obstruction to flow will alter the venous flow pattern in a manner that is readily detectable. Doppler ultrasound instrumentation can be used for detecting spontaneous venous flow signals and augmented venous flow signals. Spontaneous signals are those venous flow signals that are audible even in the absence of physical measures to increase the venous flow velocity. Augmented flow signals are those venous flow signals that are generated by the physical compression of the limb or by muscular contraction.

In the normal individual, spontaneous venous flow signals should typically be heard when the Doppler probe is located at the common femoral, superficial femoral, and popliteal veins. Additional care is required for the detection of spontaneous venous flow in the posterior tibial and saphenous veins at the ankle. The sound of spontaneous venous flow is typically of a low pitch with a wide spectrum of frequencies and may sound somewhat like a windstorm. The signal characteristically varies with the respiratory cycle—decreased with inspiration and increased with expiration. This cyclic variation in the venous flow signal is secondary to the compression of the inferior vena cave by the diaphragm during inspiration and the release of compression during expiration. With individuals that may be characterized as thoracic breathers, an opposite effect may be seen, i.e., an increase in the signal with inspiration and a decrease on expiration, secondary to the cyclic changes in intrathoracic pressure during the respiratory cycle.

In the Doppler ultrasound examination of the venous circulation of the upper extremity, the spontaneous venous flow signal also varies with the respiratory cycle but may increase or decrease.

The performance of a Valsalva maneuver effectively stops venous outflow, as the pressure exerted tends to displace venous blood out of the abdomen and back down the legs. In the patient with competent venous valves in the ileofemoral region, there will be little or no retrograde flow noted. However, if there are incompetent valves in the ileofemoral venous segment, a Valsalva maneuver will yield a prolonged period of retrograde flow in the common femoral vein as the venous blood is displaced out of the abdomen.

If one compresses the limb distal to the location of the Doppler probe, the venous blood is forced proximally from the site of compression, which augments the normal spontaneous venous flow signal. The degree of augmentation is dependent upon several factors, among which are the quantity of blood that is displaced, the vigor of compression, and the distance between the location of the probe and the site of compression. With the Doppler probe placed at the common femoral vein, distal thigh compression will cause an augmentation of the flow signal; compression of the calf may or may not augment the flow signal at the common femoral vein. Compression of the calf with the Doppler probe at the superficial femoral or popliteal veins will always yield an augmentation of the flow signal, and with the Doppler probe located at the posterior tibial vein, compression of the veins of the feet will yield augmentation.

If the compression maneuver is carried out at a point proximal to the probe, there will be a cessation of venous flow which, upon release of the compression, will yield augmented flow. In the absence of venous valves between the site of the compression and the placement of the probe, the compression manuever will give a signal characteristic of augmentation.

In the presence of venous obstruction, there will be an absence of spontaneous or augmented flow signals if the Doppler probe is placed directly over the site of the occlusion. The venous flow signal obtained with the Doppler probe placed at a point removed from the site of the occlusion varies with the extent of collateral formation between the probe and the site of occlusion. If the extent of collateralization is minimal or absent, there will be either an absence or marked reduction in flow. This effect is most frequently noted when the Doppler probe is located just distal to the site of occlusion. If the Doppler probe is placed far distal to the site of occlusion, one should detect a continuous signal that is not affected by the respiratory cycle. This continuous flow results from the high venous pressure distal to the site of occlusion, forcing venous blood through high-resistance collateral pathways, that is sufficient to negate the alterations in abdominal pressure secondary to the respiratory cycle.

Little or no augmentation of venous flow is noted when the Doppler probe is located proximal to the site of occlusion and a compression maneuver is carried out distal to the occlusion. This particular aspect of the Doppler ultrasound examination yields a false negative result in the presence of well-developed collateral vessels and a forceful compression maneuver. Additionally, false positive results are seen if the leg veins are not sufficiently filled. With the Doppler probe located distal to the site of occlusion, one may note augmentation with compression; however, the signal will be typically reduced and abrupt. If compression is done proximal to the probe and distal to the site of occlusion, augmentation will be abrupt and of low volume.

An additional factor indicative of deep venous thrombosis is an increase in flow in the superficial veins, which may be quite obvious when compared with a normal contralateral limb. If there is a suspicion of calf vein thrombosis, increased flow will be noted in the saphenous vein at the ankle. Ileofemoral thrombosis will yield increased flow through the subcutaneous inguinal veins.

The presence of incompetent valves can be detected by noting retrograde flow upon a Valsalva maneuver. Similarly, compression proximal to the Doppler probe in the presence of incompetent valves will yield a retrograde surge of blood, which will rush forward upon release of compression.

In summary, in the Doppler ulrasound examination of the venous system the clinician should be aware of the following factors: the absence of spontaneous flow, a continuous flow signal, decreased or no augmentation of flow with compression maneuvers, and the presence of increased venous flow through the superficial system.

In the presence of a thrombosed iliac vein, the common femoral vein will yield a continuous signal of reduced volume that is not altered by a Valsalva maneuver. Similar results will be obtained with the Doppler probe over more distal veins. Ileofemoral thrombosis causes an absence of a flow signal at the common femoral vein. Additionally, many collaterals in the groin region can be noted by their continuous, high-pitched flow signal. With a clot that has propagated distally in the superficial femoral vein, the flow signal at the superficial femoral may be absent, continuous, or detected only with compression, depending upon the extent of the thrombus.

Isolated thrombosis of the superficial femoral vein is rarely seen. When present, there will be an absence of spontaneous flow in the superficial femoral vein and no effect will be noted with compression maneuvers. The development of collaterals can frequently be detected adjacent to the vein.

The presence of a thrombosed popliteal vein has a variable effect on the venous flow signal in relation to the degree of proximal involvement; the signal may be absent, reduced, normal, or noticeable only upon compression. With posterior tibial thrombosis, there will be an absence of flow even with compression.

The techniques of Doppler ultrasound cannot be used for the detection of thrombi at the internal iliac or pelvic veins, the profunda femoris vein, or the venous sinuses of the calf. Difficulty will be encountered in examining the anterior tibial vein due to its deep placement within the calf. The technique will not detect a long, narrow clot that has its origin in a valvular sinus. This is indeed unfortunate as such clots are highly likely to fragment and embolize.

IMPEDANCE PLETHYSMOGRAPHY

The flow of venous blood out of the lower extremity is altered by external compression of the limb as well as by the respiratory cycle, as noted in the previous discussion of Doppler ultrasound. It is thus not surprising that the presence of an obstruction to flow in the venous

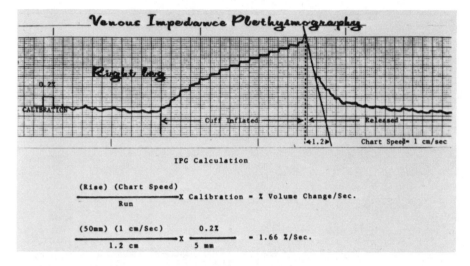

FIGURE 5-38.   Calculation of the maximum venous outflow.

system of the lower extremity would cause detectable modifications in the venous outflow rate of the lower extremity. Additionally, the presence of a thrombus in a major vein obstructing venous outflow will cause an increased pressure in the distal veins, causing distension of the vein. This increased pressure reduces the vein's capacity for further expansion in response to further increases in venous pressure, such as that produced by an occluding cuff, thereby effectively reducing the maximum venous capacity of the vein. The technique of impedance plethysmography non-invasively quantifies venous capacitance and venous outflow.

From the impedance plethysmogram, one can measure the increase in venous volume following inflation of a pneumatic cuff placed around the lower thigh. The maximum venous outflow is measured as the decrease in volume during the first three seconds following the release of the pneumatic cuff (Figs. 5-38 and 5-39).

Alternatively, the venous capacitance can be calculated and used in conjunction with the maximum venous outflow rate to score the patient's venous hemodynamics (Figs. 5-40 and 5-41).

If the results of the initial test are normal, this technique may be terminated as the patient's venous hemodynamics are normal. However, if the initial test results are equivocal or abnormal, the test should be repeated three times in succession, the final interpretation of the test procedure being based upon the best results obtained. With abnormal results, the technician should ensure that external compression, e.g., tight clothing, electrodes, or bandages, did not contribute to the positive

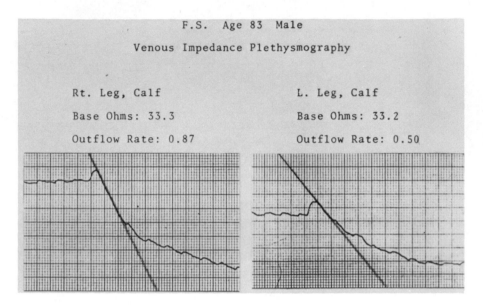

FIGURE 5-39.   Calculation of rise (venous capacitance) and fall (venous outflow).

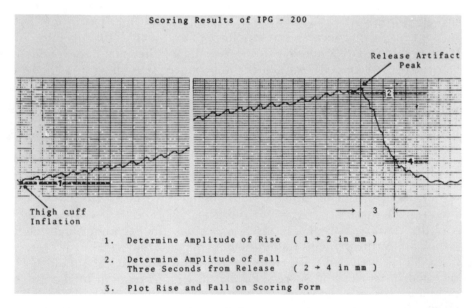

FIGURE 5-40.   A venous impedance plethysmogram showing the presence of deep venous thrombosis in the left lower extremity.

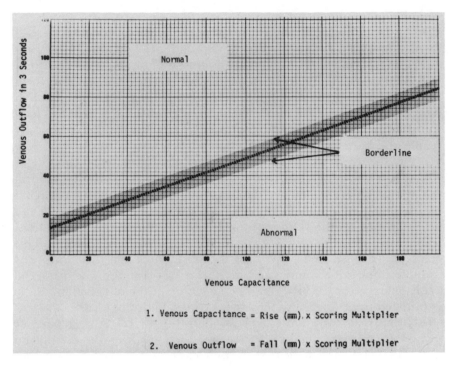

FIGURE 5-41.   The patient's calculated venous capacitance and maximum venous outflow are used to plot the position on the scoring chart.

test result. The results may additionally be influenced by factors that alter the rate of increase in venous volume—shock, marked peripheral vasoconstriction, low cardiac output, or arterial occlusive disease.

Impedance plethysmography will not detect the presence of hemodynamically insignificant thrombi or small, isolated calf thrombi. Extensive collateral formation may also mask a thrombus of long standing. Recanalization may also restore the maximum venous outflow rate to normal. A chronic obstruction when detected may be distinguished from the acute episode of thrombosis by the presence of respiratory excursions on the stripchart recording.

PHLEBORHEOGRAPHY

The technique of phleborheography is based on the principle that variations in venous pressure and volume are brought about by rhythmic respiration and such variations in venous hemodynamics can be recorded from the lower extremity. In practice, air-filled cuffs are placed around the thorax and at several levels of the lower extremity to record transmitted impulses and apply compression for the detection of venous obstruction. The presence of an acute episode of deep venous thrombosis is noted as an absence of or significant reduction in the waveform size. Repositioning the patient cannot restore the waves, as may happen in the normal individual. In the presence of a chronic thrombosis, collateral formation allows a return of the waveforms, which are typically smaller and have a rounded peak as compared with normal waves. The return of the waves with chronic thrombosis may be noted in two weeks.

In the presence of deep venous thrombosis, distal compression will yield a momentary pooling of the blood due to the thrombus reducing the maximum venous outflow rate. Such a pooling is recorded as a rise in the baseline on the volume recorder. In the absence of a thrombus, compression does not cause a change in the recording baseline. This technique may be used to localize the position of the thrombus. For example, if the calf is compressed and there is a rise in the baseline of the recording taken at the high thigh, the location of the obstruction can be determined to be above the placement of the high-thigh cuff.

In the normal individual, compression of the calf will "suck" blood out of the foot, causing a fall in the baseline obtained from the cuff at the foot. If there is no fall in the baseline or a less-than-normal fall in the foot volume baseline accompanied by a rise in baseline and absence of respiratory waves, acute deep venous thrombosis is present.

RADIOACTIVE FIBRINOGEN UPTAKE

The radioactive (^{125}I) fibrinogen uptake test is probably the most sensitive test available for the detection of the presence of thrombus that is developing and for determining whether the thrombus is extending or is lysing. Basically, the principle of the technique is that ^{125}I-fibrinogen is incorporated into the framework of a developing thrombus as ^{125}I-fibrin. The radioactive fibrin thus incorporated into the developing thrombus can be detected noninvasively using a ratemeter with a scintillation probe. Initially, ^{131}I was used to tag the fibrinogen, but this was soon abandoned for ^{125}I, due to its longer half-life (60 days for ^{125}I, compared with eight days for ^{131}I) and ^{125}I emission of lower-energy gamma radiation, allowing for the use of lighter and more portable apparatus.

After the ^{125}I-fibrinogen has been administered to the patient, the first screen is done after two hours. This delay allows for the removal of any denatured fibrinogen and establishes an equilibrium between intravascular and extravascular fibrinogen. A screen done immediately following administration will give an unusually low reading for the lower exremity and an unusually high reading for the heart region. Screens done subsequently and compared with these abnormal readings can lead to the interpretation of a normal high subsequent reading, yielding a false positive result. Following administration, screens can be done on every other day except when a thrombus is detected, in which case screens should be done every day to see if the thrombus is extending or lysing. In doing the screens, the patient's legs should be elevated to avoid false positive results due to varicose veins.

Radioactivity counts obtained from the lower extremity are usually expressed as a percentage of the radioactivity count obtained over the heart region. As the radioactivity should be washed out of the lower extremity and the heart at the same rate, the percentage should remain relatively constant from day to day. Clinically, however, the percent of radioactivity shows a tendency to increase due to the fact that the clearance of extravascular fibrinogen is slower than intravascular fibrinogen and the ratio of extravascular fibrinogen to intravascular fibrinogen is greater in the leg than in the heart. This normal increase in percentage should not exceed 2% per day.

Deep venous thrombosis is determined to be present when there is an increase of 20 or more in percent of radioactivity at the same position on two different days. Additionally, a similar increase in radioactivity between adjacent positions on the same day is indicative of deep venous thrombosis if the increase remains evident for more than 24 hours.

The ^{125}I-fibrinogen uptake test is not specific for the presence of deep venous thrombosis. A number of other pathologic states can also yield increased radioactivity counts and must be ruled out to avoid the reporting of false positive results. Such associated pathologies would include superficial thrombophlebitis, hematoma, wounds or fractures, ulceration, arthritis, and cellulitis. The presence of edema will also yield a false positive result but may be distinguished by the presence of increased radioactivity over all areas of the edema. Similar results are frequently seen following total hip replacement procedures. The technique of ^{125}I-fibrinogen uptake will not detect the presence of thrombus formation in the groin or pelvic areas because of the presence of high background radioactivity in the bladder.

PHLEBOGRAPHY

The phlebographic examination can be carried out through the use of radionuclides or radiopaque contrast agents. These techniques are presented in Chapter 6. It should be noted that contrast phlebography remains the standard for the definitive documentation of the presence of venous pathology and the technique with which all noninvasive diagnostic techniques must be compared. A particular advantage of radionuclide phlebography is the opportunity it provides for detecting pulmonary embolism while simultaneously detecting the origin of the embolus in the peripheral venous system.

SUMMARY

The clinical diagnosis of venous disease is notoriously inaccurate. The incidence of false positive and false negative results is unacceptably high—about 50 percent in most reports. The need for reliable noninvasive diagnostic techniques is readily apparent. The use of noninvasive instrumentation serves two purposes: (1) the screening of a large segment of the population for the detection of clinically silent thrombi, and (2) the diagnosis of thrombosis in patients with clinically suspected venous thrombosis.

The use of Doppler ultrasound can provide a relatively rapid examination of the venous system of the lower extremities and may additionally be useful in the evaluation of the superficial venous system and the veins of the neck and arm. Doppler ultrasound can identify both obstruction to venous outflow and the presence of venous reflux due to incompetent valves. A disadvantage of the technique is that considerable experience is required for an accurate examination; in the absence of stripchart recording, the clinician must rely on subjective interpretation of the velocity signal. Pathology of the deep femoral and internal iliac veins and the minor thrombi in the calf region cannot be detected. A false positive result may be noted if the probe is applied too heavily and occludes the underlying vein. Additionally, compression maneuvers that are done when the limb may be somewhat drained of blood will give a false positive result due to an absence of or decrease in the augmentation signal.

Plethysmographic techniques are sensitive to thrombi in the popliteal, femoral, or iliac veins. This is a particular advantage as most emboli arise from these anatomic locations. The technique has limitations similar to those of Doppler ultrasound—insensitivity to pathology of the calf veins and the deep femoral and internal iliac veins. Unlike Doppler ultrasound, plethysmography is not applicable to the superficial venous system. Particular advantages of plethysmography over Doppler ultrasound are a relatively discrete diagnostic endpoint and the quantitation of venous outflow, which can be used in comparison to determine improvement or worsening of the patient's condition. Plethysmographic techniques do not differentiate thrombotic obstruction from mechanical obstruction to flow. False positive results may be encountered in the presence of reduced outflow secondary to increased venous pressure due to congestive heart failure or constrictive pericarditis, or reduced outflow secondary to reduced inflow due to the presence of arterial occlusive disease.

The technique of phleborheography, through an analysis of the respiratory waves present in the venous circulation, can distinguish between acute and chronic venous disease. The generated tracings can be used to follow an acute episode as it progresses to chronicity or dissolution. The tracings obained sometimes present difficulty in interpretation and, as with plethysmography, patient positioning is an influential factor, as is cuff position. Thrombi present in the saphenous system, soleal veins, or isolated thrombi in the deep femoral or internal iliac veins cannot be detected. The technique of phleborheography can detect thrombi in the anterior and posterior tibial, peroneal, popliteal, femoral, and iliac veins and vena cava.

The ^{125}I-fibrinogen uptake test is the most sensitive technique available for detecting an active thrombotic process and is highly sensitive to the presence of calf vein thrombi. The technique is quite useful with patients who do not harbor a thrombus but are at high risk. Limitations are encountered in evaluating postoperative patients and the technique is of little value in evaluating the intraabdominal iliac veins or vena cava and the veins of the pelvis and proximal thigh. Positive test results are produced even in the presence of clinically insignificant thrombi such as those found in small intramuscular veins. The technique's effectiveness as a diagnostic tool is somewhat limited by the time required to obtain a positive diagnosis (up to 72 hours).

The technique of contrast and radionuclide phlebography is discussed fully in Chapter 6.

Each of the noninvasive diagnostic techniques for the evaluation of the peripheral venous system has advantages and limitations. The techniques should be considered complementary rather than contradictory. By using a combination of techniques, the advantages of one may overcome the limitations of another. For example, in using a combination of ^{125}I-fibrinogen uptake and impedance plethysmography, one has the advantage of ^{125}I sensitivity to calf thrombi and active thrombosis and the advantage of impedance in detecting more proximal thrombi. The choice of instrumentation, however, is influenced by the type of institution, number of patients who are candidates for use of the instrumentation, the availability of support personnel, etc. The primary criteria should be the selection of the technique that is sensitive to the presence of venous disease at or above the knee—the primary source of emboli.

REFERENCES

1. Matsumato N, Whisnant JP, Kurland LT, Okazaki H: Natural history of stroke in Rochester, Minnesota, 1955 through 1969: an extension of a previous study, 1945 through 1954. Stroke 4:20, 1973.
2. Baker RN, Schwartz WS, Ramseyer JC: Prognosis among survivors of ischemic stroke. Neurology 18: 933, 1968.
3. Millikan CH: The pathogenesis of transient focal cerebral ischemia. Circulation 32:438, 1965.

CHAPTER 6

DIAGNOSTIC TECHNIQUES IN PERSPECTIVE: VISUALIZATION, SCANNING, SOUNDING

INTRODUCTION

A precise delineation of the disease process is required for the proper clinical management of patients with peripheral vascular disease. Although angiography predominates as the method for the delineation of peripheral vascular disease, recently developed noninvasive techniques with the capabilities of visualizing, scanning, or sounding blood vessels dictate the need for a careful reassessment of the place of angiography in the clinical management of peripheral vascular disease. While it is unlikely that noninvasive procedures shall completely replace the use of angiography, the techniques reviewed here should provide a more rational approach to the assessment of peripheral vascular disease, particularly in elderly and high-risk patients, to avoid undue mortality and morbidity.

Angiography should be ideally reserved for patients who will undergo a reconstructive surgical procedure. Although this is still not the case, the noninvasive techniques described here should permit a more selective use of angiography, so the ratio of angiograms to vascular reconstructions approximates 1:1.

It is not within the scope of this book to provide an exhaustive discussion of angiographic techniques. It is hoped, however, that the information provided will allow the physician to make a more selective application of the technique for visualizing, scanning, or sounding. While some of the noninvasive techniques discussed may be considered developmental, they are presented to give an indication of the current and future status of this field. Some techniques obviously require instrumentation that cannot be considered feasible for the community hospital. In the future, however, major medical centers may have these techniques available for referral.

VISUALIZATION

ANGIOGRAPHY

Although a plain radiographic examination of an extremity may reveal the presence of a calcified arterial wall, such an examination is of no real value in the evaluation of the patient with peripheral vascular disease. The examination cannot provide information as to patency of the vessels (whether the vessel is patent, stenosed, or occluded) or the extent of collateral vessel development. To answer these questions, the vessels must be outlined. Angiography, through the use of injectable radiopaque agents, provides such visualization of the arterial, venous, and lymphatic systems. The development of and refinements in angiographic techniques have provided the basis for the major advancements that have recently been made in the diagnosis and management of peripheral vascular disease.

Each of the three basic techniques of angiography deals with one-third of the vascular system: arteriography (arterial), phlebography (venous), lymphography (lymphatic). Angiography demonstrates each third of the vascular system separated in time and space from the others. It should be obvious, however, that as the three systems are linked anatomically, there is a physiologic interdependence among them. Physiologic events, whether normal or pathologic, that take place in one system influence those occurring in other systems. This physiologic and anatomic inter-relationship must be considered when evaluating the indications and results of angiography.

Angiography can influence the management of a diverse array of pathologic conditions, e.g., emboli, aneurysms, atherosclerotic occulsive disease, fistulas, neoplasms. In a recently published case[1] arteriographic examination of a patient who complained of intermittent claudication demonstrated the presence of iliac artery occlusive disease. At operation, however, it was found that carcinoma of the cervix had encased the iliac artery. Such surprises at operation should not lessen the importance of angiography.

The following discussion is not intended to be an exhaustive review of angiography. Basic techniques are described, and radiopaque contrast agents are discussed, so that the physician may minimize or avoid compli-cations leading to morbidity and mortality. The emphasis is on selection of patients for angiography and the information that can be obtained. This should enable the physician to reevaluate the use of angiography, so that it can be employed more selectively than is currently the case.

Arteriography

An arteriographic examination should be carried out to provide ana-tomical information required for reaching a therapeutic decision, not for confirmation of the diagnosis, which can be satisfactorily determined noninvasively. It should be emphasized that the arteriographic demon-stration of nonoperable lesions is as valuable as the demonstration of operable lesions. An angiographic study should not be terminated until all required information is clearly demonstrated and the structure, course, and rate of flow through the vessels is clearly shown. The final decision as to the extent of the examination should obviously be tem-pered by the patient's condition. Also to be considered are the risk factors associated with the technique, including the possibility of vessel thrombosis, subintimal injection, perforation of the injected vessel, he-matoma formation, and adverse reactions secondary to the contrast media.

History and Contrast Agents. In 1895, Wilhelm K. Roentgen, a German physicist, discovered x-rays. Two months later, Haschek and Lindenthal injected contrast media into an amputated limb to provide visualization of the arteries. Many years passed, however, before the technique became used routinely in a clinical setting, primarily because of the toxicity of the agents. It was not until 1923–1924 that investigators in Germany, France, and the United States successfully accomplished percutaneous injections in living humans. The beginning of clinical arteriography may be considered to be the work of Brooks, who, in 1924, used femoral arteriography to determine the need for and level of amputation. In 1927 Moniz reported the first use of arteriography in examination of the carotid circulation, and in 1929 dos Santos reported the first use of translumbar aortography.

Much of the advancement made in arteriography since the 1920s can be attributed to the developments of suitable contrast agents. In 1929, Binz and Räth developed Selectan Neutral, and in the same year, Swick used Selectan Neutral and the less toxic Uroselectan for intravenous urography. Before this time, the contrast agents available were not adequately radiopaque or were water-soluble with high toxicity. Subsequent modifications made on these agents greatly reduced toxicity by binding iodine to benzene or pyridine rings, and water solubility was increased by the addition of acetic acid or carboxyl groups. A second iodine was added to further increase radiopacity (e.g., Diodrast and Neo-lopax) and in the 1950s radiopacity was increased by adding a third iodine (e.g., Urokon).

When a beam of x-rays is directed at a substance, some of the rays penetrate the substance while some of the rays are absorbed. The amount of the absorption of the x-rays is determined by the thickness, density, and atomic number of the matter. These factors are reflected on the x-ray film as differences in whiteness or blackness. The various parts of the body exhibit shade differences on x-ray film. For example, fatty tissue has a density of 0.92, soft tissue 1.0, bone 1.75, and air 0.0013. Bony structures display a greater radiopacity due to their higher density and calcium content. Calcium has a higher atomic number (20), as compared with elements that are abundant in other tissues (8 for oxygen, 7 for nitrogen, and 6 for carbon). Radiographic contrast agents enhance the radiopacity of soft tissues and body fluids by containing elements of high atomic number, e.g., barium 56, and iodine 53. Those agents containing iodine are the most useful in angiography.

Triiodobenzoic acid is the basic structure for all the contemporary contrast agents. Solubility is enhanced by the addition of a carboxyl group at the 1 position. Side chains at the 3 and 5 positions decrease toxicity while enhancing the agent's solubility. The various agents can be distinguished by the side chain at the 5 position (Fig. 6-1).

The agents are formed from diatrizoate, metrizoate, or iothalamate anions in combination with sodium, calcium, magnesium, or methylglucamine cations to enhance their solubility (Fig. 6-2).

Urokon was the first triiodinated compound to be given extensive evaluation and was subsequently altered to give rise to Hypaque and Renografin in the 1950s and 1960s; additional modifications gave rise to

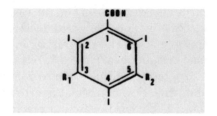

FIGURE 6-1.   The structure of triiodobenzoic acid.

Conray and Isopaque. These agents have a high iodine concentration that provides for excellent radiopacity by overcoming the diluting effect of blood. The addition of the second side chain reduced the toxicity of the agents, and the change to an iothalamate anion from a diatrizoate anion decreased the agent's viscosity, thus reducing the amount of pressure required for injection.

Radiocontrast agents may cause adverse reactions that are related to dosage or patient hypersensitivity, which is probably due to histamine release. These agents cause a direct arterial vasodilation (probably

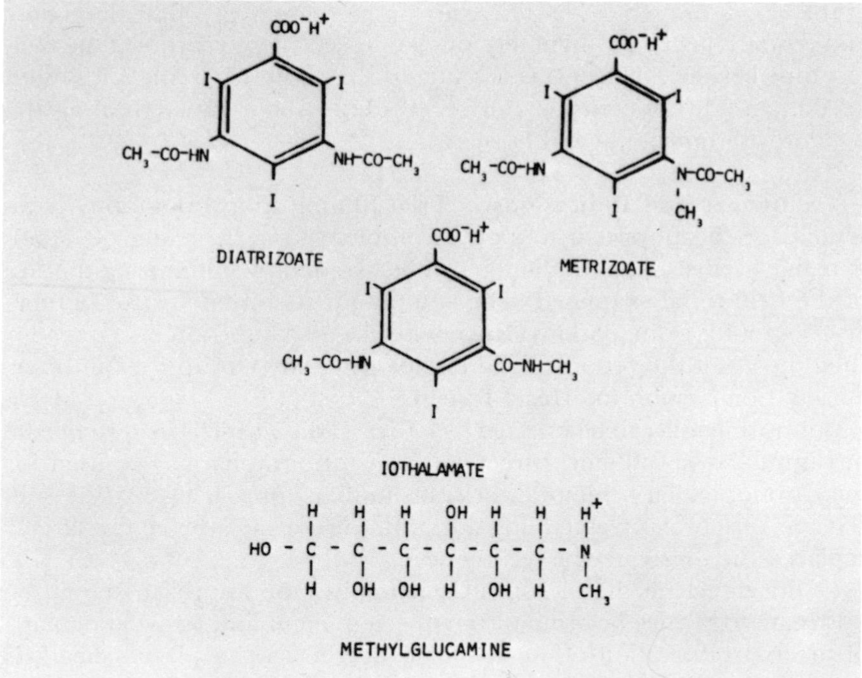

FIGURE 6-2.   Contrast agents are formed from anions (diatrizoate, metrizoate, or iothalamate) and cations (methylglucamine, calcium, sodium, or magnesium).

through a direct effect on the vascular smooth muscle) with a consequent increase in blood flow and decrease in blood pressure; there is no arterial spasm effect. The contrast agents additionally cause an increase in cardiac output, heart rate, stroke volume, chamber pressure, and circulatory blood volume. There is a decrease in hematocrit and heart rate abnormalities; abnormal heart rhythm and conduction are not uncommon. These cardiovascular reactions appear to be related to the presence of sodium in the contrast agents, as the effects are less pronounced with agents that contain a smaller sodium concentration.

The renal effects of contrast agents include osmotic diuresis, which is less pronounced with agents that have sodium than with those containing methylglucamine. There is a transient rise in renal blood flow, quickly replaced by a predominant decrease in flow, which is probably mediated by the renin-angiotensin system. Because secondary dehydration may cause a tendency toward renal failure, the patient should first be adequately hydrated.

Following carotid arteriography, adverse reactions relating to the central nervous system include convulsions, headache, and an impaired state of consciousness, as the contrast agent apparently alters the permeability of the blood–brain barrier. There are an increase in cerebral blood flow and a bradycardia and hypotension. To lessen these reactions, the contact time between the contrast agent and the cerebral circulation should be minimized; hypotension can be avoided by not premedicating the patient with morphine and Demerol.

Techniques and Indications.   Serial filming in arteriography is essential for the physician to gain a complete understanding of hemodynamic events. Excess radiation can be avoided by minimizing the size of the field to be examined. The equipment requirements for optimal arteriographic examinations shall not be discussed; the interested reader should consult the report of the Radiology Study Group for the Inter-Society Commission for Heart Disease.[2]

Contrast media can be injected by either a "direct stick" using a needle or cannula, or a catheter. Direct needle arteriography may be used for the carotid, axillary, femoral, or translumbar approaches. At the subclavian, vertebral, or ascending aorta, the use of a catheter has largely replaced the direct needle technique.

In the direct needle or cannula technique, the approach should be upstream to reduce layering of the injected agent and to avoid damage of arterial bifurcations. The use of a needle with a plastic sheath is preferred as the sheath can be advanced along the vessel, and the possibility of subintimal or extravascular injections is minimized. In the presence of an irregular artery, a guidewire may be required to advance the sheath. The plastic sheath is inserted to its hub followed by injection and filming.

The use of catheterization is increasing in popularity with the preferred approaches being via the femoral or axillary arteries. Following needle puncture, a guidewire is passed under fluoroscopic monitoring to the region for injection. Once the guidewire is properly placed, a catheter is placed over the guidewire, which is then removed. A test injection is made to ensure proper placement. If the catheter is not properly placed, the guidewire must be reinserted.

The technique of selective arteriography has been made possible through catheterization. With selective arteriography, catheter placement and rate of injection are very important factors. If the injection is too slow, the contrast agent becomes diluted, giving poor visualization, and if it is too fast, the contrast agent overflows into the parent vessel, leaving an inadequate amount for visualization of the selected vessel.

The size of catheters can be measured either in thousandths of an inch, millimeters, or the commonly used French system where 1 French (F) = $\frac{1}{3}$ millimeter. The given size of a catheter refers to its outside diameter. The most frequently used catheters are 5F and 8F. Guidewires are sized by diameter in thousandths of an inch and by length in centimeters. The most frequently encountered sizes are 0.032, 0.035, and 0.038; the 0.032 guidewire fits through the bore of an 18G needle.

Carotid arteriography.   Patients presenting with symptoms characteristic of extracranial cerebrovascular occlusive disease (transient ischemic attack, asymptomatic bruit, history of previous stroke) undergo an initial noninvasive evaluation. Based on this evaluation and the patient's clinical history, a decision as to the need for carotid arteriography can be made. Generally speaking, carotid arteriography in preparation for carotid endarterectomy is indicated for patients with transient ischemic attacks showing significant stenosis of the carotid artery, as determined noninvasively. Contraindications to carotid arteriography are profound or progressing stroke. Patients with chronic cerebral ischemia, stable stroke, or an asymptomatic bruit require a more critical assessment. Following carotid endarterectomy, the patient should be routinely followed with noninvasive testing. Carotid arteriography should be reserved for the patient who shows a sudden worsening during the follow-up period.

Those patients who undergo carotid arteriography should routinely be considered for a four-vessel study. A bilateral examination of the carotid arteries should be carried out due to the high incidence of bilateral disease. Catheterization via the femoral artery is advantageous as it provides visualization of the aortic arch as well as the carotids, vertebrals, and intracranial circulation.

For carotid arteriography, contrast agents containing methylglucamine are preferred over those with sodium. The diatrizoate agents are relatively safe although the iothalamates may be less neurotoxic. Agents with iodine concentrations in excess of 300 mg/ml are not advisable. Frequently used agents include Hypaque 60%, Reno-M-60, Renografin 60, Conray 60, and Isopaque 280 (60 or 60% is indicative of the methylglucamine concentration; 280 indicates an iodine concentration of 280 mg/ml).

Aortography.   Aortography, the arteriographic examination of the abdominal aorta, is typically carried out following a physical examination that reveals the presence of an abdominal aortic aneurysm, as the size and placement of an aneurysm affects the decision for operation, particularly in poor-risk patients. Today, however, arteriography for abdominal aortic aneurysm is gradually being replaced by ultrasonography (see "Pulse Echo Ultrasonography"). Aortography is being increasingly used in patients with gastrointestinal bleeding, low flow syndrome, or abdominal neoplasm. Selective arteriography of branches of the abdominal aorta plays an important role in the evaluation of these pathologies.

Abdominal aortography may be carried out via the transfemoral, transaxillary, or translumbar routes. The translumbar approach is increasingly used in lower-extremity arteriography. The least favorable approach is via the left axillary artery or brachial artery, due to its technical difficulty and a high rate of serious complications; it is frequently impossible due to tortuosity or uncoiling of the thoracic aorta or brachiocephalic vessels. The easiest approach is the transfemoral; however, in the presence of severe tortuosity or aortoiliac occlusive disease another approach is required.

A suprarenal injection is preferred in translumbar aortography as the position of the aorta in this region is more constant than infrarenally, and is also less likely to be diseased. There is also less chance of puncturing the aneurysm when the puncture is suprarenal. For transfemoral aortography, if the patient has bilaterally equal femoral pulses, the preferred approach is via the right femoral artery, as the right iliac artery is typically less tortuous than the left.

The characteristic arteriographic findings in the presence of an abdominal aortic aneurysm include visualization of angulation at the junction of the aorta with the aneurysm, nonvisualization of the lumbar arteries, or displacement of other arteries, in particular the superior mesenteric artery. It should be emphasized that the lumen of the aorta may be normal in appearance due to channelization of the mural thrombus, or the thrombus may completely occlude the lumen.

Aortography for abdominal aortic aneurysm is often required only if the surgeon suspects associated complications such as multiple aneurysms, the presence of an ischemic lower extremity, or an anatomical anomaly such as horseshoe kidney. In the absence of suspected complications, aortography provides little additional information that cannot be obtained intraoperatively or through the use of noninvasive instrumentation such as ultrasonography.

In aortography, a large volume of contrast agent must be rapidly injected, as it must mix with the blood rather than displace it. A contrast agent with a high iodine concentration is necessary. The methylglucamine agents are less toxic than those with sodium; however, the methylglucamine's viscosity retards a rapid injection. The preferred agents are therefore mixtures, e.g., Renografin 76 (66 percent methylglucamine, 10 percent sodium), Hypaque 75 (50 percent methylglucamine, 25 percent sodium), Vascoray (52 percent methylglucamine, 26 percent sodium). In patients of relatively small stature, 60 percent concentrations as used in carotid arteriography may prove adequate.

Peripheral arteriography. As mentioned above, arteriography should be carried out to provide precise localization of the area of disease involvement and other required anatomic information and not merely to confirm a diagnosis that is more easily and safely obtained through noninvasive means. Arteriographic examination of the extremities should thus be limited to those patients whose noninvasive test results and clinical history point to the need for operative management.

UPPER EXTREMITY.   Examples of indications for upper-extremity arteriographic examination would include scalenus anticus, castoclavicular and cervical rib syndromes, and aneurysm. For examination of the arterial system distal to the elbow, e.g., for thromboangiitis obliterans and selected patients with Raynaud's syndrome, direct needle injection is preferred and may be used as well for arteriographic studies proximal to the elbow. For examining the arm or shoulder regions as for subclavian aneurysm, transfemoral catheterization of subclavian or brachial arteries is used. In elderly patients, tortuous arteries encountered via the transfemoral route may be avoided using axillary catheterization. Delayed filling of the distal arteries may be encountered with some patients and may be overcome by an intra-arterial injection of a vasodilator.

LOWER EXTREMITY.   A good arteriographic examination of the lower extremity should demonstrate the entire arterial tree from at least the aortic bifurcation to the foot. If a distal bypass is contemplated, the arteriogram should also include the foot vasculature. An exception to the completeness of a lower extremity arteriogram would be the need to minimize the amount of contrast agent injected into poor-risk patients. In such patients, a good view of one particular segment will provide the most information with a minimum of patient risk.

Direct needle or catheterization techniques can both be used for lower-extremity arteriography. A femoral artery with a weak or absent pulse should not be punctured. In such patients, injection from the contralateral side or translumbar or transaxillary approaches should be used. There is usually bilateral disease involvement and both lower extremities should be visualized. A femoral puncture should be high to avoid damaging the origins of the superficial femoral and deep femoral (profunda femoris) arteries.

The arteriogram of the lower extremity should be assessed in three segments to aid in the determination of the operative plan: run-in, run-on, run-off. The run-in segment refers to the status of the aorta and iliac arteries (Fig. 6-3).

For this reason, femoral arteriograms should routinely include visualization of the aortic bifurcation. The run-on segment refers to the status of blood flow through the region of the femoral arteries (Fig. 6-4).

The run-off segment refers to the status of the popliteal artery and the arterial vessels distal to the trifurcation. Run-off is considered excellent

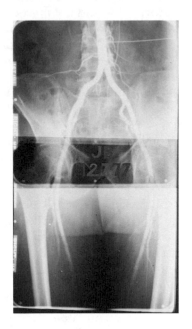

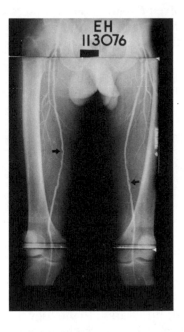

FIGURE 6-3. Arteriogram demonstrating visualization of the run-in segment, the distal aorta and iliac arteries, of arterial circulation of the lower extremities.

FIGURE 6-4. Arteriogram demonstrating visualization of the run-on segment, blood flow through the femoral regions, of arterial circulation of the lower extremities.

if the popliteal, posterior tibial, anterior tibial, and peroneal arteries are relatively normal (Fig. 6-5).

Run-off is fair if only the posterior tibial is patent, allowing blood to run off at a velocity sufficient to maintain the patency of proximal bypass (Fig. 6-6).

Run-off is poor if all three vessels are occluded. This signifies an inability to maintain a blood velocity adequate to maintain the patency of a proximal bypass (Fig. 6-7).

In some patients, the arterial inflow increase seen in an aortofemoral bypass may be of an amount sufficient to maintain good distal perfusion in the face of poor run-off. In this regard, the profunda femoris artery plays an important role. Frequently, the profunda femoris artery maintains its patency although surrounding arterial segments may be occluded. As this is an excellent route for collateral circulation, adequate distal perfusion may be restored by bringing adequate flow to the pro-

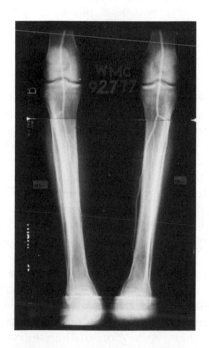

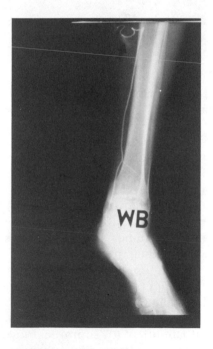

FIGURE 6-5. Arteriogram demonstrating the presence of good run-off: all three run-off vessels, the posterior tibial, dorsalis pedis, and peroneal arteries, are patent.

FIGURE 6-6. Arteriogram demonstrating the presence of fair run-off—only the posterior tibial artery is patent.

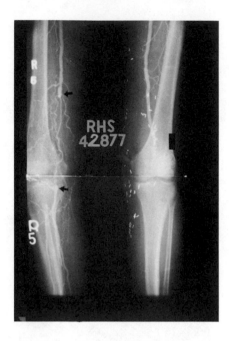

FIGURE 6-7. Arteriogram demonstrating the presence of poor run-off—all three run-off vessels, the posterior tibial, dorsalis pedis, and peroneal arteries, are occluded.

funda femoris artery. If the run-on is not obstructed, profundaplasty as a primary procedure may provide adequate distal perfusion. Profundaplasty may also be done in conjunction with aortofemoral bypass.

The assessment of the run-in is of extreme importance as a femoropopliteal bypass done in the presence of inadequate run-in is likely to fail. It is recommended that at operation, prior to placing a femoropopliteal bypass, the presence of adequate run-in should be assured using standard electromagnetic flowmetry or intra-arterial pressure measurements. This is of particular importance if preoperative non-invasive studies suggest the presence of proximal disease that is not visualized on arteriography.

When using the translumbar approach for lower-extremity arteriography, the puncture should be infrarenal, as opposed to suprarenal injection used for aortography. Infrarenal injection is advocated for lower-extremity examination as it provides adequate visualization of distal run-off. With suprarenal injection there is dilution of the contrast agent, as a large percentage of the contrast agent is diverted to the visceral branches of the aorta. An infrarenal injection also avoids any complications due to thrombosis of the superior mesenteric artery or renal artery and transverse myelitis secondary to injecting contrast media into the lumbar arteries.

For lower-extremity arteriography, contrast agents of pure methylglucamine or low-sodium concentration are preferred over pure sodium agents. An iodine concentration of 300 mg/ml or less provides adequate visualization.

Multiplane arteriography. At times, significant atherosclerotic occlusive disease may not be visualized on arteriography in the face of strongly suggestive noninvasive test results and clinical history. Such nonvisualization may be due to a superimposition of arterial branches, or bony structures or the lesion may be isolated to the posterior wall of the vessel. In such instances, an oblique projection in addition to the standard anterior-posterior projection will aid in the delineation of the disease process. A direct lateral view is not used as it superimposes the iliac vessels.

In most patients the information obtained by using multiplane arteriography will justify the necessary injection of additional contrast agent. Multiplane arteriography is recommended in the presence of noninvasive test results that are incompatible with standard projections, in patients with previous reconstructive surgery that have redeveloped symptoms, or in patients with unilateral aortoiliac occlusive disease and candidates for femorofemoral bypass.

Intraoperative arteriography. It is important that the immediate success of a bypass procedure be evaluated intraoperatively, as reoperation during the immediate postoperative period is characterized by a high mortality rate. Electromagnetic flowmetry, intra-arterial pressure measurements, and intraoperative arteriography are useful for such evaluations. One may also use intraoperative measurements of ankle pressure. We use intraoperative arteriography selectively on patients whose flow and pressure studies cannot be reconciled. The same limitations of the standard anterior-posterior projection as mentioned above apply to intraoperative arteriography. The patient should be positioned to avoid the superimposition of vessels and bony structures. The injection of the contrast agent should be made close to the area of interest and the film exposed at the end of the injection.

Pulmonary arteriography. Pulmonary arteriography may be considered the most specific test available for a definitive diagnosis of pulmonary embolism. Injection into the main pulmonary artery will detect large central pulmonary emboli but is not adequate for the detection of emboli in the segmental pulmonary arteries, due to the rapid dilution of the contrast agent during the normal cardiac cycle. Visualization of the segmental pulmonary arteries requires selective catheterization.

A 7F to 8F catheter passed via an antecubital vein under fluoroscopic control is used for selective catheterization of the pulmonary artery. Pulmonary artery pressure is measured once the catheter is properly placed and if the pressure is less than 80 mm Hg, 50 to 60 ml of contrast agent (e.g., Hypaque 75%) is injected at a rate of 25 to 30 ml/sec. Timed, serial anterior-posterior films should show the pulmonary arterial, capillary, and venous phases. Selective catheterization can then follow, if necessary, and is carried out in the regions of greatest probability based upon the patients' clinical history, chest x-ray, lung scan, and previous main trunk injection. Geometric magnification and oblique projections can enhance the exam's diagnostic capability.

Pulmonary arteriography is relatively safe; less than 5 percent of the patients have nonfatal complications. Incidences of cardiac perforation, pryogen reaction, or arrythmias are secondary to the catheterization. Incidences of bronchospasm, angioneurotic edema, and anaphylaxis are secondary to the contrast agent.

The visualization of intraluminal filling defects provides for the definitive diagnosis of pulmonary embolism. Areas of oligemia, diminished flow, or number of vessels are not characteristic as they may be secondary to other pathologic conditions, e.g., pulmonary hypertension or acute pneumonia. Pulmonary arteriography would be required in patients in shock secondary to massive pulmonary embolism or in patients prior to surgical or thrombolytic therapy. It may also be indicated in selected patients with left heart, severe chronic occlusive pulmonary disease, plural effusion, or atelectasis. In such patients the perfusion lung scan (see below) can assist in the decision for pulmonary arteriography.

Complications of Interpretation. Projectional geometry and the flow of blood are two factors that can complicate the interpretation of arteriographic films. The region of an arterial bifurcation is the most prone to the development of disease and unless it is seen in profile, the bifurcating vessels may overlap, obscuring the presence of disease. The projectional difficulty of arterial bifurcations is most frequently noted at the bifurcation of the carotid artery, the femoral artery, and at the orifice of the left vertebral artery. A similar problem is the superimposition of bony structures, which can be overcome by proper positioning of the patient, as well as by increasing the kilovoltage, which reduces the relative opacity and contrast of the bony structure but does not affect the visualization of the contrast agent.

An artery of anomalous origin may be nonfilled, giving the mistaken impression of occlusion. This is not uncommonly seen with a high origin of the radial or ulnar artery or a left vertebral artery that arises from the aorta. More commonly, such nonfilling is secondary to techniques, such as the injection of too small an amount of contrast agent or a premature film exposure. If one encounters such interpretive complications, occlusion can be diagnosed if the parent vessel is not visualized but its branches are, or if distal vessels are filled.

Sometimes the injected contrast agent may fill the venous system more rapidly than usual and may lead to the mistaken impression of an arteriovenous fistula. If a fistula is present it should be visualized and only the affected vein and its proximal drainage will be filled. In early venous filling of nonpathologic origin, all the venous tributaries will be filled.

The only definitive characteristic for distinguishing between an embolus and a thrombosed artery is the outlining of an embolus. The presence of small collateral vessels and the relative absence of distal disease is suggestive of embolus. A thrombosed artery is characterized by the presence of much greater collateral vessels.

Phlebography

The advent of noninvasive diagnostic techniques for the assessment of the venous system has let to better patient selection for phlebography and a reduction in the number of phlebographic examinations. Phlebography remains as the standard to which one must compare noninvasive techniques. The phlebographic examination does retain a definite clinical usefulness by providing a direct anatomic study of the venous system, the nature and extent of pathologic involvement, and information as to the age of the thrombus and its attachment to the vein wall.

Historical Aspects.   Berberich and Hirsch in 1923 using strontium bromide and McPheeters and Rich in 1929 using Lipiodol were the first to attempt radiographic visualization of the veins. The routine application of the technique, however, was hampered by the formation of fat emboli, hypersensitivity, thrombus formation, and severe pain. The development of agents such as Uroselectan and Abrodil reduced thrombus formation, fat emboli, and hypersensitivity. Perobrodil reduced the pain and provided excellent visualization of the veins with a minimal amount of patient morbidity.

In 1938, dos Santos used Perobrodil for the documentation of deep venous thrombosis. Similar use was made by Bauer in 1940. The technique employed is referred to as "free-flow phlebography" as both superficial and deep veins were filled. In 1942, Hellstein made use of a tourniquet to prevent filling of the superficial veins, which simplified the interpretation of phlebographic films.

Phlebography underwent a prolonged period of disuse because of its inaccurate results. The accuracy was enhanced by DeWeese and Rogoff in 1958 by using large amounts of contrast agent, long film techniques, and maintaining the patient in a semi-erect posture during the examination. This was followed by numerous variations, to the point where today practically no two centers use exactly the same technique.

Indications and Techniques. Indications for phlebography are, in part, similar to those for arteriography: in cases where noninvasive test results and clinical history are not compatible. Examples would be a patient with pulmonary embolism whose physical examination and noninvasive test results do not suggest presence of thrombus formation; a patient who fails to respond to therapy; a patient with a history of venous disease who redevelops symptoms, the suspicion of a neoplasm, or a swollen leg that cannot be diagnosed, in preparation for vena caval interruption; a patient with recurrent embolization following caval interruption, detection of incompetent perforators, and the investigation of ulceration or varicose veins. New noninvasive diagnostic techniques for the quantitation of venous reflux may soon obviate the need for phlebography in detecting incompetent perforating veins and distinguishing between primary and secondary varicose veins.

The particular phlebographic technique used is not of importance; the importance lies in the need for an excellent visualization of the venous system.

Contrast agents used are most commonly methylglucamine with an iodine concentration of less than 300 mg/ml. Iodine concentrations greater than this do little except increase the possibility of damaging the vein wall intima. Minor adverse reactions include flushing of the skin secondary to a vasodilation, occasional nausea and/or vomiting, and urticaria. If these reactions are severe, antihistamine or hydrocortisone may be required to control the reaction. Cardiovascular collapse is rare. The possibility of deep vein thrombosis secondary to phlebography is quite real; every effort should be made to remove the contrast agent from the veins by flushing with heparinized saline exercise and through massage. There is no evidence supporting embolization following phlebography on a patient with deep vein thrombosis. Injection should be monitored closely to ensure against extravasation; if it occurs, an immediate injection of hyaluronidase should prevent ulcer formation.

The use of an image-intensifier with television monitor enhances the diagnostic accuracy of the exam by allowing the determination of flow between the superficial and deep veins, aiding in the identification of incompetent perforators. Monitoring also allows timing of the exposure when the veins are noted to be filled, avoiding artifacts.

Injection is usually by a superficial foot vein toward the lateral side of the foot to avoid a too-direct contact with the long saphenous vein. Injection may be by a vein on the dorsum of the foot at the base of the big toe, where tighter skin can provide for the early detection of extravasation. The injection should be made with the patient at a 20 to 40° angle from the horizontal. Once injection is completed, the agent will normally flow into the deep system, although a series of tourniquets may be used to facilitate the flow. A tourniquet above the knee can be used to provide a better visualization of the calf veins.

The upper femoral and iliac veins can be demonstrated by the patient doing a Valsalva maneuver. This gives a rapid rise in venous pressure in the thoracic cavity that is transmitted through the inferior vena cava, causing reflux of blood in the veins of the lower extremity. This maneuver clearly demonstrates the valve cusps and profunda femoris and internal iliac veins. In some patients direct injection into the femoral vein is necessary.

Interpretive Criteria.   In a normal study, a vein should have a rather sharp border following a relatively straight course with a variable number of valves. Veins in the deep system are variable in width and may appear uniform, beaded, or sacculated. The soleal veins, where most thrombi originate, are typically seen as being short and bag-like or long and spindle-shaped.

The definitive phlebographic sign of acute venous thrombosis is a constant filling defect in an opacified vein. An acute long segment thrombus is seen centrally in the vein lumen and outlined by the contrast agent. As the thrombus "ages," it adheres to the vein walls and partially loses its outline. An additional sign of a thrombus is an abrupt cut-off of a vein that is normally opacified; there may be more proximal filling of the vein and it may be separated by nonvisualized segments.

The entire extent of a thrombus should be visualized. The presence of a thrombus with a free-floating tail is particularly indicative of possible embolization, especially if it extends into or above the popliteal vein. The ability of phlebography to determine the stage of thrombus formation is a particular advantage over noninvasive testing and emphasizes the use of angiography in the determination of the anatomical extent of the disease process.

Chronic venous thrombosis is typically visualized as a partially or completely recanalized vein with a filling defect absent. The partially recanalized vein is a narrow, tortuous, valveless vein that may or may not be accompanied by multiple collateral vessels. A completely recanalized vein is a straight, relatively wide channel without valves and duplicate vessels may also be present.

Tumors or soft tissue swelling may impinge upon a vein, simulating the presence of a thrombus. This can be distinguished from a true thrombus by the absence of an intraluminal filling defect.

Lymphography

The extracellular fluid found in the interstitial space is returned to the blood by a system of collecting ducts referred to as the lymphatic system. A constant seepage of fluid and protein through the arterial capillary membrane into the interstitial space is a normal physiologic event. The accumulation of fluid in the interstitial space is pathologic and gives rise to lymphedema—the pathologic swelling of soft tissues. This association with the lymphatic system has only recently been accepted; indeed, lymphography has been available only since the 1950s.

Anatomy and Physiology.   The lymph vessels and nodes, spleen, tonsils, thymus, adenoids, and lymph cells are collectively referred to as the lymphoreticular complex. For simplicity, the complex can be separated into three segments: the initial lymphatic vessels, which absorb fluid from the interstitial space; the collecting vessels, which transport the fluid to the venous system; and the lymph nodes, which are mechanical filters.

The initial lymphatic vessels originate as dermal capillaries, which anastomose to give a dermal plexus (there are no lymphatics in the epidermis). The dermal plexus is drained by the collecting vessels that then follow the course of the superficial veins to the lymph nodes for filtration. The filtered lymph is transported via efferent lymph vessels to the thoracic duct or right lymphatic duct. The thoracic duct deposits its lymph into the left brachiocephalic vein and the right lymphatic duct deposits its lymph into the right brachiocephalic vein.

The lymph vessels have numerous valves and the walls of the vessels have smooth muscle fibers, which assist in the movement of lymph through the system. The filtration pressure that is generated by the fluid in the interstitial space also assists in the movement of lymph, as do contracting skeletal muscle, the pulsation of adjacent arteries, and negtive intrathoracic pressures due to respiration, which affects the brachiocephalic veins. The presence of valves in the lymphatic vessels functions in preventing reflux of the lymph.

The lymphoreticular complex has two key functions: (1) the production of lymphocytes and antibodies and the phagocytosis of bacteria and particulate matter, e.g., inhaled dust; and (2) the reabsorption and transport to the blood of the interstitial fluid. Reabsorption is primarily concerned with filtered proteins of a size that prevents their direct reabsorption by the blood in the capillaries. A failure to remove these proteins, as occurs when a lymphatic vessel is occluded, results in an increased colloid osmotic pressure that increases fluid filtration, which precipitates edema. Lymphedema may also be secondary to incomplete lymphatic vessel formation or faulty valves leading to lymph reflux and dilatation of the lymphatic vessel. Important in this regard is the clotability of lymph. Lymph fluid will clot after 10 to 20 minutes' exposure to air. With the stasis of lymph as in the presence of tissue necrosis, lymph thrombosis can rapidly ensue, causing a progressive loss of the re-absorptive ability of the lymph ducts. Additional lymph thrombosis leads to valvular incompetency and additional protein accumulation in the interstitial space, causing clinical infection, which further increases edema and fibrosis.

Indications and Techniques. Lymphography should be reserved for use on those patients presenting with a swollen limb and whose physical and clinical examination has ruled out the possibility of infection, tumor, foreign body, growth abnormality, or venous disease.

Kinmoth's work in the early 1950s is the basis for today's use of lymphography. Ethiodol is the usual contrast agent used and is a mixture of 37 percent iodine in combination with ethyl esters of fatty acids obtained from poppy seed oil. As this agent does not rapidly pass through the vessel walls, a small amount of agent can outline a long segment of the system. An initial intradermal injection of water-soluble dye outlines the lymphatics, which are then identified through a small transverse incision on the dorsum of the foot. The contrast agent is slowly injected with a constant infusion pump through a 27 to 30 gauge needle at approximately 0.1 ml/min. In most patients, 10 ml of contrast agent will be sufficient for an examination of the leg and 5 ml for the arm. A spot film should be done after about 2 ml has been injected to ensure the infusion of the lymphatic and not a vein. About 45 to 120 minutes is required for full injection, after which a complete set of films can be taken. The more proximal lymphatics and lymph nodes can be observed on a delayed film at 24 hours. This will facilitate a diagnosis of lymph node disease or retroperitoneal malignancy. A similar technique can be applied to the arm.

Interpretation of Results. Superficial lymphatic vessels of the leg should be slender and of uniform caliber with conspicuous valves. There is no increase in size of the vessels as they travel proximally. In contrast to veins, the lymphatic vessels bifurcate proximally. Normally 10 to 12 lymphatic vessels enter the inguinal nodes; the presence of fewer vessels is indicative of lymphatic hypoplasia. In patients with lymphedema, about 15 percent have a diagnosis of lymphatic aplasia. The deep external, internal, and common iliac nodes should be visualized and efferent lymphatics should also be noted. Delayed films will frequently demonstrate the paravertebral and para-aortic nodes and a chest film will show the thoracic duct.

The presence of pathology is usually indicated by a "dermal back flow"—a reflux filling of the dermal lymphatics. This occurs secondary to incompetent valves and is most notable in the presence of proximal hypoplasia or obstruction.

Normal lymph nodes possess a characteristically fine, reticular homogeneous appearance. Enlarged lymph nodes or a filling defect is characteristic of pathology.

ULTRASONOGRAPHY

The use of ultrasound in medical diagnosis has seen a rapid expansion in the past five years after a comparatively slow period of development. The early use of diagnostic ultrasound relied heavily upon instrumentation that was initially designed for industrial or military use. Once instrumentation was designed for medical use, there was rapid advancement in terms of instrumentation design and clinical usefulness. Today, diagnostic ultrasound is the preferred diagnostic modality in many instances, e.g., abdominal aortic aneurysm, and is essential for high-quality patient care.

The use of ultrasound in providing information as to the presence of blood flow within a vessel has been discussed previously (Chapters 4 and 5). What we shall be concerned with here is the use of ultrasound in providing actual images of blood vessels. Three techniques shall be discussed: Doppler ultrasonic arteriography, pulse echo ultrasonography (also known as echography) and the relatively new technique of real-time high resolution ultrasonic arteriography.

Doppler Ultrasonic Angiography

Principles and Techniques.   A discussion of the Doppler principle as it pertains to acquiring information relevent to blood flow within a blood vessel has been previously presented (Chapter 3). Basically, a beam of ultrasound reflected by a moving object, e.g., red blood cells, will have its frequency shifted in proportion to the velocity of the blood cells. If the reflected beam is from a stationary object, there will not be a shift in frequency. The system for Doppler ultrasonic angiography consists of three basic units: the Doppler ultrasonic velocity detector, the transducer and spatial resolver (the position-sensing arm), and a storage oscilloscope display unit.

The Doppler ultrasonic velocity detector may be either a continuous-wave or pulse-wave Doppler with nondirectional or directional capabilities. The continuous wave unit is relatively less expensive, more readily available, and less complex than the pulse-wave Doppler unit; however, the pulsed Doppler has the advantage of being capable of echo ranging to determine the depth or location of an interface, allowing a sharper focus by limiting signals to a given plane. The continuous-wave Doppler was initially used by Reid and Spencer in 1972. With this instrumentation, a lens is used to focus a 5 MHz ultrasound beam at a depth of approximately 3 cm from its source. A field of approximately 1 mm in width and 2 to 4 cm in depth is created, from which reflected ultrasound is continuously detected, amplified, and processed for three outputs: an audio output, a directional analog output, or an output to drive a z line axis of a storage oscilloscope.

The pulsed Doppler was initially developed for noninvasive arteriography by Hokanson in 1971. It periodically emits, at 0.5 to 1.0 msec, short bursts of ultrasound at 5 MHz. As the ultrasound beam is periodic and not continuous, the use of time-gating the received signal allows the unit to detect blood flow selectively at any distance from the transducer; the continuous-wave Doppler is sensitive to blood flow everywhere in the ultrasound beam. The short bursts of ultrasound from the pulsed Doppler unit allows for detection of the Doppler shift from discrete points along the ultrasound beam by sampling the reflected signal at different times following each ultrasound transmission. The range of the reflected ultrasound beam that is detected by the receiving crystal of the transducer corresponds to the time interval for the beam of ultrasound to traverse the distance to and from the point of detected flow. The use of several time gates at the same time provides for simultaneous detection of flow at several points along the utrasound beam, corresponding to the range of the reflected beam of ultrasound. The detection of flow forms a spot on the screen of the storage oscilloscope that is stored at the appropriate position. The continual movement of the transducer and changing of its angle of incidence and range progressively constructs an image of the lumen of the blood vessel.

The spatial resolver (position-sensing arm) translates the position of the detected blood flow to the appropriate position on the oscilloscope. Potentiometers in the position-sensing arm detect movements of the transducer made in the X, Y plane which, when coupled with the range output, accurately position the point of detected blood flow as a spot at the appropriate location on the oscilloscope.

The display unit can provide information graphically or in the form of a velocity signal. As there is an inherent problem in graphically displaying blood vessel walls that are severely calcified, analysis of the velocity signal is important. The normal Doppler velocity signal is characteristically multiphasic, with a prominent systolic component with one or more diastolic sounds. The characteristic Doppler velocity signal is altered in the presence of arterial obstruction or significant stenosis. The velocity signal becomes monophasic with an attenuated systolic component and an absence of diastolic sounds when recorded distal to an arterial obstruction. In the presence of significant stenosis short of complete obstruction, the velocity signal may be noted to lose its characteristic multiphasic pattern and have a high-pitched or turbulent sound with a combination of high and low frequencies. The Doppler velocity signal may also be processed to an analog output or undergo sound spectral analysis.

As mentioned previously, a point of detected flow is appropriately located on the graphic output as a spot on the storage oscilloscope screen. This positioning of the spot on the screen is controlled using the range output and the voltage output of the potentiometers in the position-sensing arm. A spot on the oscilloscope is displayed when the voltage output of the Doppler instrument exceeds a threshold voltage greater than 200 Hz. The edge of the display is detected as the interface between the flowing blood and the blood vessel walls. The screening out of lower frequencies serves to minimize the appearance of artifacts produced by movement of the transducer or motions of the blood vessel wall. The transducer is systematically moved along the path of the blood vessel under evaluation directed by the characteristics of the audio output and the appearance of the graphic display on the oscilloscope. This procedure is repeated until the completed image is formed, at which time the graphic display may be photographed for incorporation into the patient's record.

The technique of Doppler ultrasonic angiography provides the clinician with three graphic displays: a longitudinal cross section, a transverse cross section, and a projectional view. The longitudinal cross section provides an image in the plane of movement of the transducer. The transverse cross section provides a unique visualization of the lumen of the blood vessel that cannot be produced using contrast angiography. The morphology of the blood vessel is seen as a cross section in the same plane as the transducer moved perpendicular to the longitudinal axis of the vessel. This is a most important view when evaluating arterial bifurcations, particularly when attempting to localize eccentric plaques at the carotid or femoral bifurcations. The third type of display is a projectional view where the vessel is imaged perpendicular to the beam of ultrasound. This type of display provides a visualization of the blood vessel that corresponds to that seen using contrast angiography.

Applications. Application of the technique of Doppler ultrasonic angiography has met with the most success in the evaluation of the carotid arteries, as the carotid bifurcation lies well within the range of a beam of ultrasound and the atherosclerotic process involving the carotid arteries is often localized at the bifurcation or within one to two centimeters of the orifice of the internal carotid artery. This technique is capable of detecting stenoses of 25 percent or more or complete occlusion of the vessel. Visualization of a narrowing of the carotid artery image in the presence of increased frequency and distal turbulence is highly suggestive of a stenotic lesion. In the presence of significant calcification of the vessel wall or plaque formation, a blank area is produced on the oscilloscope and this area cannot be evaluated. In this regard, velocity analysis is important and instrumentation is now available that is capable of color-coding different velocities on the oscilloscope image, providing for differentiation between normal, moderately increased, and highly increased blood velocity.

Doppler ultrasonic angiography has met with some success in examining patients for femoral artery disease and may prove more informative than contrast arteriography because of the ease of obtaining lateral views and the unique capability of obtaining transverse cross sections. The technique is also of value in evaluating points of anastomosis between arteries and prosthetic grafts that are oriented in the anterior-posterior plane; this is particularly true in evaluating the profunda femoris artery. The unique transverse cross-sectional display additionally provides a better indication as to the actual obstruction to flow.

This technique of Doppler ultrasonic angiography has also been used for follow-up in coronary artery bypass; however, the technique is limited in its usefulness in this region of the body because of the presence of the lungs which, being filled with air, seriously impede the passage of the ultrasound beam. Similar limitations are likewise encountered in attempting to visualize the aortic arch and the branches of the thoracic aorta. In the abdominal region, air located in the small and large intestines inhibits the use of this technique at this anatomical location.

In evaluating the arterial vasculature of the extremities beyond the femoral bifurcation, the technique has not been greatly successful in that the atherosclerotic process as it occurs in the extremities usually involves long segments of the arteries. Evaluating venous disease has similarly not met with much success, as long segments of veins are involved and there is a certain degree of difficulty in distinguishing between the main venous channel and prominent collateral veins.

Pulse Echo Ultrasonography (Echography)

Principles and Techniques.   In pulse echo ultrasonography, electrical energy is utilized to oscillate a crystal yielding sounds at frequencies in excess of 2 MHz at intervals of approximately 1 microsecond. This beam of ultrasound, when directed at tissues, is reflected whenever it encounters a change in tissue density or an interface with a different acoustic impedance. The greater the change in the density, elasticity, or acoustic impedance, the stronger the echo or reflection of the ultrasound beam. This reflected sound compresses the crystal in the transducer, converting the echo into a burst of electrical energy which is transported to an oscilloscope screen where it can be displayed in one of several formats: A mode, B mode, M mode, and basic variations of these modes, e.g., B scan, gray scale.

The A mode of display is the simplest format, where the echoes appear as spikes with the strength of the echo corresponding to the height or amplitude of the spike (thus the term amplitude modulation or A mode). In vascular disease, the A mode display format can be used to estimate the diameter of the aorta. At the site of maximum aortic pulsation, the transducer is applied at varying angles to obtain maximal spike height. A series of such measurements will provide a noninvasive approximation of aortic diameter.

In the B mode of display, the reflected echo is displayed as a dot on the oscilloscope screen with the brightness of the dot corresponding to the strength of the echo (thus the term brightness modulation or B mode). The M mode demonstrates structures that physically alter their distance from the transducer. The echoes travel across the oscilloscope screen at a known speed with undulating path indicating phasic changes and a straight line indicating reflection from a stationary object (thus the term motion mode or M mode). The M mode is extensively used in echocardiography.

The most extensively used display format is the B scan. This technique uses a B mode transducer moving in a particular plane obtaining numerous B mode reflections and storing them on an oscilloscope screen, thus producing a two-dimensional image. The term B scan indicates the use of the B mode and a scanning transducer. With this technique, it is relatively easy to visualize the abdominal aorta and the proximal iliac arteries. It is a most advantageous technique in examining a patient for abdominal aortic aneurysm.

One of the limitations of the B scan technique is the loss of relatively low-intensity echoes. This is due to the fact that echoes must be of a certain intensity to be visualized on the oscilloscope. This limitation has been overcome with use of gray-scale technique. With this technique, received electrical pulses are stored and at the end of the scan, the stored pulses are read and transferred to a television screen. This technique lowers the intensity threshold and is capable of producing at least eight different levels of intensity. The technique of gray-scale ultrasonography is particularly applicable in vascular disease involving the abdominal aorta and also the celiac axis and superior mesenteric artery.

Applications.   In vascular disease, perhaps the most extensive application of pulse echo ultrasonography is in the evaluation of abdominal aortic aneurysms. The clinical diagnosis of abdominal aortic aneurysm is frequently complicated by the aneurysm's small size, a tortuous aorta, the presence of lumbar lordosis, or obesity of the patient. In the elderly or patients at poor risk for surgery, serial follow-ups to monitor the size of the abdominal aortic aneurysm is required in order to evaluate the risk of surgery on a sick patient versus the risk of aneurysmal rupture. As contrast arteriography is not conducive to serial use, the noninvasive technique of pulse echo ultrasonography is particulary attractive. In addition, in the presence of a mural thrombus, the size of the aortic lumen may appear normal, with contrast arteriography failing to show the true size of the aneurysm, which can be detected using ultrasonography.

Scans of the abdomen using pulse echo ultrasonography are best carried out when the abdomen is free of excessive amounts of intestinal gas or barium, as these substances reflect an ultrasound beam almost completely. In examining the abdomen, the scan is made initially from the xiphoid process of the sternum down to past the umbilicus. A series of scans parallel to the initial scan at a distance of 1 to 2 cm is then done and, if the aorta is not extensively tortuous, one of the scans should show the aorta from its level at the tenth thoracic vertebra to its level of bifurcation around the fourth lumbar vertebra. To further outline the aorta, transverse scans can be done at two-centimeter intervals from the umbilicus to the xiphoid.

In the normal longitudinal echogram, the lumen of the aorta appears echo-free with the walls of the vessel visualized as dense lines because of their excellent reflecting properties. In the normal transverse cross section, the aorta appears as a sharply outlined circle closely associated with the anterior margin of the vertebral body. The presence of an aneurysm is usually readily apparent in both the longitudinal and transverse views; both views are necessary as the transverse diameter is often greater than the anterior-posterior diameter. The lumen of the aneurysm may show the presence of a thrombus, indicated by weak internal echoes. A periaortic hematoma due to leakage can often be identified as a lucent or "complex" collection of fluid retroperitoneally. Visualization of an intimal flap is indicative of aortic dissection. The echogram is limited in determining involvement of the renal arteries or the presence of coexistent aneurysms of the iliac arteries.

Pulse echo ultrasonography is also of value in the diagnosis of peripheral aneurysmal formation, particularly in patients with generalized arterial ectasia or abdominal aortic aneurysm, where the detection of small peripheral aneurysms may prove difficult. In such patients, examination of the femoral vessels is carried out with the patient supine and examination of the popliteal vessels is carried out with the patient prone.

Other applications of pulse echo ultrasonography would include delineating prosthetic grafts and identifying the presence of local complications such as hematoma, abscess, or false aneurysm formation. The technique may also be of value in detecting lymph node enlargement. Lymph nodes are visualized as lobulated or confluent masses in association with the aorta or inferior vena cava or mesentery. Identification of the pelvic lymph nodes is not practical because of the presence of air in the intestines. Enlarged retroperitoneal lymph nodes may actually completely surround the aorta and/or inferior vena cava, displacing these structures from their normal close proximity to the vertebral body. Many investigators have found ultrasound to be as accurate as lymphography in detecting the presence of enlarged retroperitoneal lymph nodes in patients with lymphoma and frequently the transverse cross-sectional view will be of more value than lymphography. Lymphography is required, however, in selected cases as ultrasound will not demonstrate subtle textured changes in nodes of normal size.

Recently, real-time ultrasonography has been introduced. In this technique the returning echo is displayed at a rate sufficient to allow interpretation as a continuous event. Such technique is of value in assessing pulsatile and respiratory movements of the abdominal and pelvic vessels and increasing attention is being paid to the pulsatility of abdominal aortic aneurysms in an attempt to predict rupture.

Real-Time High-Resolution Ultrasonic Arteriography. Real-time high-resolution ultrasonic arteriography is a relatively new technique (initial development of the instrumentation was begun in 1973) and may be considered to be in a developmental stage. The technique has been primarily used in the evaluation of the carotid artery, as this is a frequent and clinically important site of atherosclerotic involvement and because it lies relatively close to the skin (see below). Investigators have obtained limited success in evaluating the femoral arteries.

Conventional diagnostic ultrasound (e.g., pulse echo ultrasonography) is used for assessing structures deep within the body cavity (e.g., the abdominal aorta), and necessarily uses low-frequency ultrasound to reduce the degree of attenuation of the ultrasound beam. The use of a low-frequency ultrasound beam, while it reduces attenuation, also reduces the degree of resolution. In contrast, real-time high-resolution ultrasonic arteriography, as it is used in assessing structures lying in close proximity to the skin (e.g., the carotid arteries), uses a higher ultrasonic frequency, providing for high resolution of structures. Using this technique, resolution of approximately 0.5 millimeters can be obtained.

Using a high-frequency ultrasound B scan system (6 to 10 MHz) the image is shown at a rapid rate (15 to 30 frames per second) to give the impression of a continuous phenomenon. Visually, the arterial lumen appears as in a normal B scan; however, the relatively high frequency of the ultrasound beam in this technique provides better resolution and is an effective method of estimating the diameter and shape of the lumen. A blood velocity profile generated by a pulsed Doppler may be superimposed over this image. The B scan image and the velocity profile appear in real time and the transducer is designed in such a manner that the B scan and Doppler velocity profile are taken from the same anatomic point.

As this technique is relatively new, one can anticipate further improvements. The advantages of the technique are that it can demonstrate subtleties that are frequently better realized when seen in motion, it allows a clearer perspective of anatomical relationships, and it permits observation of blood vessel and blood flow dynamics.

The technique of real-time high-resolution ultrasonic arteriography has found some usefulness in clinical atherosclerosis research as it can decrease the time required to assess the effectiveness of dietary, medical, or surgical therapy. It does so by allowing serial evaluations of the degree of atherosclerotic involvement and quantitative measurement of the degree of arterial narrowing. Currently, such evaluations of therapy are based upon mortality rates in larger populations or upon assessing end organ damage caused by the disease.

SCANNING

The term scanning, when applied to the field of cardiovascular nuclear medicine, indicates the process of producing a two-dimensional image, referred to as the scan or scintiscan, that is representative of the rays emitted by a radioactive isotope, most frequently gamma rays, concentrated in a specific tissue of the body. The development of scanning techniques in the study of the cardiovascular system has made tremendous strides in the past several years.

Scanning of the lungs followed the detection of pericardial effusion as the second useful cardiovascular nuclear medicine technique to be developed. Its initial use in the diagnosis of pulmonary embolism was in 1963. Its continued successful use has given the clinician a better understanding of the natural history of pulmonary embolism and has provided objective documentation of the clinical usefulness of fibrinolytic agents in the medical treatment of pulmonary embolism. Since the acceptance of pulmonary scanning as a most effective diagnostic modality, the principle upon which it is based (i.e., the use of radioactive microspheres and particles to document regional blood flow) has been successfully applied to the peripheral circulation—arterial, venous, and lymphatic.

The use of radioactive tracers is advantageous in that they do not disrupt normal physiologic events. The radionuclides are used in what may be considered essentially negligible quantities that provide sufficient amounts of radioactivity to permit precise measurements. This coupled with their relatively rapid decay make the radionuclides quite safe for both the patient and the technician. The measurements of the radioactivity can be made singly or sequentially over a period of time, allowing measurements to be made in four dimensions (three spatial and one temporal) to provide a functional visualization.

The most frequently used radionuclide today is technetium-99m labeled microspheres, a gamma emitter. Three characteristics enhance the usefulness of ^{99m}Tc. It decays by means of isometric transition, which greatly reduces the radiation dosage when compared with beta emitters. Second, its half-life of 6 hours enhances its suitability for studying many physiologic processes through the use of imaging procedures. Third, a photoemission of 140 kev is high enough to penetrate body tissues but does not require extensive lead shielding. The ^{99m}Tc radionuclide is rapidly removed from the body through excretion by the intestinal mucosa and the kidneys.

PULMONARY SCANNING

Perfusion Scan

The use of pulmonary perfusion scanning technique is a safe, simple, and effective means for assessing the pulmonary blood flow in screening suspect patients for the presence of pulmonary embolism. In principle, the pulmonary blood flow distribution, i.e., the pulmonary perfusion, can be assessed if an injected radionuclide is totally or almost totally removed from the circulation in a single passage through the lung. The radionuclide particles that are injected are trapped as microemboli in the precapillary arterioles and capillaries. Such microemboli subsequently fragment, allowing passage through the alveolar capillary membrane and their reentry into the circulation to be subsequently filtered by the reticuloendothelial system of the liver and the spleen. The purposeful formation of microemboli in the lungs of patients suspected of having a pulmonary embolism may appear paradoxical; however, the margin for safety is ample in that the formation of the microemboli is transient due to relatively short half-life of the radionuclide, and the number of micro-emboli formed is much less than the number of arterioles and capillaries (about one microembolus to every 100 to 1000 arterioles and capillaries).

The radionuclide (the preferred radiopharmaceutical is ^{99m}Tc labeled albumin microspheres) is administered with the patient in the supine position to allow even distribution of the microspheres from the base to the apex of the lung. In order to completely visualize the lung, anterior and posterior and left and right lateral views are required. The use of these four views additionally allows correlation of observed perfusion defects in the various pulmonary regions.

A normal pulmonary perfusion scan is characterized by an even distri-bution of activity in all pulmonary zones with smooth margins seen in all four required views. The anterior and posterior views normally show rounded costophrenic angles; on lateral views, the costophrenic angles will appear sharp posteriorly. Additionally, on the anterior and left lat-eral views, the pericardial-cardiac silhouette is noted, while the presence of the silhouette is only suggested on the posterior view.

The pulmonary perfusion scan is highly sensitive to significant ob-struction of pulmonary blood flow. This high sensitivity, however, is coupled with a low degree of specificity. Obstruction to pulmonary blood flow, shown as a perfusion defect, may also be demonstrated with various other disease states: emphysema; bronchiectasis; bronchial asthma or chronic bronchitis leading to regional bronchospasm; regional alveolar hypoxia with reflex oligemia; pulmonary hypertension or venous ob-struction; alveolar filling processes such as pneumonia, pulmonary edema, or hemorrhage; tumors, foreign bodies, or mucus plugs leading to large or small airway obstruction; pleural effusion, bullae, cardio-megaly, or pneumothorax causing compression, displacement, or col-lapse of the lung parenchyma. In view of these many conflicting diag-noses, the specificity of the perfusion lung scan for detecting pulmonary embolism can be enhanced by considering only what can be called the "high-probability scan," i.e., only segmental or lobar perfusion defects are characteristic of pulmonary embolism. Specificity can also be in-creased by correlating chest film findings with the perfusion scan and by correlating pulmonary perfusion with pulmonary ventilation.

Ventilation Scan
Pulmonary ventilation can be measured by either of two methods: (1) a static index of ventilation per unit of lung volume, or (2) a dynamic

index of the rate at which a radioactive gas enters or leaves the lungs. With the majority of patients the clinician may encounter, an image of regional ventilation for comparison with a perfusion scan is usually all that is necessary.

Each patient who undergoes a perfusion lung scan should also undergo a ventilation scan. The pulmonary ventilation scan is done with the patient supine to facilitate the correlation of two scans. The patient is allowed to breath xenon-133 gas that has been mixed with breathing air. Scans are taken after the patient's inhalation of the xenon-133 to total lung capacity once, after the patient's rebreathing the xenon-133 from a closed system to allow the establishment of equilibrium (a period of approximately 5 minutes), and during the patient's clearance of the xenon-133 from the lungs.

The initial single inhalation to total lung capacity provides an index of ventilation. The patient should be instructed to inhale rapidly so that the distribution of the xenon-133 reflects alterations of ventilation secondary to regional changes in airway resistance. The interpretation of results in some patients is complicated by their failure to inhale rapidly or their incapability of holding their breath for the 15 to 20 seconds required to form an image on the scan. In such patients, the distribution of the radioactive xenon is not solely a function of the ventilation distribution.

The patient's rebreathing the radioactive xenon for approximately five minutes allows all normally ventilated regions to obtain equilibrium and the scan that is obtained at the end point of the state of equilibrium is representative of the volume of ventilated lung.

After the scan at equilibrium is taken, the patient is allowed to wash out the radioactive xenon. The rate at which the xenon-133 is washed out is directly related to ventilation and can be applied to the determination of the regional ventilation as a function of the ventilatory volume of that region.

In comparing the ventilation scan with the perfusion scan, the clinician can determine whether an observed region of pulmonary nonperfusion has occurred in conjunction with normal ventilation, as would be the circumstance with pulmonary embolism, or in conjunction with abnormal ventilation, as in the presence of airway obstruction. The presence, therefore, of corresponding defects in ventilation and perfusion is characteristic of disease processes such as pneumonia and other parenchymal lung diseases, and the presence of normal ventilation with perfusion defects would indicate pulmonary embolism. The interpretation of ventilation and perfusion defects may be complicated in patients with pulmonary infarction, which is associated with both abnormal pulmonary perfusion and ventilation. Chronic drug abuse or periarteritis may also lead to perfusion defects with normal ventilation.

RADIONUCLIDE ARTERIOGRAPHY

The use of radionuclides in peripheral arterial disease has been developed along two lines: (1) the evaluation of the arterial perfusion of tissues in the normal state as well as detection of changes in perfusion of tissues following physiologic (exercise, reactive hyperemia) or pharmacologic (vasodilator) manipulation; and (2) visualization of the arterial lumen. Although these topics might more properly have been included under "visualization" in this chapter they are included here (as are radionuclide phlebography and lymphography) as they more directly pertain to cardiovascular nuclear medicine.

Perfusion

The assessment of tissue perfusion through the use of radionuclides is predicated upon four basic principles: (1) the injection of the radionuclide does not alter normal arterial blood flow; (2) the first capillary bed that the radionuclide encounters traps and removes the radionuclide from the circulation; (3) the radionuclide used and the blood share the same rheological properties; (4) the radionuclide is sufficiently mixed with blood. Once injected, the radionuclide is distributed and perfusion is imaged on the scan in proportion to the muscle mass. In a normal study, therefore, the thigh is noted as having a much higher radionuclide concentration than the calf. In regions that are predominantly avascular, e.g., the joints, the radionuclide concentration is either diminished or totally absent.

In assessing tissue perfusion, the distribution of radionuclide activity can be categorized into five basic patterns: (1) the normal distribution, which is related to muscle mass with relatively little activity around the joints; (2) where the radionuclide distribution is greater and shows a relatively even distribution at the skin—predominantly seen with small vessel disease in diabetics as well as in patients with diffuse disease or previous sympathectomy; (3) asymmetrical distribution, where there is a relative hypoperfusion of a muscle mass, characteristically seen in patients with focal large vessel disease; (4) a distribution of hyperperfusion such as seen in patients with ulceration or gangrenous lesions; (5) a pattern of increased radioactivity to the bones—a hyperperfusion of bony structures that is characteristic of patients presenting with fibrous dysplasia or Paget's disease, with its well-known increase in bone vascularity.

Frequently, as has been mentioned in previous chapters with respect to noninvasive tests, peripheral vasodilation leading to increased arterial outflow is of value in detecting the presence of arterial stenoses that are not readily apparent in the resting state. Such peripheral vasodilation can be accomplished through exercise, with an occluding thigh cuff that is rapidly released to cause a reactive hyperemia, or through the use of vasodilator pharmaceuticals. Perhaps the easiest method for use in assessing tissue perfusion with radionuclides is the use of an occluding thigh cuff. Inflation of the thigh cuff above systolic pressure for a period of time followed by a sudden release causes a maximal vasodilation of the upper and lower portion of the leg. Just before releasing the cuff, an injection of ^{99m}Tc radionuclide is administered to an antecubital vein and the arrival and distribution of the radionuclide in both calves can be monitored.

In the normal scan, there is a regular symmetrical distribution of the radionuclide and a normal time-activity curve is obtained, where peak activity is obtained approximately eight seconds after the activity initially appears, following which the time-activity curve descends to a plateau. The peak activity is a characteristic response to the reactive hyperemia following cuff release. In the presence of significant proximal stenosis, the time-activity curve does not show this peak activity.

Visualization

The use of radionuclides can also be applied to visualization of the arterial tree. In addition to providing a visual image of the artery, radionuclides can provide quantitative information that can prove valuable in the diagnosis and management of patients with atherosclerotic occlusive disease. The technique can define the presence of arterial stenosis, occlusion, and aneurysmal formation.

For visualization of the arterial lumen, the radionuclide is injected as a bolus into an antecubital vein. The radionuclide usually used is ^{99m}Tc. To obtain a bolus injection, a blood pressure cuff is placed proximally to the site of injection and is inflated to a pressure above systolic. It is maintained at this pressure both before and during the injection of radionuclide. Once the injection is completed and before the needle is removed, the occlusive blood pressure cuff is rapidly deflated, at which time the injected radionuclide flows as a bolus. For approximately 100 seconds after the injection, the distribution of the radionuclide is displayed and recorded and a scan is obtained approximately five to ten minutes after injection. The data that are obtained may be displayed in the form of a histogram providing quantitative information as to arrival times and radionuclide activity in one or more areas of the arterial tree. A complete study including data analysis can be accomplished in 12 to 15 minutes.

In examining a patient for the presence of an abdominal aortic aneurysm, one should note visualization of a widened aortic lumen or, if a mural thrombus is present, a narrow and/or tortuous lumen that is encompassed by an area of relative nonradioactivity that is representative of the clot.

Using radionuclides, arterial stenoses of greater than 30 percent can be visualized. Careful attention to the arrival time of the radionuclide can enhance the diagnostic effectiveness of the radionuclide study by demonstrating a decrease in the arrival of the radionuclide activity distal to the stenosis. In a similar fashion, the technique can be used routinely to demonstrate graft patency postoperatively. The use of radionuclides can show the presence of anastomatic stenosis, graft dilatation, and stenosis of the receiving artery secondary to clamp trauma intra-operatively. The early detection of such complications prior to total graft occlusion facilitates repair and decreases the possibility of limb loss.

RADIONUCLIDE PHLEBOGRAPHY

The technique of radionuclide phlebography, particularly when applied to the above-the-knee segment, provides excellent visualization of the venous system without the disadvantages of time, expense, and patient discomfort that accompanies the use of contrast phlebography. A particular advantage of radionuclide phlebography is that it can be coupled with pulmonary radionuclide scanning, affording the opportunity of simultaneously detecting the presence of as well as the source of a pulmonary embolus. Radionuclide phlebography should not be confused with the ^{125}I-fibrinogen uptake test, which does not provide visualization but involves profile counting of radioactivity at serial points along the leg and comparing this with cardiac background activity.

The simultaneous examination of the patient for pulmonary emboli and the patency of the venous system involves the use of radionuclide-tagged particles of a size large enough to become trapped in the lungs, thus avoiding their recirculation in the arterial system. Site of active venous thrombosis in the lower extremity is excellently demonstrated using ^{99m}Tc sulfur colloid-tagged microaggregated albumin, which is selectively trapped in areas of fibrin deposits at active thrombotic sites. To a lesser degree, ^{99m}Tc human albumin microspheres provide similar results. The use of free radionuclide sodium pertechnetate provides visualization of the lumen of the veins frequently as good as that which can be accomplished using standard contrast phlebography.

Sodium pertechnetate (approximately 7.5 millicuries in 25 cc of normal saline) is rapidly injected into a vein in the dorsum of the foot. Tourniquets tightly fitted over the ankle force the sodium pertechnetate into the deep venous system. Scans are taken sequentially at five-second intervals over the thighs and then repositioned proximally to obtain visualization of the iliac venous system and the lower portion of the inferior vena cava. After photos demonstrating the iliacs and inferior vena cava are obtained, the instrumentation is repositioned over the thighs again and the tourniquet is removed, allowing the remaining radionuclide to fill the superficial and saphenous system. At the initial rapid injection, some of the sodium pertechnetate may be spared for injection later for visualization of the superficial system. After about a five-minute delay, following the initial injection and scanning, scans of the leg are repeated in similar fashion for the detection of "hot spots"—areas of increased radioactivity.

With the technique of radionuclide phlebography, five sources of information are provided for analysis: (1) appearance time, (2) major venous pattern, (3) venous collateral pattern, (4) disappearance pattern, and (5) dilution effect. In a normal study, there is no visualization of a venous collateral pattern and disappearance is relatively uniform, merging with the subsequent arterial flow phase and distribution of the radionuclide to the tissues. The diagnostic criteria for venous thrombosis include a delayed appearance time, the dilution or absence of a part of a major venous patterns, the visualization of venous collaterals, the presence of "hot spots" on the scan secondary to delayed disappearance of the radionuclide, and an overall reduction of radioactivity as noted on the scan secondary to dilution by blood from venous collaterals not containing radionuclide. It should be noted that the appearance of the radionuclide activity (within 5 seconds for the thigh and 5 to 15 seconds for the iliac veins) is not representative of circulation time, as transit time is accelerated by the forceful injection of the radionuclide distal to an occlusive cuff at the anke.

In the radionuclide phlebograph of the thigh, the femoral vein is noted as a single pathway traversing the thigh. In the presence of superficial femoral or popliteal vein thrombosis, this normal single pathway is disrupted as is the normal "wishbone" appearance of the ileo-vena caval system in the presence of ileofemoral venous thrombosis.

The presence of a comparatively prolonged transit time noted in one extremity or the visualization of multiple venous pathways in the calf is only suggestive of the presence of venous thrombosis, as the presence of valvular incompetence can yield multiple-channel visualization in the calf and visualization of superficial femoral and saphenous veins in the thigh. A definitive diagnosis of venous thrombosis can be made only in the presence of nonvisualization of a vein, either with or without the presence of collateral pathways, the appearance of collateral venous pathways in the thigh or pelvic regions, and/or the notation of "hot spots" on the delayed scan. The appearance of "hot spots" on a delayed scan suggests venous thrombosis of recent origin, as they are particularly characteristic of the presence of a nonendothelialized surface. This particular characteristic is of value in the patient with chronic venous thrombosis as it allows for the detection of newly formed thrombi.

RADIONUCLIDE LYMPHOGRAPHY

The application of the technique of radionuclide scanning to the examination of the lymphatic system can provide useful information concerning the characteristics of the flow of lymph through the lymphatic vessels and the tissue clearance. In the study of lymphatic clearance, the most frequently used technique involves the use of radioiodinated human serum albumin (^{131}I-tagged human serum albumin). With this technique, 1 to 2 μCi of the tagged serum albumin is injected subcutaneously and subsequent radioactivity is monitored immediately after injection and at delayed intervals following injection. From the data obtained, the percent of clearance is calculated for a defined period of time, as is the half-time, i.e., the period of time expressed in hours for 50 percent clearance. The results obtained by using this technique can be misleading, however, in that the radioiodinated human serum albumin clearance is realistically a simple measure of turnover time for tissue protein and an observed increase in rate of clearance of the tagged human serum albumin may be indicative of either a decrease in the lymphatic drainage or an increase in the local extracellular fluid volume. This technique of using ^{131}I-tagged human serum albumin is therefore most useful in the evaluation of the efficacy of a particular course of treatment or in a program of serial follow-up studies. A single isolated study is of no significant value.

For lymphoscintigraphy, the most useful technique entails the use of radioactive gold ([198]Au). The size of the particles in the [198]Au preparation (range of diameter: 0.02 to 2.0 μ, the majority in the range of 0.03 to 0.07 μ in diameter) is ideally suited for the study of lymphatic uptake and transport. A solution of 100 μCi of [198]Au and 75 u of hyaluronidase in a 1 percent procaine hydrochloride solution is subcutaneously injected at the dorsum of the foot. The abdominal lymphatic system can be visualized on a delayed scan taken 24 hours following injection. With lymphoscintigraphy, individual lymph nodes cannot be differentiated. Fairly well recognized, however, is a "circuit of radioactivity" associated with any one group of nodes. This technique provides a means of serial observations for documentation of lymph node size and uptake capacity; its routine use is, however, not recommended because of its high degree of beta emission and the possibility of hepatic irradiation following use of the technique.

The gamma emitter ^{99m}Tc is routinely used in radionuclide lymphography. It has the advantages of not being a beta emitter, a relatively rapid rate of disappearance from the site of injection with a comparatively rapid uptake by the lymph nodes, and the need for only a relatively small amount of injectate volume (0.2 to 0.5 ml per injection) that is well tolerated by the patient without the need for local anesthetic or hyaluronidase. Approximately 2.0 μCi of ^{99m}Tc is injected subcutaneously at the medial web spaces of each foot, following which the patient is asked to exercise. The comparatively small size of the particles allows for easy passage of the radionuclide, and scans visualizing the lymphatic system can be obtained at 90 to 150 minutes following injection.

SOUNDING

CAROTID PHONOANGIOGRAPHY

The noninvasive technique of carotid phonoangiography entails the use of a specially adapted microphone that is placed over the cervical portion of the carotid artery at three positions (more detailed studies involve more than three positions): high in the neck; in the middle of the neck corresponding to the point of the carotid bifurcation; and low in the neck. The microphone is used to make stripchart and/or magnetic tape recordings of sounds associated with bruits in the carotid arteries for analysis of the degree of stenosis present. The recordings are analyzed in reference to the first and second heart sounds as to the relative amplitude and duration of the bruit waveforms. The technique of carotid phonoangiography improves the standard technique of stethoscope auscultation of the cervical carotid for the detection of carotid bruits through the use of a permanent record, either stripchart or magnetic tape, that permits initial analysis as well as subsequent comparative follow-up studies.

Before discussing carotid phonoangiography, a brief review of the heart sounds is in order. There are four heart sounds associated with the mechanical activity of the heart. The major components of these sounds are associated with abrupt acceleration or deceleration of the blood that applies a sudden tension to the valve leaflets and/or the chordae tendinae, resulting in a vibration of the heart that is transmitted to the body wall and detected externally as a heart sound.

The first heart sound typically consists of four components. The first coincides with the initiation of contraction of the left ventricle and is probably secondary to muscle contraction in the earliest phase of ventricular systole or contraction. Atrial systole may also be contributory to the first component. The second component is a major contribution to the first heart sound and is representative of the abrupt tension placed on the mitral valve as it completes closing. During ventricular systole there is a rapid acceleration of the blood closely followed by a sudden brief deceleration that is associated with a sudden tensing of the entire atrioventricular valve structure. The third component of the first heart sound is its second major component and it has been traditionally attributed to the closure of the tricuspid valve. Most probably, however, this component is secondary to the opening of the aortic valve and the blood's initial ejection and acceleration through the aortic valve as it enters the aorta. The fourth and final component of the first sound is relatively small and corresponds to the acceleration of blood through the aorta.

The second heart sound is associated with vibrations secondary to the sudden deceleration of the columns of blood in the aorta and pulmonary artery. These vibrations arise from the column of blood, vessel walls, and closed valves rather than as primary vibrations produced when the valve leaflets hit each other when they close. The second heart sound usually has two components—aortic and pulmonary—with the aortic component occurring before the pulmonic component. This sequence of components reflects the closure of the aortic valve occurring before closing of the pulmonary valve.

The third heart sound is a low-frequency sound composed of one or two components; it occurs at the end of the rapid-filling phase of ventricular diastole. At this point, the volume of the ventricle reaches a level at which further filling requires a significantly greater pressure.

The fourth heart sound is secondary to a sudden tensing of the atrioventricular valves that is associated with a sudden acceleration and subsequent deceleration of blood produced by a vigorous atrial contraction. It is similar to the third heart sound but has a slightly lower frequency.

The presence of a bruit over the carotid artery is recognized as being indicative of the presence of carotid artery occlusive disease. The presence of a stenosis disrupts the normal laminar blood flow, giving rise to abnormal turbulent flow that creates motion in the blood vessel wall, which is transmitted transcutaneously and heard externally as a bruit. The presence of a bruit is noted primarily during systole because of the increased blood flow that occurs during cardiac contraction.

The technique calls for the patient to lie supine without the use of pillows so the head lies flat and is not flexed. The sound transducer is placed over the desired area and the sounds are recorded. A quick examination for the presence of carotid bruits would include tracings made at the highest possible position over the palpable cervical portion of the carotid; a tracing made over the site of the carotid bifurcation or the site of the bruit; and a tracing made at the base of the neck just above the clavicle. During the five seconds required to make a recording, the patient is requested to hold his breath in expiration to remove any respiratory artifacts. For a more detailed examination, include recordings made over the apex of the heart, at the suprasternal notch, at the subclavicular and supraclavicular areas, at the base of the sternocleidomastoid muscle, at the inferior and superior borders of the thyroid cartilage, at a position midway between the thyroid cartilage and the angle of the mandible, at the angle of the mandible, over the preauricular artery, and over any other location at which the bruit can be heard. A normal carotid phonoangiogram demonstrates prominent first and second heart sounds without the presence of intervening turbulence. The presence of a bruit is indicated by a noise pattern that eliminates the normal heart sound.

Bruits that arise from the great vessels in the thoracic area are also transmitted up the neck. The intensity of such a bruit, however, decreases as one progresses toward the cranium and is usually loudest immediately above the clavicle. In contrast, bruits arising from the carotid bifurcation are loudest over and above the point of the cartid bifurcation. Using the relative amplitude or intensity of a carotid bruit is not a good criterion of the source of the bruit as it reflects the placement and closeness of the microphone to the underlying artery. A good indication that the carotid bifurcation is the source of the bruit is an increase in the duration and/or the frequency (density) of the bruit as one proceeds up the neck. Basal heart murmurs are sometimes louder in proximity to the superior border of the thyroid cartilage than at positions lower in the neck because of the closeness of the carotid artery to the surface at that particular area; however, the basal heart murmur bruit is always loudest over its origin at the base of the heart.

Bruits arising from stenotic lesions of the internal carotid artery typically first appear on the recording taken over the mid-cervical area. It appears as a high-frequency systolic turbulence and is transmitted up the neck. As a localized arterial stenosis and adequate blood flow are necessary to produce turbulent flow of sufficient magnitude to create an audible bruit, complete occlusion or stenosis of 80 to 90 percent of the internal carotid artery is noted as a loss of the first heart sound above the tracing recorded from the mid-cervical area. At a stenosis of approximately 80 percent reduction in diameter, the bruit amplitude begins to decrease and is first lost visually, followed by loss of audioperception.

Stenosis of the external carotid artery at its origin in the presence of an occluded or widely patent internal carotid artery may yield a bruit that does not necessarily signify the presence of a stenotic lesion of the internal carotid artery. Although bruits arising from the internal carotid artery are not resonant while a bruit from the external carotid artery often is, the pattern of radiation of the bruit is particularly useful in distinguishing between external and internal carotid bruits. Bruits arising from the external carotid artery are typically radiated to its branches and as such can be heard over the preauricular artery; the internal carotid artery bruit is not and it can frequently be heard over the eyes.

A carotid bruit beginning at the first heart sound which then tapers off and barely extends to the second heart sound is characteristic of a 40 to 50 percent reduction in diameter of the internal carotid artery. As the percent stenosis or reduction in luminal diameter increases, the bruit tends to increase and more completely fill the interval between the first and second heart sounds. The extension of the bruit beyond the second heart sound into diastole does not always occur with progression of the stenosis, but its presence when it does occur is highly significant. The presence of a bruit that extends into diastole indicates the presence of a marked pressure gradient across a stenosis of the internal carotid artery, as blood flow in the external carotid artery during diastole is rarely associated with a bruit, regardless of the degree of localized stenosis. Bruits at the carotid bifurcation that extend into diastole often reflect more severe contralateral stenosis or total occlusion and greater blood flow on the side of the observed diastolic bruit.

Marked bruits may be encountered in the presence of a minimal percent stenosis and are secondary to increased blood flow due to, for example, the presence of an arteriovenous fistula or occlusion of the contralateral carotid artery with increased flow through the patent arteries. Young patients often have clinically insignificant bruits in the absence of actual carotid artery stenosis. Such paradoxical bruits are secondary to turbulent flow created by an arterial bifurcation. The use of computer analysis of the acoustics of the bruit signal aids in distinguishing between innocent and significant bruits. A bruit arising from the carotid bifurcation when the internal carotid artery is occluded is characteristically faint with a break frequency (a frequency beyond which intensity falls rapidly as frequency increases) that is inconsistent with the bruit amplitude. As such, a bruit of low amplitude that is barely recordable with a high break frequency may be representative of complete carotid artery occlusion.

DIAGNOSTIC TECHNIQUES IN PERSPECTIVE

Before attempting to place in perspective the diagnostic techniques discussed in this chapter, several points should be emphasized. First, the physician should beware of overenthusiastic developers and salesmen who may advocate more widespread use of a particular technique than is realistic. The physician should be just as cautious in the case of reports that refute the excellent results reported by others and claim the technique to be of little or no value. Workers unfamiliar with the instrumentation may in this way jeopardize a very useful technique. The truth probably lies somewhere between these two views. When contemplating purchase of a newly developed instrument, an extensive and meticulous survey of previously reported work with the instrument should be undertaken.

Second, the physician should not assume that a newly acquired instrument will yield as good results in his hand as those reported by physicians more experienced in the instrument's use. The physician should establish his own diagnostic accuracy. Preliminary results should be critically compared with the results obtained through contrast angiography in a preliminary series of patients. Only after the physician establishes his own level of diagnostic accuracy should the technique begin to assert itself in the management of the patient.

Perhaps the technique that is easiest to place in perspective is pulse echo ultrasonography. It is probably safe to say that it will become the standard technique for the evaluation of abdominal aortic and peripheral aneurysm; indeed, it has already become so in many centers. The use of echography in aneurysm evaluation provides for the diagnosis of aneurysm where contrast arteriography will not, such as where a normal vessel lumen may be seen on arteriography due to channelization of the thrombus. The use of ultrasound additionally provides a more realistic evaluation of aneurysmal size and its potential for growth, and it can be done repeatedly to follow the growth of the aneurysm in poor-risk patients.

The value of ultrasound lies in its safety, its capability for serial use, the fact that no special patient preparation is required, and the fact that it can be done as an outpatient procedure. Although it is known that a very high intensity of ultrasound of sufficient duration can cause soft tissue damage, the levels of ultrasound used clinically pose no such danger. A disadvantage in the evaluation of abdominal aortic aneurysm may lie in an inability to conclusively rule out renal artery involvement.

Contrast arteriography seldom shows the presence of significant disease in areas that cannot be detected by noninvasive means. It should thus be realistically limited to use for the anatomic location and extent of disease for planning the details of an operative procedure, or in the presence of equivocal noninvasive testing results or where noninvasive results are in conflict with the patient's clinical history, such as in the presence of pseudoclaudication. It should not be considered a routine diagnostic procedure—that is the domain of noninvasive techniques.

Carotid phonoangiography has a distinct advantage over the non-invasive techniques of oculoplethysmography and Doppler and photoplethysmographic examinations for the evaluation of the extracranial cerebral circulation in that it is capable of detecting the presence of cerebrovascular occlusive disease in its early stages at stenosis of approximately 35 percent. The instrumentation for carotid phonoangiography is relatively simple and inexpensive and the analysis of the results relatively easy. False positive results are rarely obtained if the evaluation is carried out at several levels in the neck. When comparing carotid phonoangiography with contrast carotid arteriography, some confusion may arise: (1) a bruit arises from a stenotic external carotid artery, (2) the internal carotid artery is completely occluded, (3) distal bruits are radiated proximally.

Carotid phonoangiography can provide an estimate of the residual lumen in the presence of a long complex lesion. The absence of a bruit cannot be considered to imply the absence of disease, as a bruit tends to disappear when there is greatly diminished flow as a lesion approaches complete occlusion. As such, the absence of a bruit should not preclude continued testing in the presence of a positive patient history.

The use of ultrasonic imaging in the carotid area can detect severe stenosis (as do oculoplethysmography, photoplethysmography, and Doppler ultrasound), can detect moderate stenosis (as does carotid phonoangiography), can distinguish between severe stenosis and complete occlusion, and possibly can demonstrate the presence of an ulcerated plaque. This latter ability is important as the current theory is that such lesions are primarily responsible for incidences of atherosclerotic embolization. As important is the fact that the technique can provide visualization in three different views. Such capabilities are advantageous in the evaluation of the carotid bifurcation. Although the technique has been applied to other anatomic regions, the carotid anatomy is particularly well suited due to its superficial placement, which permits the use of higher-frequency ultrasound, which results in improved resolution. A current problem is that the presence of calcium in the arterial wall, seen in about 50 percent of patients, can produce a shadow suggesting plaque formation in its absence. The imaging systems now available are not ready for widespread routine clinical use at this time.

It has been argued that Doppler ultrasound imaging is not competitive with a good four-vessel arteriogram. The technique does, however, provide improved patient selection and can be used as a screening procedure reserving arteriography for those patients who are operative candidates. The technique is valuable in assessing high-risk patients and can be used serially for following patients with asymptomatic carotid bruits and for following patients postendarterectomy.

The use of radionuclides can be interpreted as being indicative of relative muscle perfusion and as such can provide an estimation of the physiologic significance of the disease process. It is complementary to arteriography as it provides information not available with arteriography-microcirculatory perfusion. Radionuclide studies, however, should not be considered a replacement for contrast arteriography when anatomic documentation is required.

Radionuclides are particularly advantageous in trauma cases, especially with penetrating injuries in close proximity to a major artery. As contrast arteriography is not universally required in such cases, the use of radionuclides provides a rapid, safe, and accurate screening procedure to rule out significant traumatic arterial injury.

The technique of lymphography is useful in characterizing the exact pathologic anatomy of the swollen limb. It is of value in providing a precise classification of lymphedema as to its being congenital or idiopathic, secondary, or obstructive. The use of radionuclide lymphography is excellent for serial use and provides a physiologic approach of lymph flow dynamics. It does, however, lack anatomic definition.

The technique of contrast phlebography remains the "gold standard" for the diagnosis of venous disease. It is the most widely available technique and is carried out in most all departments of radiology. It provides the necessary anatomic details and is most advantageous for resolving equivocal noninvasive or semi-invasive results. The technique has the disadvantage of being rather painful and can result in the development of deep vein thrombosis. Contrast phlebography should be done only under well-defined circumstances, as in the presence of equivocal noninvasive results or if no noninvasive instrumentation is available. The risk of contrast phlebography is much less than the risk inherent in failure to obtain a definitive diagnosis.

Radionuclide phlebography provides a visual image that is similar to x-ray without the pain and possible deep vein thrombosis associated with contrast phlebography. The presence of persistent hot spots is indicative of the presence of an active thrombus. The use of radionuclides is limited by the need for a nuclear medicine facility. A distinct advantage is the possibility of carrying out a simultaneous examination of the peripheral venous system and pulmonary scanning permitting the simultaneous diagnosis of pulmonary embolism and the origin of the embolus. Difficulty is encountered using conventional techniques in the diagnosis of isolated internal iliac thrombosis which can result in pulmonary embolization. The diagnosis previously required interosseous phlebography. The diagnosis of the pathology can be indirectly made, as the technique can assess the patency of the internal iliac vein by its contribution to the dilution effect of the common iliac vein.

In conclusion, it should be emphasized that the results obtained by methods other than conventional contrast angiography may be totally unfamiliar to the physician. Frequently, the physician may be required to obtain new knowledge to permit the appropriate use of and interpretation of results obtained noninvasively or semi-invasively.

REFERENCES

1. Grammill S, Craighead C: Translumbar aortography updated. Surg Gynecol Obstet 140: 59, 1975.
2. Abrams H L, Adelstein S J, Elliott L P, et al: Optimal radiologic facilities for examination of the chest and the cardiovascular system. Report of the Intersociety Commission for Heart Disease Resources. Circulation 43: A-135, 1971.

CHAPTER 7

MONITORING COAGULATION DYNAMICS: THROMBOELASTOGRAPHY

INTRODUCTION

Increasing attention is being paid to the role of the blood coagulation process in peripheral vascular disease. The relationship of defects in blood coagulation to peripheral venous disease, in particular deep venous thrombosis, has been well appreciated since Virchow in 1856 included defects in the coagulation process as part of his triad of causative factors for thrombosis. Virchow's coagulation defect is now generally referred to as hypercoagulability and is known to result from trauma or operative procedures, and, more recently established, to characteristically occur in the cancer patient. Recent work suggests that the presence of an imbalance between normally occurring intravascular coagulation and endogenous fibrinolysis may be an important factor in the etiology of atherosclerosis; the absence of fibrinolytic activity may be an important contributing factor in arterial graft thrombosis; changes in blood viscosity have also been shown to be a significant etiological factor in lower-extremity vascular insufficiency. These factors, as well as the growing complexity of surgery and the increasing awareness of the occurrence of acquired coagulation defects before and during operative procedures, have made the monitoring of coagulation dynamics a necessary part of a patient's overall vascular work-up.

The technique of thromboelastography provides a measurement of dynamic changes in viscosity and elastic properties of a blood clot and gives a permanent graphic documentation, the thromboelastogram, of the various phases of the blood coagulation process from the formation of the first fibrin strands to the fibrinolytic dissolution of the clot. The instrumentation available allows the separate analysis of several blood samples simultaneously.

Thromboelastography is more sensitive to qualitative defects in fibrin or platelets than are standard clotting time techniques. Data obtained using the technique of thromboelastography are difficult to relate to data obtained using standard methods. Standard clotting techniques end with the formation of the first fibrin strand, while thromboelastography begins at this point and continues to generate data as clotting continues, ending at fibrinolytic dissolution of the clot.

INSTRUMENTATION

There are two types of thromboelastographic instruments available. One works through a mechanical-optical system using light-sensitive film, which must be developed to obtain the thromboelastogram, and the other is a direct-writing instrument with a stylus that traces the thromboelastogram on heat-sensitive paper. The obvious advantage of the direct-writing instrument is the immediate availability of the thromboelastogram. An advantage of the mechanical-optical instrument is that it allows simultaneous analysis of three samples at a time, whereas the direct-writing instrument has the capability of analyzing only two samples at a time. In our laboratory we routinely use both types of instrumentation and find them to be of equal value.

MECHANICAL-OPTICAL SYSTEM

With the mechanical-optical thromboelastograph, a single light-tight housing contains the thromboelastograph and a kymograph-like unit containing the light-sensitive film. The presence of adjustable legs allows for perfect balancing. As the thromboelastograph is running, a light source produces a beam of light that reflects off a series of mirrors to expose the light-sensitive film as well as being deflected to the upper portion of the instrument for a visual estimation of the measurements of the thromboelastogram. Three cuvette systems are located on the front of the machine (Fig. 7-1). Blood is introduced into the cuvette and a stainless steel piston attached to a torsion wire containing a mirror is lowered into the cuvette containing the sample. The cuvette rotates through a constant angle. The metal "wings" located on the torsion wire below the mirror dip into a cup of paraffin oil as the piston is lowered into the cuvette and function in stabilizing the torsion wire and to protect it from any extraneous vibrations. The piston does not move as the cuvette rotates during the initial liquid phase of the coagulation process, giving a straight line on the thromboelastogram. As fibrin strands begin to form, they attach to the piston, which then begins to rotate with the cuvette. This causes the mirror attached to the torsion wire to deflect the light and the light-sensitive film begins to show a divergence of the

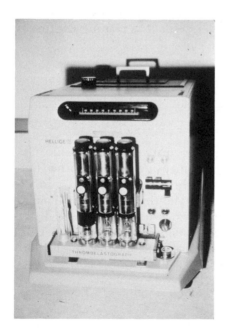

FIGURE 7-1.   The mechanical-optical thromboelastograph.

original straight line into two curved lines corresponding to the oscillations of the cuvette (Fig. 7-2). As the clot begins to "age," the fibrinolytic process begins and the divergent lines again come together, giving a straight line when the clot is completely lysed. The detection of fibrinolysis shall be discussed under "Clinical Applications."

DIRECT-WRITING SYSTEM

With the direct-writing instrument, the oscillations of the cuvette are transferred to a stylus rather than through a series of reflective mirrors. The stylus then prints out the thromboelastogram directly (Fig. 7-3). As mentioned above, with the direct-writing system, the thromboelastogram is immediately available; however, only two samples of blood can be analyzed at one time. The thromboelastograms obtained from either instrument are identical. In comparing the direct-writing instrument with the mechanical-optical instrument, one will note that with the direct-writing, the cuvette system is housed within the instrument itself and the kymograph-like portion of the mechanical-optical instrument is absent.

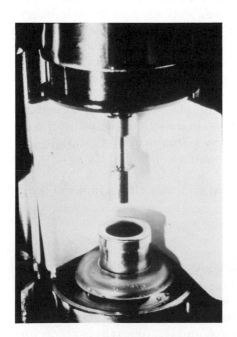

FIGURE 7-2. Close-up view of cuvette and piston of mechanical-optical thromboelastograph.

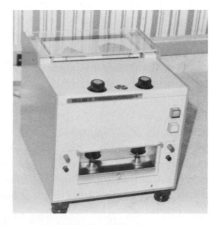

FIGURE 7-3. The direct-writing thromboelastograph.

PROCEDURE

Two slightly different techniques may be used with the thromboelasto-graph; one will be referred to as native whole blood thromboelastog-raphy and the other, celite-activated thromboelastography, which in-volves a simultaneous comparison of native and celite-activated blood samples. The procedures for each technique will be described in this section and the analysis and interpretation of each technique will be discussed under "Analysis of Results."

NATIVE WHOLE BLOOD THROMBOELASTOGRAPHY

1. The patient's arm is prepared in the usual way for drawing blood, the vein is stuck cleanly with a 22-gauge needle attached to a 5 cc plastic syringe. The tip of the needle should be approximately in the center of the lumen of the vein.
2. Withdraw approximately 3 cc of blood smoothly and evenly to pre-vent the formation of air bubbles. Start a stop watch as the first drop of blood enters the syringe. The time from the initial draw of blood to starting the thromboelastograph should be no longer than 3 minutes.
3. From the syringe, fill the cuvette with blood allowing sufficient space so placement of the piston and oil will not cause overflow of blood from the cuvette.
4. Lower the piston into the sample and place an adequate amount of mineral oil on top of the sample of blood in the cuvette, being careful not to cause overflow and not to touch the piston or the suspension wire.
5. Start the thromboelastograph to initiate oscillation of the cuvette and advance the photographic film.
6. Put dust cover in place. An adequate thromboelastogram will be ob-tained in about two hours.

CELITE-ACTIVATED THROMBOELASTOGRAPHY

When obtaining a blood sample for celite-activated thromboelastog-raphy, it is important that the sample not be "activated" before being placed in the cuvette. Syringes, pipettes, and test tubes should therefore be of a nonactivating material such as polypropylene. Using this precau-tion, any activation of the sample will therefore be due to the addition of the celite. The blood sample must be drawn quickly (within 30 seconds) but evenly so as not to cause bubbling and unnecessary turbulence.

1. With the patient's arm prepared in the usual way for drawing blood, the vein is stuck cleanly using a 19-gauge twin-flow butterfly infusion set. The needle is threaded into the vein to the needle's hub and blood flow through the catheter should be smooth and even. (If the vein is not stuck cleanly and/or blood flow through the catheter is not smooth and even, the procedure should be ended at this point and an attempt should be made to obtain a blood sample from the other arm.)

2. Discard the first 7 ml of blood to remove any tissue contaminants.

3. After checking the polypropylene syringe to make sure it contains no air, attach it to the catheter with a simple twisting motion.

4. When the first drop of blood enters the syringe a stopwatch is started. Four minutes is allowed from the initial draw to placing the sample into the cuvette.

5. With an even pressure and within approximately 30 seconds, draw 3 ml of blood into the polypropylene syringe. (If other hematological tests are required, the additional blood required for these tests may be drawn at this time.)

6. When an adequate blood sample has been obtained, remove the tourniquet and then the needle and apply a pressure bandage.

7. Remove the syringe from the catheter and place the sample (approximately 3 ml) into a polypropylene test tube, allowing the blood sample to drip down the side of the container.

8. After prewetting the pipette tip with the sample, place 360 µl into one cuvette.

9. In a second cuvette, add 330 µl of blood and 30 µl of freshly mixed celite.

10. Immediately move the thromboelastograph piston up and down three to four times in both cuvettes to ensure adequate mixing of both samples.

11. Start the machine to initiate the oscillation of the cuvette and the running of the paper.

12. Place an adequate amount of mineral oil on top of the samples of blood in the cuvette, being sure not to touch the blood or the piston wire.

13. Put the dust cover in place. An adequate thromboelastogram will be obtained in approximately 2 hours. (The placement of the oil on the blood sample and the dust cover over the cuvette unit shield the blood sample from environmental influences, e.g., the oil avoids a blood–air interface and the dust cover prevents movement of the piston by air currents.)

ANALYSIS OF RESULTS

MEASURING THE THROMBOELASTOGRAM

The first value determined is *r time* or *reaction time* in minutes (30 seconds = 1 mm). This is the initial straight line portion of the thromboelastogram and represents the time from the initial draw of the blood to the formation of the first fibrin strands. During this phase of the coagulation process, the piston offers no resistance to movement of the cuvette and therefore no oscillations are seen in the thromboelastogram. The r time is highly sensitive to thromboplastin procoagulants and is representative of the sample's intrinsic clotting. A normal r time is eight to 12 minutes or 16 to 24 mm.

The second value obtained is the *k value*, which is the period of time from initiation of the clot (the end of the r time) to a defined level of clot strength, i.e., where the diverging curved lines are 20 mm apart. The beginning of this interval is taken as the point where the curved lines are 1 mm apart. The k value is sometimes referred to as the *clot formation time* as it is a measure of the rapidity of clot development. A normal k value is 4 to 8 minutes, or 8 to 16 mm.

The final measurement of the native whole blood thromboelastogram is the *ma value* or *maximum amplitude*. This value is taken as the maximum distance between the two diverging lines. This value is a direct function of the maximum dynamic properties of fibrin and platelets and is representative of the final clot stiffness or strength. A normal ma value is approximately 50 mm (Figs. 7-4 through 7-6).

The parameters measured in evaluating the celite-activated thromboelastogram are slightly different from those enumerated above for the native whole blood thromboelastogram in that all measurements in celite-activated analysis are taken in millimeters and there is an additional parameter, the angle. Recall that celite-activated analysis involves a comparison between two simultaneous tracings from the same blood sample, one a normal thromboelastographic tracing and one a celite-activated tracing. The measurements of the two tracings are made in similar fashion and shall not be differentiated in the description to follow, save for the addition of the letter C for parameters from the celite thromboelastogram, e.g., reaction time for the native = R while the reaction time for celite = RC. Parameters from celite-activated thromboelastography are differentiated from normal whole blood thromboelastography in being designated with upper-case letters, e.g., normal whole blood maximum amplitude = ma, celite-activated maximum amplitude = Ma and MaC (Fig. 7-7).

As with native whole blood thromboelastography, the first values ob-

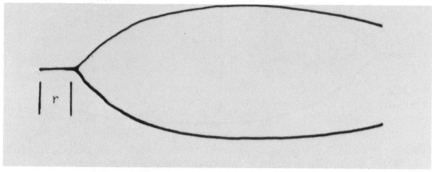

r = reaction time (8 − 12 minutes) − the period of
    latency from blood withdrawal until the clot
    begins to form. This value represents intrinsic
    clotting and is very sensitive to thromboplastin
    procoagulants.

FIGURE 7-4.   Typical native whole blood thromboelastogram showing the measurement and significance of the r value.

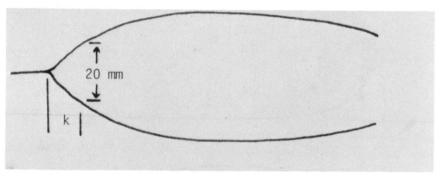

k = a measure of the rapidity of clot development and
    is the period of time from initiation of the clot
    to a defined level of clot strength.
    (4 − 8 minutes)

FIGURE 7-5.   Typical native whole blood thromboelastogram showing the measurement and significance of the k time.

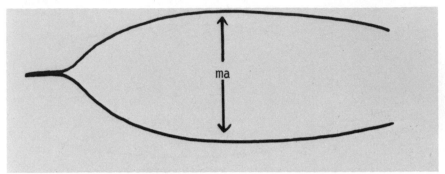

ma = maximum amplitude (approximately 50 mm) — This measurement is a direct function of the maximum dynamic properties of fibrin and platelets.

FIGURE 7-6. Typical native whole blood thromboelastogram showing the measurement and significance of the ma value.

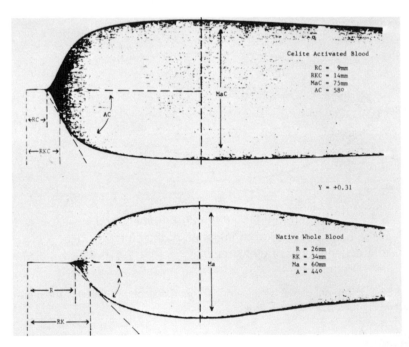

FIGURE 7-7. The technique for measuring the parameters used in evaluating the celite-activated thromboelastograph.

tained are the R and RC values. These values in millimeters are taken as the distance from the initial mark of the tracing to the point where there is a 2-mm deflection of the lines. All measurements are made from the inside of one line to the outside of the other line. With celite-activated thromboelastography, a range of normal values is really not required as the measurements obtained from two simultaneous tracings are placed into an equation that yields a *Y value,* which is the important parameter. Determination of the Y value shall be discussed in the following section.

The next values obtained are the *RK* and *RKC* values. These values are taken as the distance from the initial mark of the tracing to the point where the diverging lines are 20 mm apart. In reality, this value is an addition of the r and k values of the native whole blood thromboelastograph.

As with a native whole blood thromboelastogram the *Ma* and *MaC* values are taken as the maximum distance in millimeters between the two diverging curved lines.

The additional parameter measured in celite-activated thromboelastography is the angle, designated as *A* and *AC*. To determine the angle, a line is drawn through the reaction time straight line portion of the tracing so that it bisects a perpendicular line drawn at the point of maximum amplitude. A second line is drawn from the point at which a deflection is first noted (toward the end of the reaction time) tangent to the thromboelastogram curve. The angle formed by these two lines is measured in degrees and is taken as A and AC. The angle is indicative of the rate of clot stiffening and reflects the rate and quality of developing fibrin and platelet aggregates.

ANALYSIS OF MEASUREMENTS

The measurements obtained from a native whole blood thromboelastogram (r, k, ma) are of value without further analysis. The measurements obtained from celite-activated thromboelastography (R, RK, Ma, A, RC, RKC, MaC, AC) require further analysis before their true value is apparent. The parameters obtained from celite-activated thromboelastography have been subjected to discriminate analysis (see the work by Caprini in Selected References). From this analysis, a series of coefficients, A_1 to A_9, was obtained and assigned to each parameter allowing a maximum differentiation between two populations. The result is a linear combination of the parameters (Fig. 7-8). The value obtained by placing the parameters into the equation and carrying out the necessary multiplications, additions, and subtractions is referred to as the *Y value* and is a measure of the patient's reserve clotting potential. The interpretation of this value as it relates to the patient's status of coagulability is given in the following section.

Y = Reserve Clotting Potential

$$Y = A_1 + A_2R + A_3RK + A_4Ma + A_5A + A_6RC + A_7RKC + A_8MaC + A_9AC$$

$$A_1 = -55.55 \qquad\qquad A_6 = -2.088$$
$$A_2 = +\ 0.386 \qquad\qquad A_7 = +1.966$$
$$A_3 = -\ 0.508 \qquad\qquad A_8 = +0.17321$$
$$A_4 = -\ 0.03816 \qquad\quad A_9 = +0.877$$
$$A_5 = -\ 0.1639$$

Normal Range $= -5 \leq Y \leq +1.5$

FIGURE 7-8.   Equation used in the calculation of the Y value—the reserve clotting potential—in the celite-activated thromboelastograph.

INTERPRETATION OF RESULTS

With native whole blood thromboelastography, the characteristics typical of hypercoagulability are a shortened r time and k value and an increased ma. Such values indicate a rapidly forming clot that attains a high degree of stiffness. In a hypocoagulable state, such as during heparin therapy, the thromboelastogram is characterized by a prolonged r time and k value and a decreased ma indicative of a slow clotting process that produces a clot with a relatively low degree of stiffness. Indicative of thrombocytopenia are a normal r time, slightly prolonged k value, and decreased ma with the thromboelastogram showing a characteristically thin spindle shape (Fig. 7-9). In patients with extreme thrombocytopenia, there is also a prolongation of the r time due to a minimal amount of platelet factors available to enter into the reaction. With hemophilia, the thromboelastogram is characterized by a markedly prolonged r time and k value and a normal ma. The degree of prolongation of the r time and k value would vary with the severity of the hemophilia. The prolonged r time and k value are indicative of a slowed formation of thromboplastin, thrombin, and fibrin. In the patient with extreme thrombocytopenia, the prolonged r time and k value may be similar to values obtained with hemophilia. In such patients, the distinguishing factor is the ma value, which is relatively normal in hemophilia but decreased in thrombocytopenia.

As mentioned previously, with celite-activated thromboelastography, the important parameter is the Y value obtained from the equation presented in the preceding section (Fig. 7-8). A Y value between -5 and $+1.5$ is considered to be within normal range. Y values greater than $+2$ are considered hypercoagulable and correspond with the reduced r time and k value and increased ma obtained with native whole blood thrombo-

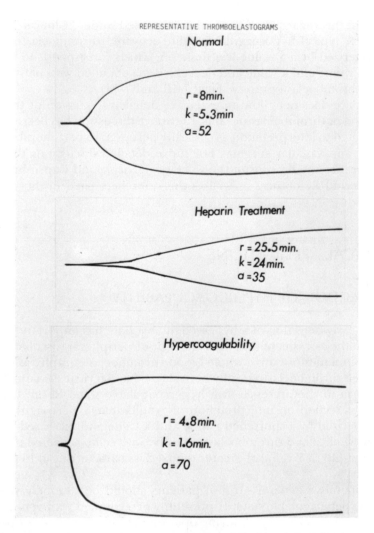

REPRESENTATIVE THROMBOELASTOGRAMS

Normal

r = 8min.
k = 5.3min
a = 52

Heparin Treatment

r = 25.5min.
k = 24min.
a = 35

Hypercoagulability

r = 4.8min.
k = 1.6min.
a = 70

FIGURE 7-9.   Representative tracings in native whole blood thromboelastography showing a normal (upper trace), one representative of heparin effect (middle trace) characterized by a prolonged r and k values and reduced ma, and one demonstrating hypercoagulability (lower trace) characterized by shortened r and k values and a large ma.

elastography. Patients found to be hypercoagulable with Y values greater than +6 indicate the need for prophylactic therapy when clinically indicated. In such patients, if heparin is instituted, a Y value ranging from −7 to −10 is indicative of a good heparin response. The use of native whole blood thromboelastography and celite-activated thromboelastography in this regard shall be further discussed under "Clinical Applications." A typical hypocoagulable celite-activated thromboelastogram is characterized by a Y value less than −5, which corresponds to the prolonged r time and k value and decreased ma obtained with native whole blood thromboelastography (Figs. 7-10 and 7-11).

As space does not allow an extensive detailed discussion of the interpretation of thromboelastograms, the above discussion has been more or less limited to interpretation as clinically pertinent to peripheral vascular disease and vascular surgery. For more detailed discussions the interested reader should consult the work of deNicola and Caprini noted in the Selected References as well as the references cited in those works.

CLINICAL APPLICATIONS

DETECTION OF HYPERCOAGULABILITY

The early detection of a hypercoagulable state has important implications in the assessment and management of peripheral vascular disease. The techniques of native whole blood thromboelastography and celite-activated thromboelastography both show characteristic deviations from the norm in the presence of a hypercoagulable state. Recall from the previous section on interpretation of results that hypercoagulability is characterized by a shortened r time and k value and increased ma with native whole blood thromboelastography; with celite-activated thromboelastography, a Y value of greater than +2 is characteristic of hypercoagulability.

Preoperative general surgical patients should be routinely screened for a hypercoagulable state. If present, when coupled with venous stasis and vein trauma incurred during operation, it may lead to postoperative deep venous thrombosis. Prophylactic measures for the prevention of venous thromboembolism may be advisable. Similarly, with medical patients confined to an extended bed rest program for any variety of reasons, the detection of a hypercoagulable state again demonstrates the patient to be at particularly high risk for deep vein thrombosis. Such early detection of factors predisposing a patient to deep venous thrombosis allows prompt institution of prophylactic measures avoiding the morbidity associated with venous thromboembolism.

The detection of hypercoagulability is also of importance in the evaluation of the patient with peripheral arterial disease. As mentioned in the introduction to this chapter, the absence of fibrinolytic activity may be an important contributory factor in the early failure of arterial bypasses.

Normal Range	:	Y value between −5 and +1.5
Hypercoagulable	:	Y value greater than +2
Requires Heparin	:	Y value greater than +6
Hypocoagulable	:	Y value less than −5
Heparin Response	:	Y value between −7 and −10

FIGURE 7-10.   The range of Y values obtained in celite-activated thromboelastography and their significance.

This possibility coupled with a hypercoagulable state would place a patient at considerable risk for early graft failure, necessitating reoperation. With the foreknowledge that a patient is hypercoagulable, the surgeon can modify the standard dosage of heparin given intraoperatively to maintain effective anticoagulation during vascular surgery, as well as possibly maintain the patient on anticoagulants during the immediate postoperative period to aid in maintaining patency of the graft. As an example, a patient was scheduled for a myocutaneous microvascular free-flap transfer to the right lower leg using the right tensor fascia lata with anastomosis of the lateral circumflex femoral artery and vein to the

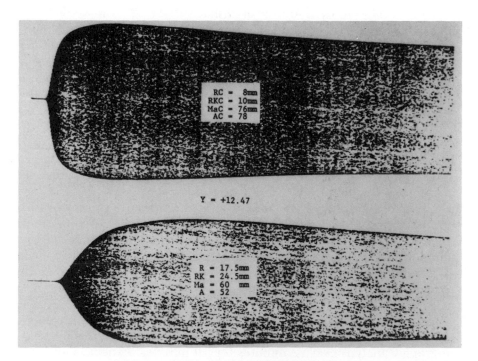

FIGURE 7-11.   Celite-activated thromboelastography showing the detection of hypercoagulability, i.e., a Y value in excess of +2.

peroneal artery and vein, an anastomosis of vessels approximately 2 mm in diameter. The patient's preoperative thromboelastogram showed hypercoagulability with a Y value of approximately +5. Following the free-flap transfer, the patency of the microvascular anastomosis was maintained with the aid of heparin administration, which maintained the patient's Y value within normal range during the critical immediate postoperative period. Several months later the patient showed excellent healing of the flap.

HEPARIN MONITORING

Considerable controversy remains as to the most advantageous mode of heparin administration for therapeutic effect, the most effective system for monitoring its effect and also as to whether heparin administration needs to be monitored at all. The technique of thromboelastography is a most effective means of monitoring the patient's response to heparin when administered in therapeutic doses, intraoperatively or prophylactically.

Therapeutic Heparin Administration

The thromboelastograph has been found to be quite useful in monitoring patient response to therapeutic heparin administration. Using native whole blood thromboelastography, therapeutic heparin dosage is adjusted on the basis of the r time—a good therapeutic heparin response is indicated by the patient's r time being prolonged to 1.5 to 2 times the normal value for that patient (Fig. 7-12). The patient is maintained on heparin for 10 full days and is monitored daily using thromboelastography. Usually, a single drawing of blood in the morning is sufficient to monitor the patient's response; however, if the heparin dosage requires alteration to bring the patient within the therapeutic range, an additional thromboelastogram is done in the afternoon.

Using this technique to monitor heparin therapy, thromboelastographic analysis has shown continuous infusion via an intravenous pump to produce a much smoother heparin response than drip or intermittent administration (Tables 7-1, 7-2, and 7-3). Using continuous infusion via a pump frequently leads to less heparin being required to maintain the patient within therapeutic range.

A patient's sensitivity to heparin administration can also be evaluated using native whole blood thromboelastography. Following intravenous administration of 1000 units of heparin, blood is drawn for thromboelastographic analysis every 2 minutes for 10 minutes. Patients showing a good sensitivity to heparin show a peak prolongation of the r time after

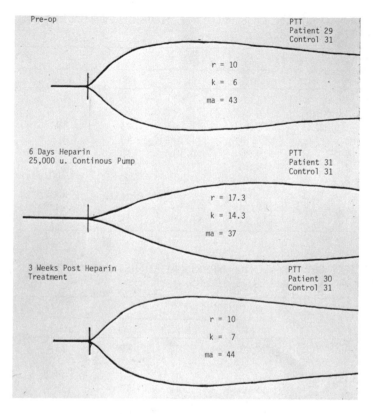

FIGURE 7-12. Native whole blood thromboelastography showing a good therapeutic heparin response—an r value that is approximately two times the patient's baseline value.

TABLE 7-1. CONTINUOUS INFUSION HEPARIN ADMINISTRATION (24,000 UNITS PER 24 HOURS).

Drip Administration			Pump Administration		
r	k	ma	r	k	ma
13.00	7.00	48	15.15	9.00	45
12.40	7.00	53	17.30	9.00	44
13.15	6.00	52	16.00	12.00	46
11.00	6.00	50	17.10	11.30	49
13.20	6.00	50	16.50	11.30	51
14.00	12.00	52	17.30	7.30	50
15.00	7.30	48			

TABLE 7-2. CONTINUOUS INFUSION HEPARIN ADMINISTRATION (24,000 UNITS PER 24 HOURS).

	TEG			PTT	
	r	k	ma	Patient	Control
Baseline	12.00	7.30	48	36	32
Days on Heparin					
1	16.30	11.00	43	32	32
3	17.00	11.30	43	35	31
4	20.00	16.30	38	47	31
7	19.00	11.30	41	38	32
8	14.40	9.00	46	29	31
9	15.00	9.00	47	43	31
10	22.30	19.30	44	43	31
11	20.30	16.00	45	61	30

TABLE 7-3. PROPHYLACTIC HEPARIN ADMINISTRATION (5,000 UNITS SUBCUTANEOUSLY EVERY 8 HOURS).

	TEG			PTT	
	r	k	ma	Patient	Control
Baseline	4.45	2.00	72	25	32
Days on Heparin					
1	90.15	73.30	44	44	28
2	55.00	51.00	57	37	30
3	47.40	41.30	60	38	31
4	73.10	34.00	63	36	32
8	72.00	49.30	60	57	30
9	37.15	28.00	52	52	30
10	68.20	30.30	63	38	27
11	46.50	21.30	50	36	27

2 to 4 minutes; patients resistant to heparin would show a peak prolongation of the r time later than 5 minutes after the heparin administration (Table 7-4).

With celite-activated thromboelastography, the schedule for monitoring heparin response is similar to that discussed above for native whole blood thromboelastography. With the celite-activated technique, the patient's heparin response is determined by the Y value—a good heparin response is a Y value in the range of -7 to -10.

The patient's heparin dosage is determined on the basis of his weight. An initial loading dose is given to the patient in the amount of 70 units/kg. His maintenance dosage is then administered via a constant infusion pump in the amount of 14.2 units/kg/hour times 24 hours. Daily

TABLE 7-4.   HEPARIN SENSITIVITY.

Minutes After Injection of 1000μ Heparin	Platelet Count	Fibrinogen	TEG		
			r	k	ma
0	310	0.32	15.20	8.30	42
2	—	—	26.45	34.30	28
4	197	—.	20.15	22.00	35
6	—	—	19.20	15.30	34
8	—	—	19.05	15.30	36
10	199	0.36	19.00	12.30	36

thromboelastographic analysis is then used to either increase or decrease the maintenance dosage until therapeutic range is obtained.

Intraoperative Heparin Administration

During vascular reconstructive procedures, heparin is routinely administered for purposes of anticoagulation in the dosage of 70 units/kg. Many centers do not monitor this administration of heparin; however, we have found native whole blood thromboelastography to be invaluable in monitoring the patient's response to the heparin, providing information as to when the patient's coagulation dynamics have returned to normal. Following the administration of the heparin, blood is drawn every 45 to 60 minutes until the patient's r time returns to normal. A good response to the heparin administration will show the r time to be prolonged to approximately 1 hour at the initial drawing 60 minutes after heparin administration. This will gradually return to normal usually by 3 hours after the heparin administration (Table 7-5). Patients very sensitive to heparin will show a greatly prolonged r time for several hours before beginning to return to baseline. A patient with such a response should be carefully monitored for bleeding complications using the thromboelastograph. We have not encountered any bleeding complications using the thromboelastograph, and have not needed to reverse the heparin effect. Patients resistant to heparin administration will not show a prolonged r time and would require additional heparin administration to maintain adequate anticoagulation (Table 7-6).

DETECTION OF FIBRINOLYSIS

The decrease in the distance between the two diverging lines of the thromboelastograph following the maximum amplitude is indicative of fibrinolysis. To quantify the percent fibrinolysis, one measures the max-

TABLE 7-5.   INTRAOPERATIVE MONITORING OF HEPARIN WITH
THROMBOELASTOGRAPHY. (GOOD RESPONSE.)

	r	k	ma
Pre-Heparin	9.5	6.3	60
Post-Heparin			
(5,000 units IV)			
2 minutes	>5 hours	—	—
7 minutes	>4 hours	—	—
30 minutes	>4 hours	—	—
1 hour	67.00	117.00	>28
2 hours	24.00	30.30	41
3 hours	12.00	7.30	55

TABLE 7-6.   INTRAOPERATIVE MONITORING OF HEPARIN WITH
THROMBOELASTOGRAPHY. (POOR RESPONSE.)

	r	k	ma
Pre-Heparin	7.40	2.00	58
Post-Heparin			
(5,000 units IV)			
60 minutes	19.00	12.00	36
120 minutes	11.30	8.30	39
(+5,000 units IV)			
45 minutes	50.00	>100.00	17
90 minutes	28.00	28.00	24
180 minutes	3.00	18.00	28

imum amplitude and then measures the amplitude at four 10-millimeter
intervals after the maximum amplitude to obtain values for a_1, a_2, a_3, and
a_4. These values are then analyzed to determine the percent fibrinolysis
(Fig. 7-13). A value of zero to five percent fibrinolysis is considered
normal. Values above this range are indicative of increased fibrinolytic
activity.

MONITORING INTERMITTENT
PNEUMATIC COMPRESSION

Attempts to prevent deep venous thrombosis have taken many directions. Considerable attention has been paid to chemical modes of prevention (e.g., low-dose heparin, aspirin, dextran). These have been the
subject of many reports of conflicting views as to the efficacy of their use.
Most physical measures such as leg elevation, early ambulation, and

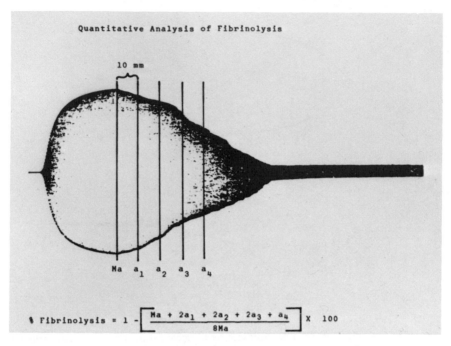

FIGURE 7-13.   Representation of the method for evaluating a thromboelastogram to obtain a quantitative measure of fibrinolytic activity.

passive exercise have not been found to be very effective. For some time now, we have used external intermittent pneumatic compression for prevention of postoperative deep venous thrombosis and have had excellent results (zero percent incidence of DVT in over 400 general and orthopedic surgical patients who have remained on the system until fully ambulatory). The beneficial effect of physically "pumping" blood out of the lower extremity by intermittently compressing the peripheral venous heart of the calf muscle has been adequately demonstrated. We routinely monitor all patients using external intermittent pneumatic compression with thromboelastography and have seen a qualitative enhancement of fibrinolytic activity in a significant number of patients (Fig. 7-14). Recently, a selected group of patients has been monitored with thromboelastography before and after two hours' external intermittent pneumatic compression applied to one arm. Euglobulin lysis time and fibrin degradation products analysis were also carried out. The results obtained demonstrated a marked enhancement in fibrinolytic activity in a significant number of patients that was not detectable using euglobulin

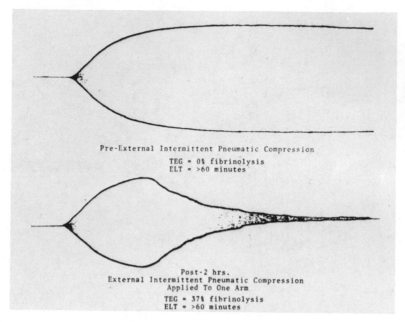

Pre-External Intermittent Pneumatic Compression
TEG = 0% fibrinolysis
ELT = >60 minutes

Post-2 hrs.
External Intermittent Pneumatic Compression
Applied To One Arm
TEG = 37% fibrinolysis
ELT = >60 minutes

FIGURE 7-14.   Use of thromboelastography to demonstrate the fibrinolytic effect of external intermittent pneumatic compression. Following application of external intermittent pneumatic compression to one arm for only 2 hours, this patient's thromboelastograph shows enhanced fibrinolytic activity.

lysis time or fibrin degradation products. The work adequately demonstrates external intermittent pneumatic compression to have a biochemical effect by stimulating the naturally occurring fibrinolytic activity of the vein wall in addition to its physical effect of "pumping" the blood out of the leg and shows thromboelastography to be more sensitive to the presence of fibrinolytic activity than standard hematological tests such as euglobulin lysis time and fibrin degradation products.

CHAPTER 8

RISK FACTORS IN ATHEROSCLEROSIS

INTRODUCTION
PATHOLOGY OF ATHEROSCLEROTIC LESIONS
THEORIES OF ATHEROSCLEROTIC PATHOGENESIS
UNMODIFIABLE RISK FACTORS
MODIFIABLE RISK FACTORS
- Environmental Factors
- Physiologic Factors

INTRODUCTION

The premature development of atherosclerosis has a demonstrated association with factors that place the individual at high risk. For convenience, these factors may be broadly classified into three categories: genetic factors, environmental factors, and physiologic factors. Genetic factors are those risk factors that cannot be modified and would include the individual's age, sex, and family history. Environmental factors are those risk factors tht are subject to modification and can be eliminated or at least controlled. Such factors would include smoking, the use of oral contraceptives, and exercise. Physiologic factors are those risk factors that can be brought under control and would include hyperlipidemia, hypertension, diabetes mellitus, obesity, and stress.

The control of atherosclerosis is possible only by prevention, i.e., the identification of the specific risk factors that are operant in the individual and the control or elimination of those factors where possible. Such a program for prevention is both beneficial and feasible.

This chapter reviews each risk factor and the interaction of these risk factors in the development of the artherosclerotic process. The pathology and pathogenesis of the atherosclerotic process are discussed briefly.

Although mention may be made of possible modes for altering these factors, the clinician is referred to more definitive works as suggested in the Selected References.

PATHOLOGY OF ATHEROSCLEROTIC LESIONS

The atherosclerotic lesion is considered to be a change in the intimal layer of the arterial wall due to the abnormal excess accumulation, in variable proportions, of lipids, complex carbohydrates, blood and blood products, fibrous tissue, and calcium deposits. Such changes in the intimal layer are associated with changes in the medial layer of the arterial wall as well. A typical atherosclerotic lesion is initially a yellow/yellowish-gray fatty streak developing in the arterial wall intima. This fatty streak may then progress to a firm fibrous plaque that is characteristically gray to pearly white. This stage may be subsequently transformed to an atheromatous plaque that shows fatty softening. Finally, a complicated lesion may form with thrombus formation, ulceration, hemorrhage, or calcareous deposits. It should be mentioned that this stepwise progression does not occur universally; not every fatty streak progresses to an atheromatous plaque.

Histologically, The World Health Organization in its report on atherosclerotic lesions (Technical Report Series #143) has listed eight abnormalities that are seen during the development of an atherosclerotic lesion: (1) the deposit consists of various lipids, primarily cholesterol and cholesterol esters with phospholipids and triglycerides. These lipid deposits may be seen intracellularly as foam cells (altered smooth muscle cells) or extracellularly in the arterial intima and inner media. (2) Fibroplasia may be present and the plaque may become amorphous in parts. The fibroplasia is in the form of reticulin, collagen fibers, mucopolysaccharides, and hyalin and may be confined to the subendothelial region of the intima. (3) The intimal surface may have a fibrin-like film attached or it may have a covering of endothelium. (4) The thickness of the intimal layer may be increased due to the accumulation of complex carbohydrates. (5) There may be calcification in the area of the lipid deposit. This calcification may be noticeable on plain x-rays. (6) There may be changes in the medial layer of the artery, e.g., smooth muscle fiber disintegration. (7) Amorphous glycoprotein or crystals of cholesterol may be seen. (8) Endothelial loss from the surface of the plaque results in the formation of mural thrombi, hemorrhage, or ulceration.

The atherosclerotic process is usually diffuse in nature, but there is a tendency for the more extensive plaque to be localized, causing segmental occlusion of a major artery, thus making surgical intervention feasible in most cases. The opposite occurrence, that of numerous diffuse lesions in small arteries, does not lend itself to surgical intervention. The formation of plaque may interfere with the nutritive blood flow to the vessel and this may lead to softening rather than "hardening" of the artery. At a point, the plaque become self-perpetuating in that the turbulence and pressure that occur secondary to the original plaque formation contribute to secondary plaque formation.

THEORIES OF ATHEROSCLEROTIC PATHOGENESIS

A number of theories as to the pathogenesis of atherosclerotic lesions have been hypothesized and been extensively discussed in the literature. It appears that no single theory accounts for the entire pathogenic process but rather the theories interact with each other and contribute different factors at various stages of the disease process.

The *lipid infiltration theory* was first postulated by Virchow in 1862. The thinking today is that ultramicroscopic gaps in the arterial endothelium allow for the filtration and accumulation of certain elements from the serum in the arterial wall. Such elements would include the low-density and very-low density lipoproteins (see "Hyperlipidemia," under "Physiologic Factors"). This process appears to be continuous and not a matter of simple mechanical filtration. These lipoproteins accumulate inside and outside of the smooth muscle cells of the artery. When there is an abnormally high accumulation of these lipoproteins, the system for their metabolism becomes saturated, allowing for further lipoprotein accumulation. The accumulation of the metabolites damages the smooth muscle cells, stimulating cellular division and ultimately leading to a fibrocalcific reaction. Concentration of cholesterol will also yield a fibrocalcific reaction. The effects of smoking seem to operate in accordance with this theory, as the carbon monoxide in smoke increases the carboxyhemoglobin levels and leads to local hypoxia which, in turn, alters the permeability of the artery. Additionally carbon monoxide may inhibit cytochrome oxidase. Nicotine, another component of cigarette smoke, may impair oxidative enzymes in the arterial wall. Hypertension may also influence this theory in providing for a higher filtration pressure.

The *thrombogenic theory* of atherosclerosis was initially postulated as the *encrustation theory* by Rokitansky in 1852. With this theory, microthrombi composed of fibrin, platelets, serum lipids, and red blood cells are formed on the arterial endothelial surface and become incorporated into the intima. Recent studies favor the role of platelet aggregates in this theory. The possibility of increased platelet adhesiveness and inhibition of fibrinolysis by hyperlipidemia adds support to this idea.

The importance of vascular hemodynamics is contained in the *vascular dynamic theory* of atherogenesis. Support for the importance of hemodynamics comes from the preference of atherosclerotic plaque formation for regions of arterial branching. Other important factors would include turbulent flow and eddy currents, wave reflection, and viscous drag. Blood pressure may increase the possibility of plaque formation in cooperation with the lipid infiltration theory by increasing intraluminal filtration pressure and possibly altering the vessels' permeability to lipoproteins. Hemodynamic factors may additionally affect the intimal surface in a fashion that would predispose to microthrombi formation in agreement with the thrombogenic theory. Areas of hypotension may also predispose to plaque formation due to a decrease in lateral or hydrostatic pressure, which may yield intimal thickening, altered vessel permeability, or microthrombi formation.

The *capillary hemorrhage theory* as postulated by Winternitz in 1938 states that the lipids in atherosclerotic lesions are secondary to rupture of capillaries in the lumen or vasa vasorun of the vessel. This theory may have importance in the additional accumlation of lipids and fibrosis following the initial formation of the plaque.

Each of the above theories of atherosclerotic pathogenesis appears to contribute to the overall process. The lipid infiltration theory appears to provide the best explanation for the early development of the atherosclerotic lesion. The thrombogenic theory may be the most important in the secondary progression of the lesion. The importance of hemodynamic factors in each theory is also significant.

UNMODIFIABLE RISK FACTORS

The unmodifiable risk factors in atherosclerosis include the patient's age, sex, and family history. As the development of atherosclerosis, or any disease entity, is dependent upon time, an individual's age is obviously associated with the formation of atherosclerotic lesions, although they do not always occur.

The individual's sex may be considered a risk factor as the consensus is that males are more susceptible to atherosclerosis than females. The greater susceptibility in males has variously been attributed to the protective effect of estrogen which exhibits a minor influence on α and β lipoproteins, differences in hematocrit, differences in smoking, or the fact that females may lead a more sheltered existence. There is no scientific proof lending great support to any of these factors. Interestingly though, the difference in the occurrence of angina in males and females shows a rapid convergence following menopause.

A family history of premature atherosclerosis increases an individual's susceptibility, although it does not necessarily presage development of the disease. It is not clear to what extent such a family tendency is influenced by other risk factors.

MODIFIABLE RISK FACTORS

Modifiable risk factors in the development of atherosclerosis include (1) environmental factors that can theoretically be eliminated, such as smoking, physical inactivity, oral contraceptives, and (2) physiologic factors that can be controlled, such as hyperlipidemia, hypertension, diabetes mellitus, obesity, and stress.

ENVIRONMENTAL FACTORS

Smoking

Since the Surgeon General's report on the effect of smoking on health in 1964, smoking has been established as a significant contributing factor in the development of lung cancer, bronchitis, emphysema, and atherosclerosis. Studies have shown that the younger the age group, the higher the incidence of atherosclerosis among smokers. The youngest men smoking two or more packs of cigarettes per day have been found to be at the highest risk. When smoking is combined with other risk factors, the incidence of atherosclerosis is futher increased. Pipe or cigar smokers have a lower incidence of atherosclerosis than cigarette smokers, with a mortality rate that is almost as low as that for nonsmokers. If, however, the pipe or cigar smoke is inhaled, the mortality rate is about equal to that for cigarette smokers.

The extent of an atherosclerotic lesion appears to be directly proportional to the amount of smoking; additionally, hyaline thickening of the coronary arterioles appears to be unique in cigarette smokers.

Nicotine and carbon monoxide are the two components of tobacco smoke that have the most important effects on the cardiovascular sytem. The principal actions of nicotine are through adrenergic stimulation. Within approximately ten minutes following a cigarette, there is an increase in norepinephrine and epinephrine plasma levels. Even more quickly, there is an acceleration of the pulse rate, an increase in blood pressure, and a diffuse vasoconstriction. Additionally, nicotine increases the adherence of platelets and precipitates a sudden elevation in circulating free fatty acids.

Carbon monoxide's primary effects are the development of a functional anemia through a displacement of oxygen from hemoglobin and the development of local tissue hypoxia by causing a shift in the oxygen-hemoglobin dissociation curve to the left, increasing the affinity of hemoglobin for oxygen. In a patient with a circulatory system already compromised by atherosclerosis, the carbon monoxide in cigarette smoke further reduces the delivery of oxygen to tissues, thus effectively increasing the risk of severe ischemia. Such local tissue hypoxia may become chronic, causing polycythemia, whose increased thrombogenicity when combined with nicotine's increase in platelet adherence further compounds the harmful effects of cigarette smoking. Carbon monoxide is postulated to increase the permeability of the arterial wall by the formation of areas of relative anoxia. Additionally, carboxyhemoglobin disrupts the hepatic clearance of the cholesterol risk products formed by the breakdown of chylomicrons and very-low-density lipids which, if not cleared by the liver, are easily absorbed into the smooth muscle cells that comprise the wall of the arteries. The monitoring of the patient's carboxyhemoglobin level can provide more accurate information about the patient's smoking habits than personal estimates. While patients may take up pipe or cigar smoking to avoid cigarettes, they may continue to inhale, thus maintaining the concentration of carboxyhemoglobin at a harmful level.

Once smoking is stopped, the increased pulse rate returns to normal, the skin becomes warmer as diffuse vasoconstriction is replaced, and the increased adrenergic stimulation returns to baseline. This process is relatively rapid. In the long term, the risk of mortality and morbidity from cerebrovascular accidents, myocardial infarction, and peripheral vascular disease is reduced. In studies on patients who have undergone arterial bypass procedures, a definite relationship has been shown between graft patency and cigarette smoking—patients whose grafts failed were found to have high levels of carboxyhemoglobin (normal: 0.5 to 2.0 percent). Additionally, preliminary reports on the use of computer-generated arteriographic images have shown that cessation of smoking leads directly to a regression of plaques in the femoral artery. It appears obvious that cessation of smoking may be the single most important factor in the management of the patient with atherosclerosis. It is thought that even in the presence of normal triglycerides and cholesterol levels, cigarette smoking accelerates the atherosclerotic process.

Exercise

Autopsy studies have not shown a relationship between the occurrence of atherosclerosis and the level of physical activity. What is readily apparent as regards coronary artery disease, however, is a high early mortality rate for physically inactive individuals following a first myocardial infarction. Autopsy studies have further demonstrated that physically active individuals have fewer myocardial scars and occlusions than physically inactive individuals in spite of relatively comparable atherosclerotic involvement. It appears that exercise does not prevent the development of atherosclerosis, but does function in preventing its clinical manifestations. From experimental studies involving the heart, it has been hypothesized that exercise reduces the harmful effects of an atherosclerotic plaque by promoting the development of collateral circulation. Such conclusions are readily applicable to individuals with peripheral vascular disease; the clinical manifestations of peripheral vascular disease should be reduced in the physically active individual due to increased collateral circulation.

With exercise, at the cellular level the skeletal muscle attains a greater oxygen utilizaton capacity secondary to increased size and number of mitrochondria, increased concentration of the enzymes of oxidative phosphorylation, and myoglobin. Angiography shows an enhanced arterial supply to the skeletal muscle.

Oral Contraceptives

The use of oral contraceptives has been shown to yield an increase in thromboplastin and a number of other coagulation factors in the ciculation, as well as increasing platelet aggregation. Paradoxically, estrogen in the contraceptive is thought to be the agent responsible for the increase in the thrombogenicity, even though in normal amounts estrogen may function as a protective agent against the development of atherosclerosis. Large doses of estrogen (as would be contained in contraceptives) have been experimentally demonstrated to have an inflammatory effect on atherosclerotic lesions.

The most evident vascular pathology associated with the use of oral contraceptives is the development of deep venous thrombosis; stroke and myocardial infarction are also more prevalent. Other side effects are a sometimes pronounced increase in blood pressure, and an increase in serum cholesterol and triglycerides.

PHYSIOLOGIC FACTORS

Hyperlipidemia

In the past few years, research on lipid disorders has shown a definite association between the presence of excessive amount of plasma lipids and the development of atherosclerosis. This tendency is exacerbated in modern societies by a diet high in animal fat and carbohydrates. Although one might naturally suppose that a diet low in animal fat and carbohydrates would decrease the incidence of atherosclerosis, there is no hard scientific proof that this is the case, although such a diet will reduce the amount of circulating lipids.

Due to their insolubility in water, lipids are present in serum in combination with proteins. The resultant lipoprotein complexes can enhance the development of atherosclerosis. The classification of the various lipoprotein complexes is based upon their response to ultracentrifugaton: β lipoproteins, which are low density, pre-β lipoproteins, which are of a very low density, and α lipoproteins, which are of a high density. The chylomicron is an additonal group that is formed in the intestine by the complexing of exogenous triglycerides with protein. The resulting chylomicron is then transported to the plasma by the lymphatics. Very-low-density lipoproteins (VLDL) are formed primarily in the liver by the combination of protein with endogenous triglycerides synthesized from fatty acids and carbohydrates. Low-density liproproteins (LDL) are primarily cholesterol and high-density lipoproteins (HDL) are primarily phospholipid. The transformation from VLDL to LDL is via the formation of an intermediate low-density lipoprotein (ILDL). The biochemical composition of the various lipoproteins is shown in Table 8–1.

Studies have shown the presence of LDL and fibrinogen in atherosclerotic lesions. Conspicuously absent is any significant amount of HDL. Based on the belief that HDL functions in the transport of cholesterol from the cell to the liver for catabolysis, it has been postulated that increased HDL levels may protect against atherosclerosis. The incidence of atherosclerosis is closely associated with increased LDL levels (LDL is 50 percent cholesterol). LDL levels greater than 160 mg percent are to be considered pathologic.

In vitro studies have demonstrated the formation of precipitate or a coacervate when LDL, fibrinogen, and acid mucopolysaccharide, an ingredient of the arterial wall are combined in solution. Such studies suggest that an atherosclerotic lesion forms in a subintimal space where these factors may react. From this it follows that LDL and fibrinogen levels in the arterial wall are precipitating factors in the formation of atherosclerotic lesions and that the higher the levels of these factors, the higher the risk of atherosclerosis. It has additionally been shown that patients with combined aortoiliac/femoropopliteal occlusive disease have higher levels of triglycerides and cholesterol as compared with patients with aortoiliac or femoropopliteal occlusive disease occurring singly.

There are five types of hyperlipidemia based upon which of the lipoproteins in the plasma are increased. The five types can usually be differentiated by the appearance of the plasma following overnight refrigeration at 4C (Table 8–2).

Type I hyperlipidemia is referred to as exogenous hyperlipidemia and

TABLE 8-1. BIOCHEMICAL COMPOSITION OF LIPOPROTEIN GROUPS.*

Chylomicron (75–100 ηm)	Very-Low-Density Lipoproteins (30–80 ηm)	Intermediate Low-Density Lipoproteins (25–40 ηm)	Low-Density Lipoproteins (20 ηm)	High-Density Lipoproteins (7.5–10 ηm)
90% Triglycerides	60% Triglycerides	40% Triglycerides	50% Cholesterol	50% Protein
5% Cholesterol	18% Phospholipid	30% Cholesterol	25% Protein	25% Phospholipid
3% Phospholipid	12% Cholesterol	20% Phospholipid	15% Phospholipid	20% Cholesterol
2% Protein	10% Protein	10% Protein	10% Triglycerides	5% Triglycerides

*Adapted from Levy RI, Morganroth J, Rifkind BM: Treatment of hyperlipidemia. N Engl J Med 290:1295, 1974.

TABLE 8-2. MAIN FEATURES OF HYPERLIPIDEMIA.

Type	Chylomicrons	VLDL	ILDL	LDL	Plasma* Supernate	Plasma* Infranate
I	Markedly increased	Normal or decreased	—	Normal or decreased	Creamy	Clear
IIA	Absent	Normal	—	Increased	Clear	Clear
IIB	Absent	Increased	—	Increased	Noncreamy	Turbid
III	Absent	Increased	Increased	Increased	Slightly creamy	Turbid
IV	Absent	Increased	—	Normal or increased	Clear	Clear to turbid†
V	Increased	Increased	—	Normal or increased	Creamy	Turbid

*Plasma refrigerated at 4C overnight.
†Infranate turbid in the presence of very high VLDL levels.

is characterized by the presence of a markedly elevated level of plasma chylomicrons with normal or decreased LDL or VLDL levels and a plasma with a creamy supernate and clear infranate following refrigeration. This type of hyperlipidemia is relatively rare and has no association with artherosclerosis.

Type II hyperlipidemia is commonly seen and is categorized into two subtypes: IIA and IIB. Type IIA is referred to as hyperbetalipoproteinemia or hypercholesterolemia and is characterized by an increased level of LDL, a normal VLDL level, an absence of chylomicrons, and a clear refrigerated plasma. Type IIB is referred to as combined or mixed hyperlipidemia and is characterized by increased LDL and VLDL levels, an absence of chylomicrons, and a plasma with a noncreamy supernate and an infranate that ranges from clear to turbid in the presence of very elevated VLDL levels. Type II hyperlipidemia may occur at any time from infancy to young adulthood and is known to accelerate and accentuate ischemic heart disease.

Type III hyperlipidemia is characterized by increased plasma levels of ILDL, VLDL, and LDL, an absence of chylomicrons, and a plasma that upon refrigeration yields a slightly creamy supernate and turbid infranate. Patients with Type III hyperlipidemia may be glucose-intolerant and hyperuricemic (increased blood uric acid levels). This type of hyperlipidemia is infrequently seen. It tends to be found early in adult life and, when present, increases the incidence of peripheral vascular disease and coronary atherosclerosis.

Type IV hyperlipidemia is also referred to as endogenous hyperlipidemia or hypertriglyceridemia. The plasma is characterized by increased VLDL levels, normal or increased levels of LDL, an absence of chylomicrons, no creamy supernate, and clear to turbid infranate in the presence of very high VLDL. As with Type III, these individuals often exhibit glucose intolerance and are hyperuricemic. This type of hyperlipidemia is quite common, most often seen in middle-aged adults, and increases the incidence of peripheral vascular disease and coronary artery disease.

Type V hyperlipidemia is referred to as mixed hyperlipidemia. It is characterized by increased plasma VLDL levels, normal or increased LDL levels, increased chylomicrons, and a creamy supernate and turbid infranate. These individuals frequently exhibit glucose intolerance, hyperuricemia, and an intolerance to dietary intake of fats. Type V hyperlipidemia is infrequently seen and, when present, is usually found in young adults. Type V hyperlipidemia is not thought at this time to be associated with the incidence of atherosclerosis.

Table 8–2 lists the features of the five types of hyperlipidemia.

It is recommended that serum triglyceride and cholesterol level determinations be carried out at least three times over a period of two weeks, each time following a 12–16-hour fast to minimize postprandial chylomicronemia. The specific type of hyperlipidemia may be easily determined by examining the patient's plasma following overnight refrigeration at 4C. If necessary, the type of hyperlipidemia can be ascertained using ultracentrifugation or electrophoresis. Attention should also be paid to the presence of hypothyroidism, alcoholism, liver or renal disease, or diabetes mellitus, as they may cause secondary hyperlipidemia, which can be corrected by management of the primary illness.

Several factors must be kept in mind when interpreting lipoprotein determinations. First, commercial laboratory determinations of plasma lipid levels, depending upon the analytical procedure employed, may be reported at 10 to 40 percent higher than actual level. Second, there is an increase with age in the concentration of plasma lipids and lipoproteins. Generally speaking, patients under age 55 with accurate plasma cholesterol levels in excess of 250 mg percent or a plasma triglyceride level exceeding 200 mg percent should undergo therapy for hyperlipidemia. Third, plasma lipoprotein levels are influenced by diet, illness, drugs, or fluctuations in body weight. For example, it has been reported that plasma cholesterol and LDL levels may fall as much as 60 percent immediately following myocardial infarction. There is no dividing level of plasma cholesterol above which one will develop atherosclerosis; individuals with cholesterol levels that approach the upper limit of normal are at much higher risk than individuals with cholesterol levels in the lower range of normal.

The treatment of the hyperlipidemic patient is particularly important in the presence of a family history of premature peripheral vascular disease or coronary heart diesease. Once the type of hyperlipidemia has been determined, the primary mode of therapy is dietary adjustment. Increased chylomicron levels are due to excessive dietary fat intake and can be brought within range by retricting one's intake of saturated and unsaturated long chain fatty acids. Increased VLDL levels can be corrected through a program of weight reduction. Also, as VLDL are 60 percent triglycerides, it may be necessary to reduce triglyceride precursors (e.g., alcohol and carbohydrates). Increased ILDL levels can also be controlled through a weight reduction program, a decrease in carbohydrate and alcohol intake, and a moderate restriction on intake of cholesterol and saturated fatty acids. Increased LDL levels can be controlled by a reduction in cholesterol intake and an increase (of approximately 2 grams) in the dietary intake of polyunsaturated fatty acid. If dietary adjustment and weight control do not prove effective, drug therapy may be instituted while continuing the dietary regulation and weight control. In view of the absence of convincing evidence that control of lipoprotein and lipid blood levels will improve the prognosis of a patient with atherosclerosis, it is possible that such therapy is beneficial only in the absence of symptoms.

Hypertension

It remains to be determined whether hypertension is a causative agent of atherosclerosis or whether it enchances the effects of preexisting atherosclerotic lesions. Hypertension is particularly important in the presence of hyperlipidemia especially in view of the lipid infiltration theory of the pathogenesis of atherosclerosis. Hypertension may influence the permeability of the arterial wall or, due to increased filtration pressure, contribute to the increased accumulation of lipids in the arterial intima. Although hypertension is rarely seen as the original cause of aneurysmal disease, systemic hypertension may play a role in the progression of aneurysmal disease due to an elevation in lateral tension on the arterial wall.

It is generally conceded that control of hypertension will diminish the incidence of vascular disease and consequently congestive heart failure, cerebral hemorrhage, dissecting aneurysm, and renal disease. It is unlikely, however, that control of hypertension will halt the progression of atherosclerotic disease. This is pointed up by studies showing that the incidence of myocardial infarction was not influenced by the control of hypertension.

Diabetes

Of the two types of diabetes—juvenile onset and adult onset—atherosclerosis is characteristically associated with the latter. Juvenile-onset diabetes is usually diagnosed before middle age, does not respond to attempts at control using oral agents, and has a predisposition to ketosis. Such patients usually die from renal pathology or infection rather than cardiovascular problems. Adult-onset diabetes is usually diagnosed at middle age, responds to control using oral agents, and shows no tendency toward ketosis.

The presence of diabetes usually leads to a more diffuse atherosclerotic involvement in a greater number of arteries. Such an extensive involvement significantly inhibits the development of collateral circulation and frequently makes surgical intervention difficult. There is an acceleration of the atherosclerotic process in the coronary and cerebral circulations as well as the circulation in the below-knee segment of the lower extremity, Diabetes also promotes peripheral neuropathy and microangiopathy-proliferative endothelial lesions of the arterioles and capillaries. The presence of peripheral neuropathy is secondary to loss of nerve fibers and demyelination of the nerve. Microangiography may be a result of an abnormal accumulation of glycoprotein that is not influenced by the presence or absence of insulin, or the absence of insulin may precipitate increased glycoprotein synthesis by the basement membrane. It is possible that continually high levels of blood sugar damages the walls of the arteries and capillaries, allowing greater infiltration of lipids, as diabetics typically have elevated levels of plasma lipids and rate of cholesterol synthesis.

It remains to be answered as to whether control of adult-onset diabetes by diet, insulin, or oral medication will halt the atherosclerotic process. Until the question is answered satisfactorily, the most reasonable approach for the clinician is to maintain control of the patient's diabetes as well as aggressively manage all other risk factors the patient may harbor.

Obesity

Obese individuals typically have an increased incidence of diabetes and hypertension and as a consequence have a high incidence of atherosclerosis. Although obese individuals without other risk factors do not necessarily develop atherosclerosis, the presence of obesity is still considered a risk factor, albeit a minor one.

Perhaps more significant than obesity's effect on atherosclerosis is its effect on other disorders. Obesity may precipitate venous insufficiency, thrombophlebitis, cirrhosis, or osteoarthritis. There are additional cardiovascular effects such as increased demand upon the heart and an expanded blood volume.

Stress

Although the association of stress with the atherosclerotic process has been extensively studied, inherent shortcomings in testing techniques do not permit a definitive statement of the relationship. Stressful emotional stimuli yields a discharge of norepinephrine, which causes a vasoconstriction of the peripheral vessels. The cerebral and cardiac vasculature is not so affected. In the normal, healthy individual, the long-term effect does not appear to be harmful. In the individual with cardiovascular problems, however, the increased oxygen requirements and peripheral vascular resistance brought about by the vasoconstrictory response can precipate congestive heart failure, angina, or myocardial infarction. The importance of stress in relation to the atherosclerotic process may lie in its association with a tendency for increased smoking and alcohol consumption.

CHAPTER 9

SPECIFIC CLINIC APPLICATIONS

UPPER-EXTREMITY OBSTRUCTION/
   ACUTE ARTERIAL OCCLUSION
AORTOILIAC OCCLUSIVE DISEASE
FEMOROPOPLITEAL OCCLUSIVE DISEASE
MULTIPLE SEGMENT INVOLVEMENT
SELECTION OF LEVEL OF AMPUTATION
AORTIC ANEURYSM
OPERATIVE EVALUATION OF MESENTERIC BLOOD
   FLOW
● Resection of Abdominal Aortic Aneurism
● Colon–Esophageal Bypass
● Colon Resection
VENOUS THROMBOSIS AND HEPARIN THERAPY

UPPER-EXTREMITY OBSTRUCTION/
ACUTE ARTERIAL OBSTRUCTION

This 62-year-old black male presented with a complaint of a one and one-half year history of pain in the left hand radiating to the left forearm and occasionally to the shoulder, and a two-week history of swelling of the distal left forearm with a tingling pain over the fingers.

The patient's physical examination was unremarkable save the left upper extremity, which was found to have a slightly swollen and warm but not tender distal left forearm. The left hand demonstrated elevation pallor and dependent rubor. There was questionable atrophy of the hypothenar muscle and a remarkable absence of pulsation over the left radial artery. Radiographic examination of the thoracic outlet disclosed bilateral cervical ribs and advanced cervical spondylolithesis. Doppler ultrasound examination disclosed reduced left brachial, radial, and ulnar arterial pressure on the left as compared with the right and photoplethysmography demonstrated an absence of distal pressures and flow waveforms on the left (Fig. 9-1).

The patient had a sudden onset of a painful, cyanotic, and very cold left hand and underwent emergency exploration of the left forearm. An intraoperative arteriogram revealed thrombosis of the brachial artery at its bifurcation into the radial and ulnar arteries (Fig. 9-2).

Thromboembolectomy was carried out and, immediately, postoperatively, the pulsation over the left radial artery returned. During the postoperative period, the radial pulsation disappeared and Doppler ultrasound showed an absence of blood pressure at the brachial, radial, and ulnar arteries. The patient underwent reexploration where an intraoperative arteriogram demonstrated the presence of a subclavian aneurysm (Fig. 9-3).

Thromboembolectomy of the axillary, brachial, radial, and ulnar arteries, partial claviculectomy, resection of the scalenus anticus muscle, and resection of the subclavian aneurysm with modified human umbilical vein were carried out. Postoperatively, photoplethysmography demonstrated return of digital pulsatile flow and Doppler demonstrated adequate arterial pressure. The patient has remained asymptomatic for over 3 years (Fig. 9-4).

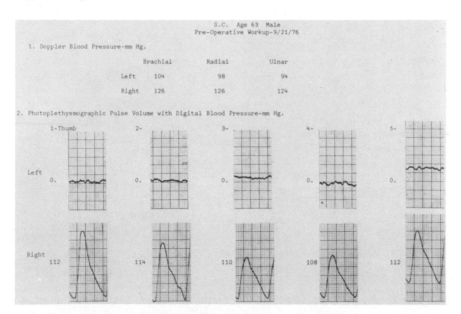

FIGURE 9-1.   Patient's preoperative noninvasive workup showing Doppler ultrasound systolic pressures and photoplethysmographic waveforms and pressures at the fingers.

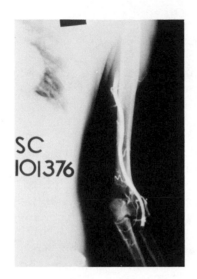

FIGURE 9-2.   Patient's arteriogram showing an acute
occlusion of the brachial artery
on the left.

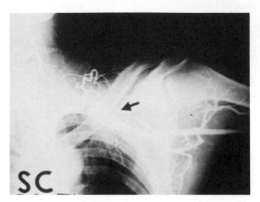

FIGURE 9-3   Subsequent intraoperative arteriogram revealing the presence of a subclavian artery aneurysm to be the source of
the peripheral embolization.

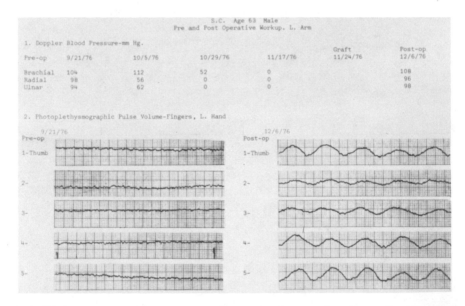

FIGURE 9-4.   Preoperative–postoperative comparison noninvasive studies showing
the restoration of pulsatile digital waveforms on photoplethysmography and adequate Doppler ultrasound systolic pressures following resection of the aneurysm and
thromboembolectomy.

AORTOILIAC OCCLUSIVE DISEASE

This 58-year-old white male presented with a chief complaint of a pain behind his right knee when walking. On admission, the patient was evaluated using segmental Doppler systolic pressures with the following results:

Location	Right	Left
Brachial	142	140
High thigh	102	164
Above knee	96	148
Calf	94	152
Posterior tibial	94	138
Dorsalis pedis	98	132

The 40 mm Hg drop in arterial pressure between the brachial and high-thigh readings on the right and a 60 mm Hg drop between left and right high thigh readings is indicative of severe aortoiliac occlusive disease on the right. Segmental systolic pressures below the high thigh show no significant gradient, indicating the absence of distal disease on the right. Noninvasive electromagnetic flowmetry showed similar results for the right leg. Peak pulsatile flow for the thigh was 93 ml/min (24 percent of normal) with a very jagged and irregular waveform indicative of the presence of only collateral flow; the right calf showed a vastly reduced peak pulsatile blood flow of 15 ml/min (12 percent of normal) with a flat waveform.

The noninvasive diagnosis of severe aortoiliac occlusive disease was confirmed by arteriography, which revealed a total obstruction of the origin of the right common iliac artery with flow reconstituted distally by collaterization through the lumbar arteries (Fig. 9-5). The area of obstruction extended to the distal abdominal aorta. The patient was scheduled for an aorto-right femoral bypass.

Intraoperatively following the bypass, standard electromagnetic flowmetry showed a functional graft with excellent pulsatile flow (207 ml/min) and pulsatile waveform showing a rapid acceleration and deceleration denoting good run-in and run-off (Fig 9-6).

Postoperatively, the patient's segmental Doppler systolic pressure profile was restored to normal:

Location	Right	Left
Brachial	128	124
High thigh	166	158
Above knee	162	150
Calf	158	154
Posterior tibial	156	152
Dorsalis pedis	126	130

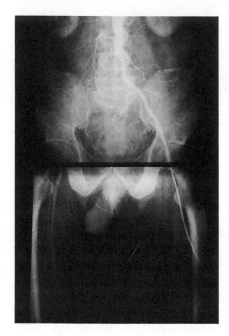

FIGURE 9-5. Preoperative arteriogram showing a total occlusion of the right common iliac artery at its origin.

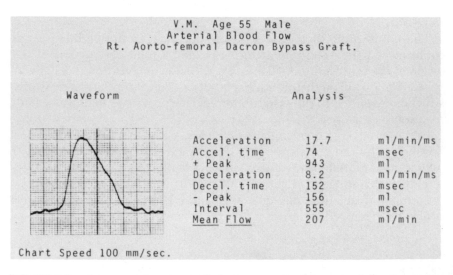

FIGURE 9-6. Intraoperative standard electromagnetic flowmetry following aorto-right femoral artery bypass (Dacron). The bypass graft shows an excellent flow value of 207 ml/min and an excellent pulsatile waveform.

Similarly, noninvasive electromagnetic flowmetery showed excellent peak pulsatile flow, 405 ml/min for the thigh and 132 ml/min for the calf and excellent pulsatile waveforms showing normal rapid acceleration and deceleartion. The patient is doing well more than two years post-operatively (Fig. 9-7).

FEMOROPOPLITEAL OCCLUSIVE DISEASE

This 78-year-old white male presented with a complaint of chronic ulceration of the medial and lateral aspects of the right ankle. The patient's Doppler segmental systolic pressure profile showed the following:

Location	Right	Left
Brachial	122	126
High Thigh	146	147
Above Knee	124	133
Calf	76	130
Ankle	77	145
Index	0.63	1.15

The high thigh pressures are of a magnitude to rule out aortoiliac occlusive disease. On the right, the above knee pressure is reduced and a large reduction is seen in the calf pressure, indicating the occlusive process to be between the above knee and calf sites. Noninvasive electromagnetic flowmetry showed a peak pulsatile right thigh flow of 200 ml/min with the waveform showing good acceleration, indicating an absence of proximal aortoiliac occlusive disease. The deceleration was relatively prolonged, indicating the presence of distal disease. Peak pulsatile flow for the right calf was 50 ml/min with acceleration and deceleration very prolonged. On the left, the segmental pressure profile was normal and noninvasive electromagnetic flowmetry showed normal peak pulsatile flows for the thigh, 356 ml/min, and for the calf, 127 ml/min.

On arteriography, femoropopliteal occlusive disease was noted at the level determined noninvasively (Fig. 9-8). Good run-in was noted with reconstitution of the popliteal and with acceptable run-off.

The patient was scheduled for a right femoropopliteal bypass using modified human umbilical vein. Following placement of the graft, intraoperative standard electromagnetic flowmetry studies showed the bypass to have an excellent pulsatile waveform and a mean flow of 561 ml/min (Fig. 9-9).

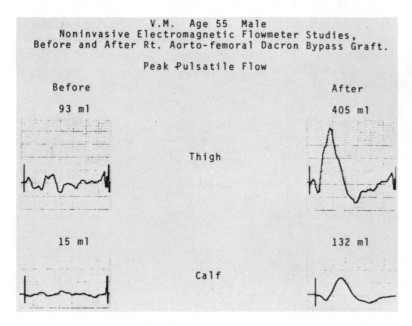

V.M. Age 55 Male
Noninvasive Electromagnetic Flowmeter Studies,
Before and After Rt. Aorto-femoral Dacron Bypass Graft.

Peak Pulsatile Flow

Before   After

93 ml   405 ml

                        Thigh

15 ml   132 ml

                        Calf

FIGURE 9-7. Preoperative–postoperative comparison study using noninvasive electromagnetic flowmetry showing excellent postoperative peak pulsatile flow and pulsatile flow waveforms for both the thigh and calf segments.

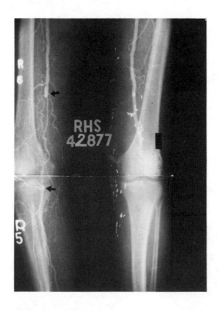

FIGURE 9-8. Preoperative femoral arteriogram showing femoropopliteal occlusive disease at the level predicted noninvasively.

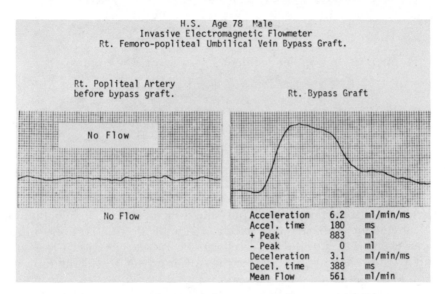

FIGURE 9-9. Intraoperative standard electromagnetic flowmetry showing excellent pulsatile waveforms for the modified human umbilical vein femoropoliteal bypass graft and an excellent mean flow.

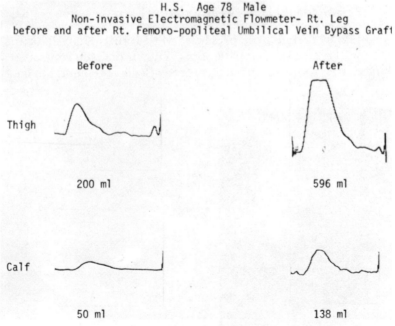

FIGURE 9-10 Preoperative–postoperative comparison of noninvasive electromagnetic flowmetry study. Note the excellent agreement of invasive and noninvasive electromagnetic flowmetry flow values (compare with Figure 9-9).

Postoperatively Doppler segmental systolic pressure improved:

Location	Right	Left
Brachial	133	127
High thigh	160	143
Above knee	146	135
Calf	72	126
Ankle	104	136
Index	0.78	1.07

The patient's noninvasive electromagnetic flowmetry studies showed excellent improvement in peak pulsatile flow for the thigh, 596 ml/min, in agreement with standard electromagnetic flowmetry done intraoperatively. The waveform's acceleration and deceleration were both rapid. The peak pulsatile flow for the calf improved to 138 ml/min with a rapid acceleration and deceleration (Fig. 9-10).

The patient's modified human umbilical vein femoropopliteal bypass has remained functional more than 3 years postoperatively.

MULTIPLE SEGMENT INVOLVEMENT

This 65-year-old white male presented with frank gangrene of the left fourth toe (Fig. 9-11). The patient is a known diabetic controlled with Diabinase, well recovered from a cerebrovascular accident. He had pre-

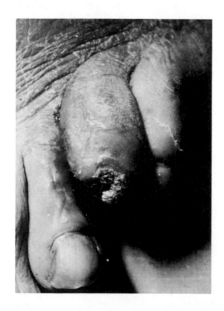

FIGURE 9-11.   Patient's gangrenous toe at the time of admission.

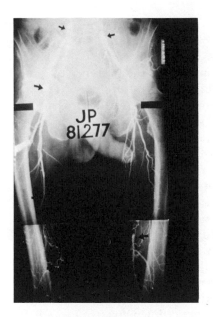

FIGURE 9-12.   Preoperative arteriogram of run-in segment.

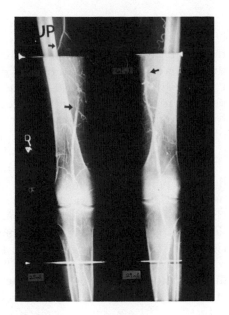

FIGURE 9-13.   Preoperative arteriogram
of run-on and run-off segments showing
the presence of bilateral femoropopliteal
occlusive disease with adequate run-off
vessels.

viously had bilateral sympathectomy over two years ago for impending
gangrene of the second and third toes on the left and over one year ago
for severe claudication on the right. Lumbar sympathectomy was effective in both instances.

Upon admission, frank gangrene was noted of the left fourth toe and
there was an absence of pulses in both lower extremities. The patient
underwent a bilateral femoral arteriogram (Fig. 9-12). The arteriogram
was reported as showing relatively normal pelvic arteries with bilateral
occlusion of the superficial femoral arteries with good run-off (Fig. 9-13).

The patient's segmental Doppler systolic pressure profile gave the
following results:

Level	Right	Left
Brachial	136	128
High thigh	120	122
Above knee	84	108
Calf	74	70
Posterior tibial	70	64
Dorsalis pedis	72	64

The Doppler systolic pressure indices at the high thigh (right, 0.88, left, 0.95) showed the presence of aortoiliac occlusive disease. Pressure drops between the high thigh and above knee segment of 36 mm Hg on the right and 14 mm Hg on the left demonstrate the presence of femoropopliteal occlusive disease. On the left, a 38 mm Hg pressure drop between the above knee and calf segements indicates the presence of femoropopliteal occlusive disease on the symptomatic side. The presence of equal posterior tibial and dorsalis pedis pressures on the right and left signifies the probable patency of both of these run-off vessels.

Noninvasive electromagnetic flowmetry showed vastly reduced thigh flows (23 percent of normal on the right and only 16 percent of normal on the left). The thigh waveform shapes show a prolonged deceleration characteristic of distal femoropopliteal occlusive disease. Calf peak pulsatile flow was similarly greatly reduced (19 percent of normal on the right and 22 percent of normal on the left). The pulsatile blood flow waveform for the calves is practically flat, indicating severe proximal disease (Fig. 9-14). Other noninvasive tests showed similar poor results and the patient was scheduled for reconstructive surgery.

Intraoperatively, standard electromagnetic flowmetry confirmed the presence of severe aortoiliac occlusive disease and an aorto-bilateral femoral bypass was carried out to bring adequate inflow to the profunda femoris artery.

Postoperatively, the patient's segmental Doppler systolic pressures showed deterioration and a minimal improvement was seen in noninvasive electromagnetic flowmetry for the thigh, where there was improvement in the pulsatile waveform acceleration but deceleration remained prolonged and jagged, indicating remaining distal disease. There was no change in calf peak pulsatile flow or waveform shape. The patient remained symptomatic and was scheduled for femoropopliteal bypass (Figs. 9-15 and 9-16).

Following femoropopliteal bypass, the patient's noninvasive electromagnetic flowmetry studies of peak pulsatile thigh and calf blood flow showed excellent improvement, with thigh and calf waveform shape becoming qualitatively normal and thigh and calf peak pulsatile blood flow values approaching normal (Fig. 9-17).

Similar excellent improvement was also noted in the segmental Doppler systolic pressure profile, toe temperature, and photoplethysmographic pulsatile recordings at the toes (Fig. 9-18).

The patient's gangrene showed complete healing and the patient remains asymptomatic with maintained patency of the aorto-bilateral femoral and left femoropopliteal bypasses (Fig. 9-19).

This particular patient demonstrates the use of noninvasive vascular diagnostic techniques in the detection of multilevel occlusive disease. It is important to dectect the presence of latent aortoiliac occlusive disease in that a lower-extremity bypass (femoropopliteal, femorotibial, etc.) done in the presence of inadequate inflow is usually doomed to failure. In such patients, sequential aortofemoral-femoropopliteal bypass should be carried out. This particular patient additionally demonstrates that a "normal" arteriogram may indeed be shown to be in error by noninvasive diagnostic techniques. This instance reemphasizes the importance of looking at all available diagnostic information prior to planning a patient's course of treatment.

Segmental Doppler Systolic Pressures		
	Rt.	Lt.
Brachial	136	128
High Thigh	120	122
Thigh Pressure Index	0.88	0.95
Above Knee	84	108
Calf	74	70
Posterior Tib.	70	64
Ischemic Index	0.51	0.50
Dorsalis Ped.	72	64
Ischemic Index	0.53	0.50

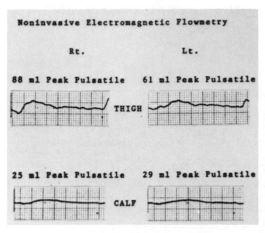

Noninvasive Electromagnetic Flowmetry

Rt.   Lt.

88 ml Peak Pulsatile   61 ml Peak Pulsatile   THIGH

25 ml Peak Pulsatile   29 ml Peak Pulsatile   CALF

FIGURE 9-14.   Preoperative noninvasive workup. Doppler systolic segmental pressures and noninvasive electromagnetic flowmetery both demonstrate the presence of combined aortoiliac-femoropopliteal occlusive disease, which was documented intraoperatively using standard electromagnetic flowmetry.

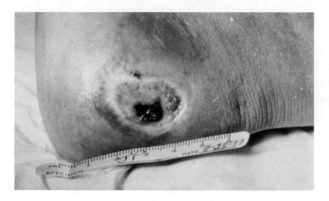

FIGURE 9-15. Following an aorto-bilateral femoral bypass, the patient remained symptomatic on the left.

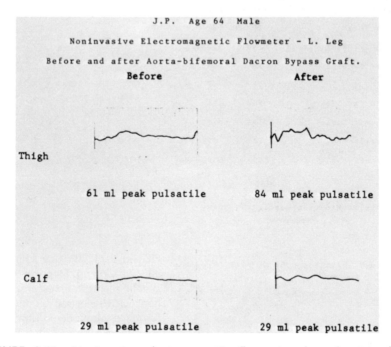

FIGURE 9-16. Noninvasive electromagnetic flowmetry showed minimal improvement on the left. Note the jagged and prolonged deceleration for the waveform of the thigh segment, indicating the presence of remaining distal disease, which is shown by a relatively flat waveform obtained for the calf segment.

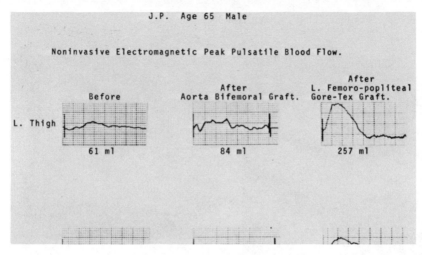

FIGURE 9-17. Comparison of noninvasive electromagnetic flowmetry before and after aortofemoral and femoropopliteal bypasses on the patient's symptomatic left side. There was minimal improvement following aortofemoral bypass. Following the sequential femoropopliteal bypass graft that bypassed the distal obstruction, the patient's flow values approached normal.

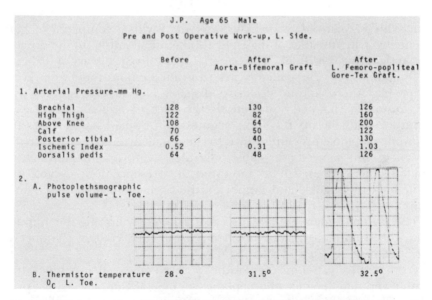

FIGURE 9-18. Following sequential aortofemoral-femoropopliteal bypass, segmental Doppler systolic pressures, digital temperatures, and photoplethysmography showed excellent improvement.

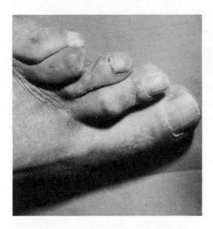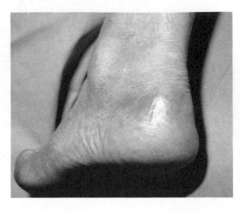

FIGURE 9-19.   The patient's gangrenous lesions showed complete healing on the toe (**left**) and on the heel (**right**).

SELECTION OF AMPUTATION LEVEL

1. This 57-year-old black male presented with a complaint of gangrene involving the toes of the right foot and extending up the dorsum of the right foot (Fig. 9-20). The patient had a 20-year history of diabetes.

On admission, the patient's arteriogram demonstrated nonreconstructable atherosclerotic occlusive disease. Noninvasive studies with thermistor thermometry showed the absence of any significant temperature gradient up the foot; segmental Doppler systolic pressure showed acceptable pressures down to the ankle; arterial impedance plethysmography showed acceptable pulsatile waveforms for the thigh-to-ankle segment. These studies indicated the presence of acceptable pulsatile flow to the ankle and supported the probable healing of a Syme's amputation (Fig. 9-21).

The patient underwent a Syme's amputation. Following the amputation, the stump was placed in an environmental control chamber to facilitate healing (Fig. 9-22).

Postoperatively, noninvasive studies showed an excellent temperature profile and maintenance of acceptable segmental Doppler systolic pressures. Photoplethysmography done on the stump showed excellent pulsatile waveforms for the superior and inferior surfaces of the stump. The patient showed excellent healing and rehabilitation and is doing well 5 years later (Figs. 9-23 and 9-24).

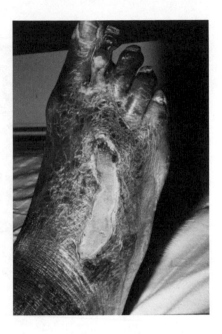

FIGURE 9-20.   The patient's gangrenous foot at the time of admission.

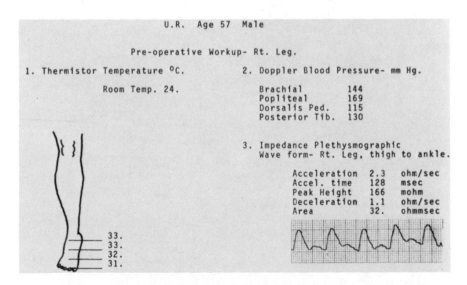

FIGURE 9-21.   The patient's preoperative noninvasive workup showed an absence of temperature gradient, good segmental Doppler systolic pressures to the ankle, and an acceptable arterial impedance plethysmographic study. On this basis, a Syme's amputation was done.

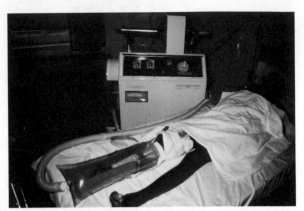

FIGURE 9-22.   Postoperatively, healing of the Syme's amputation was facilitated by placing the stump in an environmental control chamber, which also functions in preventing edema.

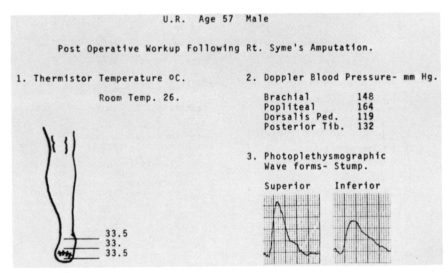

FIGURE 9-23.   Postoperatively, photoplethysmography demonstrated pulsatile blood flow on the superior and inferior surfaces of the stump and maintenance of adequate segmental Doppler systolic pressures and temperatures.

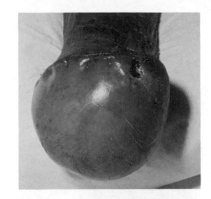

FIGURE 9-24A. The patient's Syme's amputation showed excellent healing.

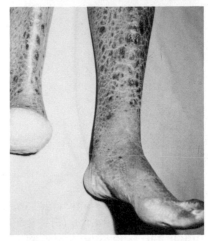

FIGURE 9-24B. Five years after amputation, the stump remains healed.

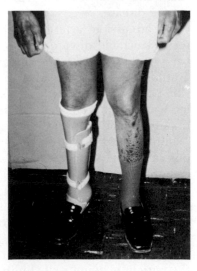

FIGURE 9-24C. The patient was well rehabilitated following amputation.

317

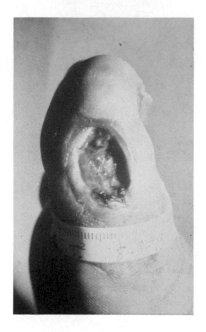

FIGURE 9-25.   The patient's gangrenous toe at the time of admission.

2. This 66-year-old white male presented with a complaint of gangrene of the right toe (Fig. 9-25). The patient is a known diabetic and unilateral below-the-knee amputee secondary to atherosclerotic occlusive disease.

On admission, arteriography demonstrated the presence of a nonreconstructable disease process. The patient was scheduled for lumbar sympathectomy. Postsympathectomy, noninvasive photoplethysmographic determination of skin perfusion pressure showed acceptable skin perfusion pressure for the stump as well as on the symptomatic right leg with acceptable skin perfusion pressure down the leg and over the dorsum of the foot (Figs. 9-26 and 9-27).

Photoplethysmographic determination of metatarsal pressures demonstrated the presence of pulsatile flow waveforms for all toes and acceptable pressures. (Fig. 9-28).

On the basis of these data obtained postlumbar sympathectomy, it was decided that there would probably be primary healing of an amputation of the gangrenous right great toe. The patient was scheduled for amputation of the great toe.

There was primary healing of the great toe amputation (Fig. 9-29) and the patient is doing well almost 2 years postoperatively.

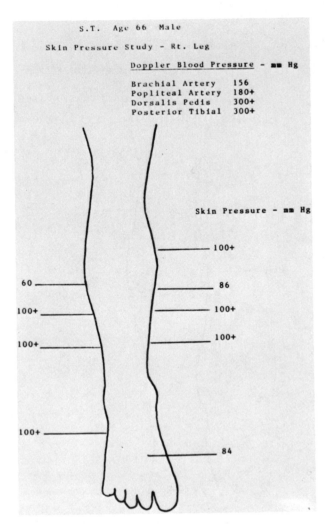

S.T.   Age 66   Male

Skin Pressure Study - Rt. Leg

Doppler Blood Pressure - mm Hg

Brachial Artery   156
Popliteal Artery   180+
Dorsalis Pedis   300+
Posterior Tibial   300+

Skin Pressure - mm Hg

100+

60
86

100+
100+

100+
100+

100+

84

FIGURE 9-26.   Skin perfusion pressure study on the patient's symptomatic right leg demonstrates acceptable skin perfusion pressure down the leg and over the dorsum of the foot.

AORTIC ANEURYSM

This 58-year-old white male presented with a complaint of an annoying pain in his right foot. The patient had no other complaints.

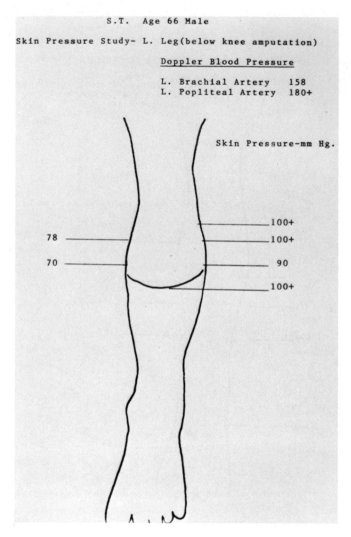

S.T.   Age 66 Male

Skin Pressure Study- L. Leg(below knee amputation)

Doppler Blood Pressure

L. Brachial Artery   158
L. Popliteal Artery   180+

Skin Pressure-mm Hg.

78
70

100+
100+
90
100+

FIGURE 9-27.   Skin perfusion pressure study, on the patient's amputated limb showing good skin perfusion pressure, indicating a viable and healthy stump.

Segmental Doppler systolic pressures showed an ischemic index of 0.97 on the right and 0.83 on the left, demonstrating the presence of minimal atherosclerotic occlusive disease. Photoplethysmographic examination at the toes showed reduced metatarsal pressures and pulsatile waveforms recorded at the toes (Table 9-1).

The finding suggested the possibility of peripheral embolization. On

PHOTOPLETHYSMOGRAPHIC WAVEFORMS AT THE TOES

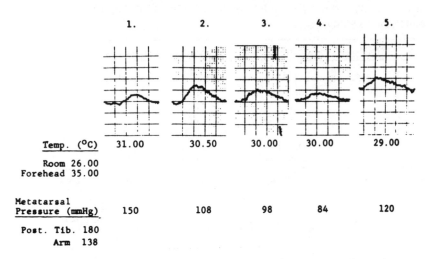

	1.	2.	3.	4.	5.
Temp. (°C)	31.00	30.50	30.00	30.00	29.00

Room 26.00
Forehead 35.00

Metatarsal Pressure (mmHg)	150	108	98	84	120

Post. Tib. 180
Arm 138

FIGURE 9-28. Photoplethysmography and thermistor thermometry showed acceptable pulsatile waveforms, pressures, and temperature at the digits, indicating probable healing following amputation of the patient's gangrenous toe.

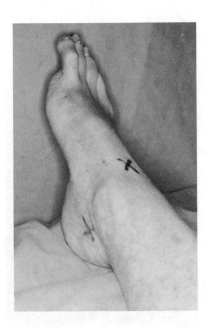

FIGURE 9-29. Following amputation of the involved digit, the patient showed excellent subsequent healing.

TABLE 9-1. INDICATION OF POSSIBLE PERIPHERAL EMBOLIZATION
REVEALED BY PRESENCE OF PRESSURE GRADIENT BETWEEN ANKLE
AND TOE PRESSURES.

		Segmental Doppler Systolic Pressures	
		Rt.	Lt.
	Brachial	122	112
	High Thigh	128	114
	Above Knee	128	118
	Calf	126	90
	Post. Tibial	124	100
	Dors. Pedis	116	106

	Photoplethysmographic Pressures at Toes	
	Right	Left
Toe	Ankle/Metatarsal	Ankle/Metatarsal
1	72/55	75/64
2	74/20	74/69
3	55/80	46/55
4	105/25	83/64
5	104/54	80/37

arteriography, a saccular abdominal aortic aneurysm was revealed (Fig.
9-30). The patient underwent resection of the abdominal aortic aneurysm. Postoperatively, the patient's metatarsal pressure improved, as
did the pulsatile waveforms. The patient had an uneventful recovery.

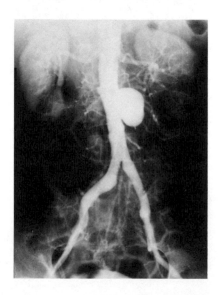

FIGURE 9-30. Arteriography demonstrated the presence of a saccular abdominal aortic aneurysm to be the source of
the peripheral emboli.

OPERATIVE EVALUATION OF MESENTERIC BLOOD FLOW

RESECTION OF ABDOMINAL AORTIC ANEURYSM

A 59-year-old white male was diagnosed as having an abdominal aortic aneurysm and was scheduled for elective aneurysmectomy.

Intraoperatively, the patient's inferior mesenteric artery arising from the saccular abdominal aortic aneurysm was extremely large (Fig. 9-31). Measurement of arterial pressure at the inferior mesenteric artery revealed a stump pressure of 30 mm Hg (Fig. 9-32).

The size of the inferior mesenteric artery and the magnitude of the stump pressure suggested the need for reimplantation of the inferior mesenteric artery following resection of the aneurysm. Doppler blood velocity studies on the serosal surface of the left colon showed excellent pulsatile flow prior to temporary interruption of inferior mesenteric artery blood flow, which was maintained and enhanced following interruption of blood flow (Fig. 9-33).

On this basis, the inferior mesenteric artery was not reimplanted following graft placement and the operation was concluded. The patient's postoperative course was uneventful and he is doing well almost 2 years postoperatively.

Colon–Esophageal Bypass

This 59-year-old white male presented with a three-month history of retrosternal pain and discomfort with dysphagia. He was known to have esophageal carcinoma and had been undergoing cobalt treatment. At admission, a barium swallow disclosed a 50 percent reduction of the lumen in the mid-third portion of the esophagus. There was a definite suspicion of a recurring or persistent tumor and the patient was scheduled for a colon–esophageal bypass.

A portion of the right colon was selected for the bypass. Intraoperatively, Doppler ultrasound tracings were obtained over the ileocolic artery, at the mesenteric–cecum junction, and over the serosal surface of the cecum. To evaluate the blood supply to this portion of the colon, the ileocolic artery and midcolic artery were isolated and noncrushing vascular clamps were used to temporarily interrupt their blood flow. The serosal surface of the right colon continued to show pulsatile flow during temporary arterial occlusion, indicating that sacrifice of these arteries would not compromise the right colon's blood supply (Fig. 9-34).

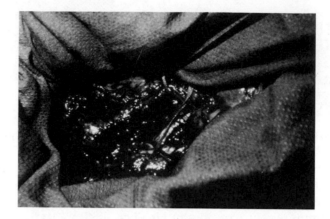

FIGURE 9-31.   At operation, a very large inferior mesenteric artery was found.

The portion of the right colon was transposed and Doppler ultrasound showed pulsatile flow at the proximal and distal portions of the transposed colon as well as the site of anastomosis, ensuring viability of the transposed colon. The operation was concluded after gastrostomy. The patient's postoperative course was unremarkable and he is doing well more than 1 year postoperatively (Fig. 9-35).

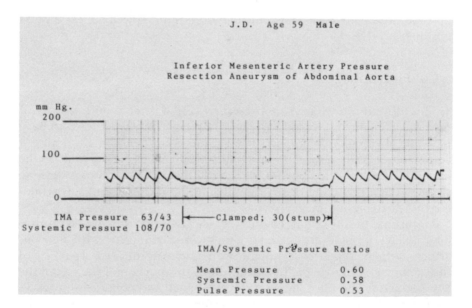

FIGURE 9-32.   A stump pressure of 30 mm Hg was obtained which, in conjunction with the size of the inferior mesenteric artery, suggested the need for reimplantation following aneurysm resection.

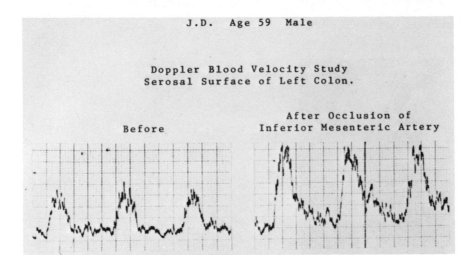

FIGURE 9-33. Enhanced Doppler waveforms recorded over the surface of the left colon following temporary clamping of the inferior mesenteric artery indicating presence of adequate collateral circulation, allowing sacrifice of the inferior mesenteric artery with impunity.

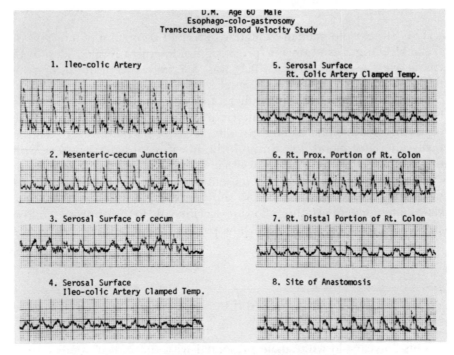

FIGURE 9-34. Doppler ultrasonic waveforms showing the presence of adequate collateral flow to the right colon prior to transposition and at the site of anastomosis after transposition, indicating a viable colon.

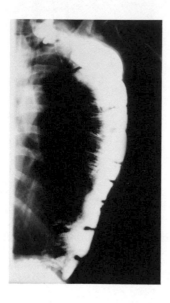

FIGURE 9-35.   More than one year post-operatively the patient is doing well and a barium swallow shows a functional colon–esophageal bypass.

COLON RESECTION

This 81-year-old male presented with a chief complaint of a history of rectal bleeding. On admission, proctosigmoidoscopy revealed a lesion 12 cm above the anal verge, which was diagnosed as infiltrating adenocarcinoma, and the patient was scheduled for colon resection.

During operation, Doppler ultrasound showed acceptable pulsatile blood flow for the inferior mesenteric artery and over the serosal surface of the left colon. Noncrushing vascular clamps were then used to temporarily interrupt blood flow through the inferior mesenteric artery with the Doppler probe remaining over the serosal surface of the left colon. During interruption of inferior mesenteric artery flow, the serosal surface of the left colon continued to show acceptable pulsatile blood flow via collateral channels, thus allowing sacrifice of the inferior mesenteric artery with impunity (Fig. 9-36). The patient's postoperative course was unremarkable.

VENOUS THROMBOSIS AND HEPARIN THERAPY

This 55-year-old white male presented with three ulcerations on the lower one-third of the right leg. The patient has had a 10-year history of chronic ulceration of the right leg with intermittent healing and breaking

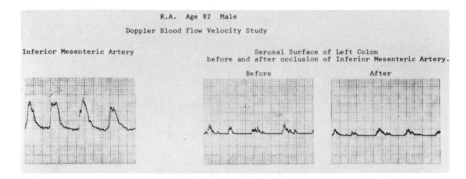

R.A.   Age 82   Male

Doppler Blood Flow Velocity Study

Inferior Mesenteric Artery

Serosal Surface of Left Colon
before and after occlusion of Inferior Mesenteric Artery.

Before   After

FIGURE 9-36.   Pulsatile Doppler waveforms over the surface of the left colon during temporary clamping of the inferior mesenteric artery during colon resection, demonstrating the presence of adequate collateral flow.

down of ulcers. On admission, a regimen of treatment with Betadine and antibiotic cream yielded improvement in the ulcer. Venous impedance plethysmography done at this time was positive on the right (Fig. 9-37). This was confirmed by venography showing thrombus formation without complete obstruction and highly suggestive of involvement of the distal aspect of the posterior tibial, anterior tibial, and peroneal veins (Fig. 9-38). The patient was started on heparin therapy.

Prior to heparin administration, the patient's partial thromboplastin time was 25 with a control of 32. With thromboelastography, the patient's r value was 9.2. The patient received an initial loading dose of 10,000 units of heparin at 12:00 P.M. and was placed on a regimen of 5,000 units every 6 hours. Four hours following the initiation of heparin therapy, the patient's thromboelastogram showed a very strong heparin effect with an r value of 34 (Fig. 9-39). Partial thromboplastin time showed little difference from control (patient 33 and control 32).

On the weekend, one day following heparin administration of 5,000 units every 6 hours, the patient's PTT showed little difference from the control (patient 38 and control 33). On this basis, heparin administration was increased to 7,500 units every 6 hours and one day following this regimen, the patient's PTT again showed little difference from control (patient 35.5 and control 31.0). Two days following heparin 7,500 units every 6 hours, the patient's thromboelastogram was a straight line with an r value in excess of 4 hours suggestive of imminent hemorrhagic complications. At this time, PTT continued to show no difference from control (patient 32 and control 33). At this time, the route of administration and dosage of heparin was changed to 20,000 units over 24 hours via a constant infusion pump. Several hours following this change, the patient's thromboelastogram remained a straight line; however, the r

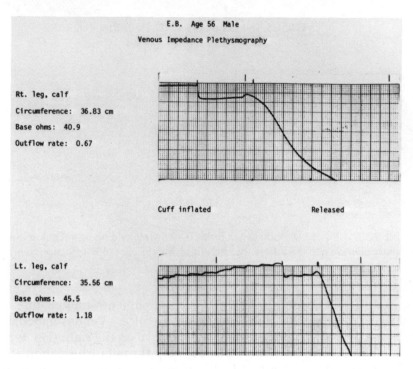

E.B. Age 56 Male

Venous Impedance Plethysmography

Rt. leg, calf

Circumference: 36.83 cm

Base ohms: 40.9

Outflow rate: 0.67

Cuff inflated   Released

Lt. leg, calf

Circumference: 35.56 cm

Base ohms: 45.5

Outflow rate: 1.18

FIGURE 9-37.   Venous impedance plethysmogram demonstrating the presence of deep venous thrombosis on the right.

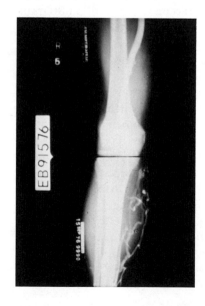

FIGURE 9-38.   Venogram confirming the presence of deep venous thrombosis on the right.

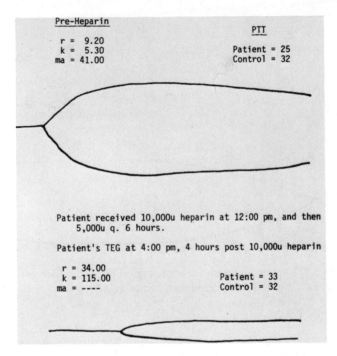

Pre-Heparin

r = 9.20
k = 5.30
ma = 41.00

PTT

Patient = 25
Control = 32

Patient received 10,000u heparin at 12:00 pm, and then
    5,000u q. 6 hours.

Patient's TEG at 4:00 pm, 4 hours post 10,000u heparin

r = 34.00
k = 115.00
ma = ----

Patient = 33
Control = 32

FIGURE 9-39.   Patient's thromboelastogram prior to heparin therapy (upper trace) and four hours following the initial loading dose of 10,000 units of heparian (lower trace).

TABLE 9-2. PATIENT'S THROMBOELASTOGRAM 2 DAYS FOLLOWING 7,500 UNITS OF HEPARIN EVERY 6 HOURS WAS A STRAIGHT LINE WITH AN r TIME GREATER THAN 4 HOURS. PTT SHOWED NO HEPARIN EFFECT. THE MODE OF ADMINISTRATION WAS CHANGED TO A CONTINUOUS INFUSION PUMP, 20,000 UNITS OF HEPARIN OVER 24 HOURS , AND THE r TIME WAS REDUCED TO 3 HOURS. PTT FINALLY SHOWS A HEPARIN EFFECT.

2 days post heparin 7,500 units every 6 hours

TEG	PTT	PT
r = >4 hours	Patient = 32	Patient = 12.30
k = —	Control = 33	Control = 10.80
ma = —		

Administration changed to 20,000 units continuous infusion pump

TEG	PTT
r = >3 hours	Patient = 53
k = —	Control = 33
ma = —	

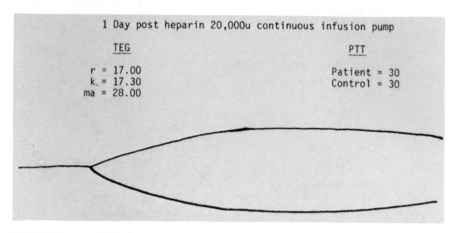

FIGURE 9-40. Thromboelastogram showing a good heparin response one day following continuous infusion pump administration of 20,000 units of heparin over 24 hours.

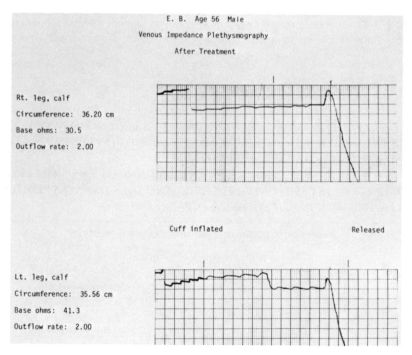

FIGURE 9-41. Following heparin therapy, the patient's venous impedance plethysmogram returned to normal.

value began to come down, showing an r time greater than 3 hours. At this point, the patient's PTT finally showed a difference from control (patient 53 and control 33) (See Table 9-2).

One day post heparin 20,000 units via continuous infusion, the patient's thromboelastogram showed a good heparin effect with an r value of 17 (Fig. 9-40); the patient's PTT, however, showed no difference from control (patient 30 and control 30). The patient remained on continuous heparin infusion with no hemorrhagic complications.

Following heparin therapy, a venous impedance plethysmogram was bilaterally normal (Fig. 9-41). The patient was discharged on Coumadin and is doing well amost 4 years later.

VASCULAR INSTRUMENTATION SOURCES

TREADMILL

Del Mar Avionics
1601 Alton Avenue
Irvine, California 92714

Quintron Instruments
2121 Ferry Avenue
Seattle, Washington 98121

Warren E. Collins, Inc.
220 Wood Road
Braintree, Massachusetts 02184

MULTIPLE MEASUREMENT SYSTEMS

PVR (Photoplethysmograph, strain-gauge plethysmograph,
    stripchart recorder)
    Life Sciences Incorporated
    270-T Greenwich Avenue
    Greenwich, Connecticut 06830

Vasculab (Photoplethysmograph, strain-gauge plethysmo-
    graph, stripchart recorder)
    Medasonics
    PO Box M, 340 Pioneer Way
    Mountain View, California 94042

AVD (Automatic inflation-deflation system, Doppler, in-
    guinal compression device, pressure gauges, stripchart
    recorder telemetry system)
    Narco Diagnostics, Inc.
    Commerce Drive
    Fort Washington, Pennsylvania 19034

THERMOMETRY

Portable Digital Thermometers
    Bailey Instruments
    515 Victor Street
    Saddle Brook, New Jersey 07662

YSI-Tele-Thermometers
    Yellow Springs Instrument Co.
    PO Box 279
    Yellow Springs, Ohio 45387

BLOOD PRESSURE ACCESSORIES (CUFFS, MANOMETERS, INFLATORS, ETC.)

D. E. Hokanson, Inc
3324-72nd Avenue, S.E.
Mercer Island, Washington 89040

Tyco Instrument Division
Data Instruments, Inc.
4 Hartwell Place
Lexington, Massachusetts 02173

W. A. Baum, Co., Inc.
Copiague, New York 11726

ELECTROMAGNETIC BLOOD FLOWMETER (INTRAOPERATIVE)

Clinical Blood Flowmeter
    Biotronex Laboratory, Inc.
    9153 Brookville Road
    Silver Springs, Maryland 20910

Square-Wave Electromagnetic Flowmeter
    Carolina Medical Electronics, Inc.
    PO Box 307
    King, North Carolina 27021

Electromagnetic Flowmeter
    Hunter Instruments
    18704 Bryant Street
    Northridge, California 91324

Electromagnetic Blood Flowmeter
   In-Vivo Metric Systems
   PO Box 217
   Red Wood Valley, California 95470

Narcomatic Electromagnetic Flowmeter
   Narcomatic Biosystems, Inc.
   PO Box 12511, 7651 Airport Boulevard
   Houston, Texas 77017

Statham Electromagnetic Blood Flowmeters
   Statham Instruments
   Division of Gould, Inc.
   2230 Statham Boulevard
   Oxnard, California 93030

ELECTROMAGNETIC BLOOD FLOWMETER (NONINVASIVE)

Electromagnetic Noninvasive Blood Flowmeter
   Doll Research Inc.
   18 East 78th Street
   New York, New York 10021

PHOTOPLETHYSMOGRAPH

Photoplethysmograph
   Biotronex Laboratory, Inc.
   9153 Brookville Road
   Silver Spring, Maryland 20910

Photopulsephotoplethysmograph
   Medasonics
   PO Box M, 340 Pioneer Way
   Mountain View, California 94042

OCULOPNEUMOPLETHYSMOGRAPH

Pneuma-Tonometer
   Digilab
   Bio Rad Laboratories
   237 Putnam Avenue
   Cambridge, Massachusetts 02139

Gee-O.P.G.
    Electro-Diagnostic Instruments
    819 South Main Street
    Burbank, California 91506

OPG
    Life Sciences, Inc.
    270-T Greenwich Avenue
    Greenwich, Connecticut 06830

Narco Oculoplethysmograph
    Narco Diagnostics, Inc.
    Commerce Drive
    Fort Washington, Pennsylvania 19034

Zira International OPG
    Zira International, Inc.
    2817 North Country Club Road
    Tucson, Arizona 85716

ELECTRICAL IMPEDANCE PLETHYSMOGRAPH

Bilateral Impedance Rheograph
    Electronic Instruments Division
    Beckman Instruments, Inc.
    3900 River Road
    Schiller Park, Illinois 60176

Codman IPG
    Codman and Shurtleff, Inc.
    Randolph, Massachusetts 02368

Minnesota Impedance Cardiograph
    Surcona, Inc.
    Edmund Boulevard
    Minneapolis, Minnesota 55406

ULTRASONIC DOPPLER

  Spectral Analysis
Sona-Graphs
    Kay Elemetrics Corporation
    12 Maple Avenue
    Pine Brook, New Jersey 07058

Angioscan Real Time Vascular Doppler Ultrasound Spectral Display
  Unigon Industries, Inc.
  PO Box 9999
  Mount Vernon, New York 10551

CAROTID PHONOANGIOGRAPHY

CPA
  Life Sciences, Inc.
  270-T Greenwich Avenue
  Greenwich, Connecticut 06830

CPA
  Narco Diagnostics, Inc.
  Commerce Drive
  Fort Washington, Pennsylvania 19034

DOPPLER ULTRASOUND

Blood Velocity Meter
  Bach-Simpson Ltd.
  PO Box 5484
  London, Ontario, Canada N6A4L6

Ultrasound Stethoscope
Versatone Doppler
  Medasonics
  PO Box M, 340 Pioneer Way
  Mountain View, California 94042

Narco Blood Flow Detector
  Narco Diagnostics, Inc.
  Commerce Drive
  Fort Washington, Pennsylvania 19034

Directional Doppler, Single and Dual Frequency
  Parks Electronics Laboratory
  PO Box BB
  Beaverton, Oregon 97005

Doppler Pocket Blood Flow Detector
Directional Doppler Blood Velocimeter
  Sonicaid
  PO Box 714
  Fredericksburgh, Virginia 22401

THROMBOELASTOGRAPH

Thromboelastograph D
PO Box 65, Dept. TR
Glenview, Illinois 60025

PNEUMOPLETHYSMOGRAPH

Vasograph
Electro Dignostic Instruments
819 South Main Street
Burbank, California 91506

PRG (Phleborheograph)
Grass Medical Instruments
Quincy, Massachusetts 02169

PVR (Pulse Volume Recorder)
Life Sciences, Inc.
270-T Greenwich Avenue
Greenwich, Connecticut 06830

STRAIN-GAUGE PLETHYSMOGRAPH

D. E. Hokanson Mercury Strain Gauge Plethysmograph
D. E. Hokanson, Inc.
3324-72nd Avenue, S.E.
Mercer Island, Washington 98040

Strain-Gauge Plethysmograph
Medisonics
PO Box M, 340 Pioneer Way
Mountain View, California 94042

Universal Plethysmograph
Medimatic
18103 Sky Park South
Irvine, California 92711

Mercury Strain-Gauge Plethysmograph
Parks Electronics Laboratory
PO Box BB
Beaverton, Oregon 97005

ULTRASONIC ARTERIOGRAPHY

Dopscan Ultrasonic Arterial Scanning System
 Carolina Medical Electronics, Inc.
 PO Box 307
 King, North Carolina 27021

Ultrasonic Arteriograph
 D. E. Hokanson, Inc.
 3324-72nd Avenue, S.E.
 Mercer Island, Washington 98040

Echoflow Color-Coded Arterial Imaging System
 Diagnostic Electronics Corp.
 Box 580
 Lexington, Massachusetts 02173

SELECTED REFERENCES

ANGIOGRAPHY

Abrams HL (ed): Angiography, ed 2. 2 volumes, Waltham, Mass: Little Brown Co, 1971

Arteriography

Beales JS, Adcock JA, Frawley JS, et al: The radiological assessment of disease in the profunda femoris artery. Br J Radiol 44:854, 1971

Berne FA, Lawrence WR, Carlton WA: Roentgenographic measurement of arterial narrowing. Am J Roentgenol Radium Ther Nucl Med 110:757, 1970

Clark OH, Moore WS, Hall AD: Radiographically occluded, anatomically patent carotid arteries. Arch Surg 102:604, 1971

Dardik H, Ibrahim IM, Koslow A, Dardik II: Evaluation of intraoperative arteriography as a routine for vascular reconstructions. Surg Gynecol Obstet 147:853, 1978

Dardik II, Ibrahim IM, Sprayregen S, et al: Routine intraoperative angiography. An essential adjunct in vascular surgery. Arch Surg 110:184, 1975

Engleman RM, Clements JM, Herrmann JB: Routine operative arteriography following vascular reconstructions. Surg Gynecol Obstet 128:745, 1969

Foster JH: Arteriography: cornerstone of vascular surgery. Arch Surg 109:605, 1974

Gammill SG, Craighead C: Translumbar aortography updated. Surg Gynecol Obstet 140:59, 1975

Haimovici H: Patterns of arteriosclerotic lesions in the lower extremity. Arch Surg 95:918, 1967

Hass WK, Fields, WS, North RR, et al: Joint study of extracranial arterial occlusion II. Arteriography, techniques, sites, and complications. JAMA 203:159, 1968

Haut G, Amplatz, K: Complication rates of transfemoral and transthoracic catheterization. Surgery 63:594, 1968

Kingsley O: A simplified method of demonstrating the profunda femoris artery. Br J Radiol 49:641, 1976

Lang E: A survey of the complications of percutaneous retrograde arteriography. Seldinger technic. Radiology 81:257, 1963

Lang E: Prevention and treatment of complications following arteriography. Radiology 88:950, 1967

Lindgren P, Tornell G: Blood circulation during and after peripheral arteriography. Acta Radiol 49:425, 1958

Moore WS, Hall AD: Unrecognized aortoiliac stenosis. Arch Surg 103:633, 1971

Newsome HH: A simple approach to improved visualization and identification of the vessels of the lower part of the leg. Surg Gynecol Obstet 148:927, 1979

Plecha FR, Pories WJ: Intraoperative angiography in the immediate assessment of arterial reconstruction. Arch Surg 105:902, 1972

Renwick S, Royle JP, Martin, P: Operative angiography after femoropopliteal arterial reconstruction — its influence on early failure rate. Br J Surg 55:134, 1968

Rosenthal JJ, Gaspar MR, Movius HJ: Intraoperative arteriography in carotid thromboendarterectomy. Arch Surg 106:806, 1973

Sethi GK, Scott SM, Takaro T: Multiple-plane angiography for more precise evaluation of aortoiliac disease. Surgery 78:154, 1975

Phlebography

Albrechston U, Olsson CG: Thrombotic side-effects of lower limb phlebography. Lancet 1:723, 1976

Brobelius A, Lorinc P, Nylander G: Phlebographic techniques in the diagnosis of acute deep venous thrombosis in the lower limb. Am J Roentgenol 111:794, 1971

Carlson PA: Phlebography of the lower extremities and plevic region. Am J Surg 118:632, 1969

Halliday P: Phlebography of the lower limb. Br J Surg 55:220, 1968

Lipchik ED, De Weese JA, Rogoff SM: Serial long term phlebography after documented lower leg thrombosis. Radiology 120:563, 1976

Rabinov K, Paulin S: Roentgen diagnosis of venous thrombosis in the leg. Arch Surg 104:134, 1972

Rogoff SM, De Weese JA: Phlebography of the lower extremity. JAMA 172:1599, 1960

Sander RJ, Glaser JL: Clinical uses of venography. Angiology 20:388, 1969

Thomas ML: Phlebography. Arch Surg 104:145, 1972

Thomas ML, McAllister V, Tonge K: The radiological appearance of deep venous thrombosis. Clin Radiol 45:199, 1971

Lymphography

deRoo T: Atlas of Lymphography. Philadelphia, JB Lippincott, 1975.

Kinmonth JB: The Lymphatics: Diseases, Lymphography and Surgery. Baltimore, Williams & Wilkins Co, 1972

Storen EJ, Myhre HO, Stiris G: Lymphangiographic findings in patients with leg edema after arterial reconstructions. Acta Chir Scand 140:385, 1974

Thompson LK, Futrell JW, Anlyan WG: Lymphangiography: direct and indirect using an iodinated emulsion. Plast Reconstr Surg 37:125, 1966

Miscellanous

Ansell G: Adverse reactions to contrast agents. Invest Radiol 5:374, 1970

Freisinger GC, Schaffer J, Criley JN, et al: Hemodynamic consequences of the injection of radiopaque material. Circulation 31:730, 1965

Rockoff SD, Brasch R, Kuhn G, Chraplyoy M: Contrast media as histamine liberators. Invest Radiol 5:503, 1970

ARTERIAL PLETHYSMOGRAPHY

Couch NP, van de Water JM, Dmochowski JR: Noninvasive measurement of arterial flow-impedance cardiograph and ultrasonic Doppler flowmeter. Arch Surg 102:435, 1971

Kroh BG, Dunne E, Magidson O, et al: The electrical impedance cardiogram in health and disease. Am Heart J 76:377, 1968

Griffin LH, Wray CH, Vaughn BL, Morentz WH: Detection of vascular occlusions during operation by segmental plethysmography and skin thermometry. Ann Surg 173:389, 1971

Moore TC, Riberi A, Kajikuri H, Schumacker HB: Use of impedance plethysmography in evaluation of peripheral vascular response to arteriography. Surgery 44:345, 1958

Nyboer J: Electrical Impedance Plethysmography, ed 2. Springfield, Ill, Charles C Thomas, 1970

Nyboer J, Murray P, Sedensky JA: Blood flow indices in amputated and control limbs by mutual electrical impedance plethysmography. Am Heart J 87:704, 1974

O'Connell TF, Kennedy JH, Steelquist JH: The surgical treatment of arterial emboli with special reference to the use of a standardized segmental plethysmograph. Ann Surg 148:731, 1958

Sakaguchi S, Tomita T, Endo I, Ishitobi K: Functional segmental plethysmography—clinical application and results. Angiology 21:714, 1970

van de Water JM, Dove GB, Mount BE, Linton LA: Application of bioelectric impedance to the measurement of arterial flow. J Surg Res 15:22, 1973

van de Water JM, Dmochowski JR, Dove GB, Couch NP: Evaluation of an impedance flowmeter in arterial surgery. Surgery 70:954, 1971

van de Water JM, Mount BE, Chandler KE, et al: Noninvasive measurement of pulsatile blood volume changes: its usefulness in peripheral vascular disease. Am J Surg 132:590, 1976

van de Water JM, Mount BE, Roettinger WF, Trudell LA: Noninvasive assessment of the peripheral vascular system. Arch Surg 112:679, 1977

BIOMEDICAL INSTRUMENTATION (GENERAL)

Cromwell L, Weilbell FJ, Pfeiffer EA: Biomedical Instrumentation and Measurements, ed 2. Englewood Cliffs, NJ, Prentice-Hall, Inc, 1980

Roberts C (ed): Blood Flow Measurements. Baltimore: Williams & Wilkins Co, 1972

Thomas HE: Handbook of Biomedical Instrumentation and Measurements. Reston, Va, Reston Publishing Co, Inc, 1974

Webster JG (ed): Medical Instrumentation. Application and Design. Boston, Houghton Mifflin Co, 1978

CAROTID PHONOANGIOGRAPHY

Blackshear WM, Thiele BL, Harly JD, et al: A prospective evaluation of oculo-plethysmography and carotid phonoangiography. Surg Gynecol Obstet 148:201, 1979

Duncan GW, Gruber JO, Dewey CF Jr, et al: Evaluation of carotid stenosis by phonoangiography. N Engl J Med 293:1124, 1975

Gross WS, Verta MJ, Van Bellen B, et al: Comparison of noninvasive diagnostic techniques in carotid artery occlusive disease. Surgery 82:271, 1977

Kartchner MM, McRae LP: Auscultation for carotid bruits in cerebrovascular insufficiency. JAMA 210:494, 1969

Lees RS, Dewey CF Jr: Phonoangiography: a new noninvasive diagnostic method of studying arterial disease. Proc Natl Acad Sci USA 67:935, 1970

Townes HW, Bowers JM, Braun HA: Characteristics of innocent and stenotic cervical bruits. Am Heart J 79:734, 1970

Ziegler DK, Zileti T, Dick A, et al: Correlation of bruits over the carotid artery with angiographically demonstrated lesions. Neurology 21:860, 1971

CEREBROVASCULAR EVALUATION

Cerebral Doppler

Barnes RW, Wilson MR: Doppler Ultrasonic Evaluation of Cerebrovascular Disease. A Programmed Audiovisual Instruction. Iowa City, University of Iowa Press, 1975

Barnes RW, Russell HE, Bone GE, Slaymaker EE: Doppler cerebrovascular examination: improved results with refinements in technique. Stroke 8:468, 1977

Bone GE, Barnes RW: Clinical implications of the Doppler cerebrovascular examination: a correlation with angiography. Stroke 7:271, 1976

Bone GE, Barnes RW: Limitations of the Doppler cerebrovascular examination in hemispheric cerebral ischemia. Surgery 79:577, 1976

LoGerfo FW, Mason GR: Directional Doppler studies of supraorbital artery flow in internal carotid stenosis and occlusion. Surgery 76:723, 1974

Lye CR, Sumner DS, Strandness DE Jr: The accuracy of the supraorbital Doppler examination in the diagnosis of hemodynamically significant carotid occlusive disease. Surgery 79:42, 1976

Machleder HI: Evaluation of patients with cerebrovascular disease using the Doppler ophthalmic test. Angiology 24:374, 1973

Machleder HI, Barker WF: Stroke on the wrong side. Use of the Doppler ophthalmic test in cerebral vascular screening. Arch Surg 105:943, 1972

Maroon JC, Campbell RL, Dyken ML: Internal carotid artery occlusion diagnosed by Doppler ultrasound. Stroke 1:122, 1970

Moore WS, Bean B, Burton R, Goldstone J: The use of ophthalmosonometry in the diagnosis of carotid artery stenosis. Surgery 82:107, 1977

Muller HR: The diagnosis of internal carotid artery occlusion by directional Doppler sonography of the ophthalmic artery. Neurology 22:816, 1972

Cerebral Photoplethysmography

Barnes RW, Garrett WV, Slaymaker EE, Reinertson JE: Doppler ultrasound and supraorbital photoplethysmography for noninvasive screening of carotid occlusive disease. Am J Surg 134:183, 1977

Barnes RW, Clayton JM, Bone GE, et al: Supraorbital photoplethysmography. Simple accurate screening for carotid occlusive disease. J Surg Res 22:319, 1977

Garrett WV, Slaymaker EE, Barnes RW: Noninvasive perioperative monitoring of carotid endarterectomy. J Surg Res 26:225, 1979

Sahbejami H: Photoelectric plethysmography and carotid compression. Med Ann Dist Columbia 39:138, 1969

Oculoplethysmography

Gee W, Oller DW, Wylie EJ: Noninvasive diagnosis of carotid occlusion by ocular pneumoplethysmography. Stroke 7:18, 1976

Johnston GG, Bernstein EF: Quantitation of internal carotid artery stenosis by ocular plethysmography. Surg Forum 26:290, 1975

Kartchner MM, McRae LP, Morrison FD: Noninvasive detection and evaluation of carotid occlusive disease. Arch Surg 106:528, 1973

Kartchner MM, McRae LP, Crain V, Whitaker B: Oculoplethysmography: an adjunct to arteriography in the diagnosis of extracranial carotid occlusive disease. Am J Surg 132:728, 1976

McDonald PT, Rich NM, Collins GJ, et al: Ocular pneumoplethysmography. Detection of carotid occlusive disease. Ann Surg 189:44, 1979

Combined Approach

Ackerman RH: Noninvasive carotid evaluation. Curr Concepts Cerebrovasc Dis 15:7, 1980

Brewster DC, Schlaen H, Raines JK: Rational management of the asymptomatic carotid bruit. Arch Surg 113:927, 1978

Herrmann JB, Korgaonker M, Cutler BS: Limitations of noninvasive evaluation of carotid occlusive disease. Arch Surg 114:1049, 1979

Kartchner MM, McRae LP: Noninvasive evaluation and management of the "asymptomatic" carotid bruit. Surgery 82:840, 1977

Kempczinski RF: A combined approach to the noninvasive diagnosis of carotid artery occlusive disease. Surgery 85:689, 1979

Lee BY, Thoden WR, Trainor FS, Kavner D: Noninvasive evaluation of peripheral arterial disease in the geriatric patient. J Am Geriatr Soc 28:352, 1980

Malone JM, Bean B, Laguna J, et al: Diagnosis of carotid artery stenosis. Comparison of oculoplethysmography and Doppler supraorbital examination. Ann Surg 191:347, 1980

McDonald PT, Rich NM, Collins GJ, et al: Doppler cerebrovascular examination, oculoplethysmograph and ocular pneumoplethysmography. Use in detection of carotid disease: A prospective clinical study. Arch Surg 113:1341, 1978

Moore WS: Diagnosis of carotid artery stenosis. Ann Surg 191:347, 1980

Satiana B, Cooperman M, Clark M, et al: An assessment of carotid phonoangiography and oculoplethysmography in the detection of carotid artery stenosis. Am J Surg 136:618, 1978

DOPPLER ULTRASOUND

Arterial

Allan JS, Terry HJ: The evaluation of an ultrasonic flow detector for the assessment of peripheral vascular disease. Cardiovasc Res 3:503, 1969

Balas P, Segditsas T, Koutsopoulos D: The value of the ultrasonic flowmeter in the diagnosis of arterial disease. Angiology 21:451, 1970

Barnes RW, Wilson MR: Doppler Ultrasonic Evaluation of Peripheral Arterial Disease: A Programmed Audiovisual Instruction. Iowa City, University of Iowa Press, 1976

Barnes RW, Shanik GD, Slaymaker EE: An index of healing in below-knee amputation: leg blood pressure by Doppler ultrasound. Surgery 79:13, 1976

Bell G: Systolic pressure measurements in occlusive vascular disease to assess run-off preoperatively. Scand J Clin Lab Invest 31 (suppl 128):173, 1973

Benchimol A, Desser KB: Clinical application of the Doppler ultrasound flowmeter. Am J Cardiol 29:540, 1972

Bollinger A, Schlumph M, Butti P, Gruntzig A: Measurement of systolic ankle blood pressure with Doppler ultrasound at rest and after exercise in patients with leg artery occlusions. Scand J Clin Lab Invest 31 (suppl 128):123, 1973

Carter SA: Clinical measurement of systolic pressure in limbs with arterial occlusive disease. JAMA 207:1869, 1969

Carter SA: Response of ankle systolic pressure to leg exercise in mild or questionable arterial disease. N Engl J Med 287:578, 1972

Carter SA: The relationship of distal systolic pressures to healing of skin lesions in limbs with arterial occlusive disease with special reference to diabetes mellitus. Scand J Clin Lab Invest 31 (suppl 128):239, 1973

Dean RH, Yao JS, Stanton PE, Bergan JJ: Prognostic indicators in femoropopliteal reconstructions. Arch Surg 110:1287, 1975

Dean RH, Yao JS, Thompson RG, Bergan JJ: Predictive value of ultrasonically derived arterial pressure in determination of amputation level. Am Surg 41:731, 1975

Fronek A, Coel M, Bernstein EF: Quantitative ultrasonographic studies of lower extremity flow velocities in health and disease. Circulation 53:957, 1976

Fronek A, Johansen K, Dilley RB, Bernstein EF: Ultrasonigraphically monitored post-occlusive reactive hyperemia in the diagnosis of peripheral arterial occlusive disease. Circulation 48:149, 1973

Garrett WV, Slaymaker EE, Heintz SE, Barnes RW: Intraoperative predictor of symptomatic result of aortofemoral bypass from changes in ankle pressure index. Surgery 82:504, 1977

Hartley CJ, Strandness DE Jr, Reid JM, Rogers WE: The effects of atherosclerosis on the transmission of ultrasound. J Surg Res 9:575, 1969

Hobbs JT, Yao JS, Lewis JD, Needham TN: A limitation of the Doppler ultrasonic method of measuring ankle systolic pressure. J Vasc Dis 3:160, 1974

Johnson WC: Doppler ankle pressure and reactive hyperemia in the diagnosis of arterial insufficiency. J Surg Res 18:1, 1975

Kazamias TM, Gander MP, Franklin DL, Ross J Jr: Blood pressure measurement with Doppler ultrasonic flowmetry. J Appl Physiol 30:585, 1971

Keitzer WH, Lichti EL, Brossart FA, DeWeese MS: Use of the Doppler ultrasonic flowmeter during arterial vascular surgery. Arch Surg 105:302, 1972

Lennihan R Jr, Mackereth MA: Ankle pressures in arterial occlusive disease involving the legs. Surg Clin North Am 53:657, 1973

Nicolaides AN, Gordon-Smith IC, Dayandas J, Eastocott HHG: The value of Doppler blood velocity tracings in the detection of aortoiliac disease in patients with intermittent claudication. Surgery 80:774, 1976

Rittenhouse EA, Maixner W, Burr JW, Barnes RW: Directional arterial flow velocity: a sensitive index to changes in peripheral vascular resistance. Surgery 79:350, 1976

Seegar JM, Lazarus HM, Alba D Jr: Preoperative selection of patients for lumbar sympathectomy by use of the Doppler index. Am J Surg 134:749, 1977

Stegall HF, Kardon MB, Kenmmerer WT: Indirect measurement of arterial blood pressure by Doppler ultrasonic sphygmomanometry. J Appl Physiol 25:793, 1968

Strandness DE Jr, McCutcheon EP, Rushmer RF: Application of a transcutaneous Doppler flowmeter in evaluation of occlusive arterial disease. Surg Gynecol Obstet 122:1039, 1966

Strandness DE Jr, Schultz RD, Sumner DS, Rushmer RF: Ultrasonic flow detection: a useful technic in the evaluation of peripheral vascular disease. Am J Surg 113:311, 1967

Yao JS, Bergan JJ: Predictability of vascular reactivity relative to sympathetic oblation. Arch Surg 107:676, 1973

Yao JS, Bergan JJ: Application of ultrasound to arterial and venous diagnosis. Surg Clin North Am 54:1, 1974

Yao JS, Hobbs JT, Irvine WT: Ankle systolic pressure measurements in arterial diseases affecting the lower extremities. Br J Surg 56:676, 1969

Intestinal Viability

Cooperman M, Martin EW, Carey LC: Assessment of anastomotic blood supply by Doppler ultrasound in operations upon the colon. Surg Gynecol Obstet 149:15, 1979

Cooperman M, Pace WG, Martin EW, et al: Determination of viability of ischemic intestine by Doppler ultrasound. Surgery 83:705, 1978

Hobson RW, Wright CB, Rich NM, Collins GJ: Assessment of colonic ischemia during aortic surgery by Doppler ultrasound. J Surg Res 20:231, 1976

Kurstin RD, Soltanzedah H, Hobson RW, Wright CB: Ultrasonic blood flow assessment in colon-esophageal bypass procedures. Arch Surg 112:270, 1977

Lee BY, Trainor FS, Kavner D, McCann WJ: Intraoperative assessment of intestinal viability with Doppler ultrasound. Surg Gynecol Obstet 149:671, 1979

Wright CD, Hobson RW: Prediction of intestinal viability using Doppler ultrasound technics. Am J Surg 129:642, 1975

Venous

Alexander RH, Folse R, Pizzorno J, Coon R: Thrombophlebitis and thromboembolism: results of a prospective study. Ann Surg 180:833, 1974

Barnes RW, Ross EA, Strandness DE Jr: Noninvasive quantification of deep venous incompetence: primary versus secondary varicose veins. Surg Forum 28:252, 1974

Barnes RW, Ross EA, Strandness DE Jr: Differentiation of primary from secondary varicose veins by Doppler ultrasound and strain gauge plethysmography. Surg Gynecol Obstet 141:207, 1975

Barnes RW, Russell HE, Wilson MR: Doppler ultrasonic Evaluation of Venous Disease: A Programmed Audiovisual Instruction. Iowa City, University of Iowa Press, 1975

Barnes RW, Russell HE, Wu KK, Hoak JC: Accuracy of Doppler ultrasound in clinically suspected venous thrombosis of the calf. Surg Gynecol Obstet 143:425, 1976

Barnes RW, Slaymaker EE: Postoperative deep vein thrombosis in the lower extremity amputee: a prospective study with Doppler ultrasound. Ann Surg 183:429, 1976

Barnes RW, Wu KK, Hoak JC: Differentiation of superficial thrombophlebitis from lymphangitis by Doppler ultrasound. Surg Gynecol Obstet 142:23, 1976

Evans DS: The early diagnosis of deep vein thrombosis by ultrasound. Br J Surg 57:726, 1970

Evans DS: The early diagnosis of thromboembolism by ultrasound. Ann R Coll Surg Engl 49:225, 1971

Evans DS, Cockett FB: Diagnosis of deep vein thrombosis with an ultrasonic Doppler technique. Br Med J 2:802, 1969

Folse R, Alexander RH: Directional flow detection for localizing venous valvular incompetence. Surgery 67:114, 1970

McCaffrey J, Williams O, Stathis M: Diagnosis of deep venous thrombosis using a Doppler ultrasonic technique. Surg Gynecol Obstet 140:740, 1975

Meadway J, Nicolaides AN, Walker CJ, O'Connell JD: Value of Doppler ultrasound in diagnosis of clinically suspected deep vein thrombosis. Br Med J 4:552, 1975

Miller SS, Foote AV: The ultrasonic detection of incompetent perforating veins. Br J Surg 61:653, 1974

Sigel B, Felix WR, Popky GL, Ipsen J: Diagnosis of lower limb venous thrombosis by Doppler ultrasound technique. Arch Surg 104:174, 1972

Sigel B, Popky GL, Mapp EM, et al: Evaluation of Doppler ultrasound examination. Its use in diagnosis of lower extremity venous disease. Arch Surg 100:535, 1970

Sigel B, Popky GL, Wagner DK, et al: A Doppler ultrasonic method for diagnosing lower extremity venous disease. Surg Gynecol Obstet 127:339, 1967

Strandness DE Jr, Sumner DS: Ultrasonic velocity detector in the diagnosis of thrombophlebitis. Arch Surg 104:180, 1972

Sumner DS, Baker DW, Strandness DE Jr: The ultrasonic velocity detector in a clinical study of venous disease. Arch Surg 97:75, 1968

Yao JS, Gourmos C, Hobbs JT: Detection of proximal vein thrombosis by Doppler ultrasound flow-detection method. Lancet 1:1, 1972

ELECTROMAGNETIC FLOWMETRY

Intraoperative

Barner HB, Kaminski DL, Codd JE, et al: Hemodynamics of autogenous femor-popliteal bypass. Arch Surg 109:291, 1974

Bernhard VM: Intraoperative monitoring of femorotibial bypass grafts. Surg Clin North Am 54:77, 1974

Dillon ML, Reeves JW, Postlethwait RW: Cartid artery flows and pressures in twenty-two patients with cerebral vascular insufficiency. Surgery 58:951, 1965

Gessner V: Effects of the vessel wall on electromagnetic flow measurements. Biophys J 1:627, 1961

Golding AL, Cannon JA: Application of electromagnetic blood flowmetry during arterial reconstruction. Results in conjuction with Papaverine in 47 cases. Ann Surg 164:662, 1966

Hobson RW, Rich NM, Wright CB, Fedde CW: Operative assessment of carotid endarterectomy: internal carotid arterial back pressure, carotid arterial blood flow, and carotid arteriography. Ann Surg 41:603, 1975

Lee BY, Trainor FS: Peripheral Vascular Surgery: Hemodynamics of Arterial Pulsatile Blood Flow. New York, Appleton, 1973

Lee BY, Castillo HT, Madden JL: Quantification of the arterial pulsatile blood flow waveform in peripheral vascular disease. Angiology 21:595, 1970

Lee BY, LaPointe DG, Madden JL: Evaluation of lumbar sympathectomy by quantification of arterial pulsatile waveform. Vasc Surg 5:61, 1971

Lee BY, Madden JL, McDonough WB: Use of square-wave electromagnetic flowmeter during direct arterial surgery, before and after lumbar sympathectomy in peripheral vascular surgery. Vasc Surg 3:218, 1969

Lee BY, Trainor FS, Madden JL: Significance of arterial blood flow in reconstructive arterial procedure. Surg Gynecol Obstet 132:803, 1971

Lee BY, Trainor FS, Kavner D, McCann WJ: Evaluation of modified human umbilical vein as an arterial substitute in femoropopliteal reconstructive surgical procedures. Surg Gynecol Obstet 147:721, 1978

Lee BY, Assadi C, Madden JL, et al: Hemodynamics of arterial stenosis. World J Surg 2:621, 1978

Terry HJ, Taylor GW: Quantitation of flow in femoropopliteal grafts. Surg Clin North Am 54:85, 1974

Weissenhofer W, Schmidt R, Schenk WG: Technique of electromagnetic blood flow measurements: notes regarding a potential source of error. Surgery 73:474, 1973

Noninvasive

Lee BY, Trainor FS, Kavner D, Madden JL: A clinical evaluation of a noninvasive electromagnetic flowmeter. Angiology 26:317, 1975

Lee BY, Trainor FS, Thoden WR, et al: Use of noninvasive electromagnetic flowmetry in the assessment of peripheral arterial disease. Surg Gynecol Obstet 150:342, 1980

Lee BY, Trainor FS: Arterial flow in the lower leg correlated with plasma levels of two formulations of papaverine hydrochloride. Angiology 39:310, 1978

^{125}I-FIBRINOGEN

Browse NL: The ^{125}I-fibrinogen uptake test. Arch Surg 104:160, 1972

Browse NL, Clapham WF, Croft DN, et al: Diagnosis of established deep vein thrombosis with the ^{125}I-fibrinogen uptake test. Br Med J 4:325, 1971

Charles ND: ^{125}I-Fibrinogen scanning. Lancet 1:1191, 1973

Flanc C, Kakkar VV, Clarke MB: The detection of venous thrombosis of the legs using ^{125}I-labelled fibrinogen. Br J Surg 55:742, 1968

Hume M, Gurewich V: Peripheral venous scanning with ^{125}I-tagged fibrinogen. Lancet 1:845, 1972

Kakkar VV: The diagnosis of deep vein thrombosis using the ^{125}I-fibrinogen test. Arch Surg 104:152, 1972

Kakkar VV, Nicolaides AN, Renney JTG, et al: ^{125}I-Labelled fibrinogen test adapted for routine screening for deep-vein thrombosis. Lancet 1:540, 1970

Negus D, Pinto DJ, LeQuesne LP, et al: ^{125}I-Labelled fibrinogen in the diagnosis of deep vein thrombosis and its correlation with phlebography. Br J Surg 55:835, 1968

PHLEBORHEOGRAPHY

Cranely JJ, Gay AY, Grass AM, Simeone FA: A plethysmographic technique for the diagnosis of deep venous thrombosis of the lower extremities. Surg Gynecol Obstet 136:385, 1973

Cranely JJ: Phleborheography. RI Med J 58:111, 1975

Cranely JJ, Canos AJ, Sull WJ, Grass AM: Phleborheographic technique for diagnosing deep venous thrombosis of the lower extremities. Surg Gynecol Obstet 141:331, 1975

PHOTOPLETHYSMOGRAPHY

Anderson NM, Sekelj P: Light absorbing and scattering properties of non-haemolyzed blood. Phys Med Biol 12:178, 1967

Barnes RW, Garrett, WV, Hummel BA, et al: Photoplethysmographic assessment of altered cutaneous circulation in the post-phlebitic syndrome. AAMI Proceedings, Washington, DC, 1978, p 25

Baudet J, LeMaire J, Guimberteau J: Ten free groin flaps. Plast Reconstr Surg 57:589, 1976

Creeche BJ, Miller S: Evaluation of circulation in skin flaps. In Grabb W, Meyer B (eds): Skin Flaps. Boston, Little, Brown & Co, 1975, p 32

Hertzman AB: The blood supply of various skin areas estimated by the photoelectric plethysmograph. Am J Physiol 124:338, 1938

Lee BY, Trainor FS, Kavner D, et al: Assessment of the healing potentials of ulcers of the skin by photoplethysmography. Surg Gynecol Obstet 148:232, 1979

Muir IFK, Fox RH, Stranc WE, Stewart FS: The measurement of blood flow by a photoelectric technique and its application to the management of tubed skin pedicles. Br J Plast Surg 21:14, 1968

PHYSIOLOGY

Abramson DI: Circulation of the Extremities. New York, Academic Press, 1967

McDonald DA: Blood Flow in Arteries. London, England, Edward Arnold, 1960

McHenry LC: Cerebral Circulation and Stroke. St. Louis, Warren H Green 1978

Shephard JT: Physiology of the Circulation in Human Limbs in Health and Disease. Philadelphia, WB Saunders, 1963

Strandness DE Jr: Peripheral Arterial Disease: A Physiologic Approach. Boston, Little, Brown & Co, 1969

Strandness DE Jr, Summer DS: Hemodynamics for Surgeons. New York, Grune and Stratton, 1975

Strandness DE Jr, et al (eds): Collateral Circulation in Clinical Surgery. Philadelphia, WB Saunders, 1969

RADIONUCLIDE SCANNING

Pulmonary Scanning and Angiography

Dalen JE, Books HL, Johnson LW, et al: Pulmonary angiography in acute pulmonary embolism: indications, techniques, and results in 367 patients. Am Heart J 81:175, 1971

DeNardo CL, Goodwin DA, Ravasini R, et al: The ventilation lung scan in the diagnosis of pulmonary embolism. N Engl J Med 282:1334, 1970

Johnson PM: The role of lung scanning in pulmonary embolism. Semin Nucl Med 1:161, 1971

Kelly MJ, Elliott LP: The radiologic evaluation of the patient with suspected pulmonary thromboembolic disease. Med Clin North Am 59:3, 1974

Secker-Walker RH, Siegal BA: The use of nuclear medicine in the diagnosis of lung disease. Radiol Clin North Am 11:215, 1973

Radionuclide Arteriography

Bergan JJ, Yao JS, Henkin RE, et al: Radionuclide aortography in the detection of arterial aneurysms. Arch Surg 109:80, 1974

Diamond AB, Meng C, Wolanske AC, et al: Radionuclide demonstration of traumatic arterial injury. Radiology 109:623, 1973

Dibos PE, Muhletaler CA, Natarajan TK, et al: Intravenous radionuclide arteriography in peripheral occlusive disease. Radiology 102:181, 1972

Griep RJ, Wise G, Marty R: Detection of carotid artery obstruction by intravenous radionuclide angiography. Radiology 97:311, 1970

Moss CM, Delaney HM, Rudavsky AZ: Isotope angiography for detection of embolic arterial occlusion. Surg Gynecol Obstet 142:57, 1976

Moss CM, Rudavsky AZ, Vieth FJ: The value of scintiangiography in arterial disease. Arch Surg 111:1235, 1976

Moss CM, Rudavsky AZ, Vieth FJ: Isotope angiography: techniques, validation and value in the assessment of arterial reconstruction. Ann Surg 184:116, 1976

Radionuclide Phlebography

Barnes RW, McDonald GB, Hamilton GW, et al: Radionuclide venography for rapid dynamic evaluation of venous disease. Surgey 72:706, 1973

Henkin RE, Yao JS, Quinn JL, Bergan JJ: Radionuclide venography (RNV) in lower extremity venous disease. J Nucl Med 15:171, 1974

Yao JS, Henkin RE, Conn J Jr, et al: Combined isotope venography and lung scanning. A new diagnostic approach to thromboembolism. Arch Surg 107:146, 1973

Radionuclide Lymphography

Dunson GL, Thrall JH, Stevenson JS, et al: ^{99m}Tc Minicolloid for radionuclide lymphography. Radiology 109:387, 1973

Herting SE, Fredericksen PB, Jagt T, Jeppesen P: Lymph node scanning with colloidal radioactive gold. Acta Radiol 10:359, 1970

Sage HH, Gozun BV: Lymphatic scintigrams: a method for studying the functional patterns of lymphatics and lymph nodes. Cancer 11:200, 1958

Walker LA: Localization of radioactive colloids in lymph nodes. Clin Med 36:440, 1950

RISK FACTORS AND PATHOGENESIS

Frank CW, Weinblatt E, Shapiro S, Sager RV: Physical inactivity as a lethal factor in myocardial infarction among men. Circulation 34:1022, 1966

Friedman SA, Holling HE, Roberts B: Etiologic factors in aortoiliac and femoropopliteal vascular disease. N Engl J Med 271:1382, 1964

Gordon T, Kannel WB: Predisposition to atherosclerosis in the head, heart, and eyes: the Framingham Study. JAMA 221:661, 1972

Haimovici H: Atherogenesis: recent biological concepts and clinical implications. Am J Surg 134:174, 1977

Javid H: Development of carotid plaque. Am J Surg 138:224, 1979

Juergens JL, Barker NW, Hines EA Jr: Arteriosclerosis obliterans: review of 520 cases with special reference to pathogenic and prognostic factors. Circulation 21:188, 1960

Levy RI, Morganrath J, Rifkind BM: Treatment of hyperlipidemia. N Engl J Med 290:1295, 1974

Phillips R: Cardiovascular Therapy—A Systematic Approach. Philadelphia, WB Saunders, 1979

Report of the Inter-Society Commission for Heart Disease Resources. Primary Prevention of Atherosclerotic Diseases. Circulation 42:A 53, 1970

Rosen AJ, DePalma RG, Victor Y: Risk factors in peripheral atherosclerosis. Arch Surg 107:303, 1973

Ross R, Glomset JA: The pathogenesis of atherosclerosis. N Engl J Med 295:369, 1976

Schenk EA: Pathology of occlusive disease of the lower extremities. Cardiovasc Clin 5:287, 1973

Stamler J: Cardiovascular diseases in the United States. Am J Cardiol 10:319, 1962

Wissler RW: Development of the atherosclerotic plaque. Hosp Pract 8:61, 1973

Wray R, DePalma RG, Hubay CA: Late occlusion of aortofemoral bypass grafts: influence of cigarette smoking. Surgery 70:969, 1971

Vavrik M: "High risk" factors and atherosclerotic cardiovascular diseases in the aged. J Am Geriatr Soc 22:203, 1974

STRAIN GAUGE PLETHYSMOGRAPHY

Barnes RW, Collicott PE, Mozersky DJ, et al: Noninvasive quantitation of maximum venous outflow in acute thrombophlebitis. Surgery 72:971, 1972

Barnes RW, Collicott PE, Mozersky DJ, et al: Noninvasive quantitation of venous reflux in the postphlebitic syndrome. Surg Gynecol Obstet 136:767, 1973

Barnes RW, Collicott PE, Sumner DS, Strandness DE Jr: Noninvasive quantitation of venous hemodynamics in the postphlebitic syndrome. Arch Surg 107:807, 1973

Holm JS: A simple plethysmographic method for differentiating primary from secondary varicose veins. IEEE Trans Biomed Eng 22:25, 1975

Nielson PE, Bell G, Lassen NA: The measurement of digital systolic blood pressure by strain gauge technique. Scand J Clin Lab Invest 29:371, 1972

Parrish D, Strandness DE Jr, Bell JW: Dynamic response characteristics of a mercury-in-Silastic strain gauge. J Appl Physiol 19:363, 1964

Strandness DE Jr, Bell JW: Peripheral vascular disease. Diagnosis and objective evaluation using a mercury strain gauge. Ann Surg 161 (suppl):1, 1965

Whitney RJ: The measurement of volume changes in human limbs. J Physiol 121:1, 1953

TEMPERATURE AND THERMOGRAPHY

Bergquist D, Dahlgren S, Efsing O, et al: Thermographic diagnosis of deep vein thrombosis. Br Med J 4:684, 1975

Branemark PI, Nilsson K: Thermographic and microvascular studies of the peripheral circulation. Bibl Radiol 5:130, 1969

Burton AC: The range of variability of blood flow in human fingers and the vasomotor regulation of body temperature. Am J Physiol 127:437, 1939

Burton AC: Temperature of skin: measurement and use as an index of peripheral blood flow. Meth Med Res 1:146, 1948

Capistrant TD, Gumnit RJ: Thermography following a carotid transient ischemic episode. JAMA 211:656, 1970

Cooke ED, Pilcher MF: Deep vein thrombosis: preclinical diagnosis by thermography. Br J Surg 61:971, 1974

Davidson TW, Ewing KI, Fergason J, et al: Detection of breast cancer by liquid crystal thermography. A preliminary report. Cancer 29:1123, 1972

Felder D, Russ E, Montgomery H, Horowitz O: Relationship in the toe of skin surface temperature to mean blood flow measured with a plethysmograph. Clin Sci 13:251, 1954

Karpman HL, Kalb IM, Sheppard JJ: The use of thermography in a health care system for stroke. Geriatrics 27:96, 1972

Lee BY, Trainor FS, Madden JL: Liquid crystal tape: its use in the evaluation of vascular disease. Arch Phys Med Rehabil 54:96, 1973

Mawdsley C, Samuel E, Sumerling MD, Young GB: Thermography in occlusive cerebrovascular diseases. Br Med J 3:521, 1968

Trandel RS, Lewis DW, Verhonick PJ: Thermographical investigation of decubitis ulcers. Bull Prosthet Res, Fall, 1975, p 137

Windsor T, Windsor D: Thermography in cardiovascular disease. Appl Radiol, Nov-Dec 1975, p 117

THROMBOELASTOGRAPHY

Caprini JA, Kurtides S, Dorsey JM: Coagulation changes in acutely bleeding patients. Arch Surg 104:559, 1972

Caprini JA, Zuckerman L, Cohen E: Thromboelastographic analysis of patients with cancer. A preliminary report. Diagnostica 30:4, 1974

Caprini JA, Zuckerman L, Cohen E, et al: The identification of accelerated coagulability. Thromb Res 9:167: 1976

Cohen E, Caprini JA, Zuckerman L, et al: Evaluation of three methods to identify accelerated coagulability. Thromb Res 10:587, 1977

DiNicola P: Thromboelastography. Springfield, Ill, Charles C Thomas, 1957

Ettinger MG: Thromboelastographic studies in cerebral infarction. Stroke 5:350, 1974

Howland WS, Castro EB, Fortner JB, Gould P: Hypercoagulability: thromboelastographic monitoring during extensive hepatic surgery. Arch Surg 108:605, 1974

Lee BY, Madden JL, Trainor FS, et al: Detection and prevention of deep vein thrombosis in the general surgical patient. In Madden JL, Hume M (eds): Venous Thromboembolism: Prevention and Treatment. New York, Appleton, 1976, p 61

Lee BY, Taha S, Trainor FS, et al: Monitoring heparin therapy with thromboelastography and activated partial thromboplastin time. World J Surg 4, 323, 1980

Lee BY, Thoden WR, Sarabu MR, et al: Fibrinolytic activity of external intermittent pneumatic compression. Contemp Surg, in press, 1980

Lee BY, Trainor FS, Kavner D, et al: Noninvasive prevention of thrombosis of deep veins of the thigh using intermittent pneumatic compression. Surg Gynecol Obstet 142:705, 1976

Lee BY, Trainor FS, Kavner D, McCann WJ: Monitoring of heparin therapy. Surg Gynecol Obstet 149:843, 1979

Lee BY, Trainor FS, Thoden WR, Kavner D: Prevention of venous thromboembolism using external intermittent pneumatic compression. Contemp Surg 15:67, 1979

ULTRASONOGRAPHY

Doppler Ultrasonic Angiography

Barnes RW, Bone GE, Reinertson JE, et al: Noninvasive ultrasonic carotid angiography: prospective validation by contrast arteriography. Surgery 80:328, 1976

Day TK, Fish PJ, Kakkar VV: Detection of deep vein thrombosis by Doppler angiography. Br Med J 1:618, 1976

Fish PJ, Corrigan T, Kakkar VV, Nicolaides AN: Arteriography using ultrasound. Lancet 1:1269, 1972

Hokanson DE, Mozersky DJ, Sumner DS, Strandness DE Jr: Ultrasonic arteriography: a new approach to arterial visualization. Biomed Eng 6:420, 1971

Hokanson DE, Mozersky DJ, Sumner DS, et al: Ultrasonic arteriography. A noninvasive method of arterial visualization. Radiology 102:435, 1972

Mozersky DJ, Hokanson DE, Sumner DS, Strandness DE Jr: Ultrasonic visualization of the arterial lumen. Surgery 72:253, 1972

Mozersky DJ, Hokanson DE, Baker DW, et al: Ultrasonic arteriography. Arch Surg 103:663, 1971

Ried JM, Spencer MP: Ultrasonic Doppler technique for imaging blood vessels. Science 176:1235, 1972

Pulse Echo Ultrasonography (Echography)

Davis RP, Neiman HL, Yao JS, Bergan JJ: Ultrasound scan in diagnosis of peripheral aneurysms. Arch Surg 112:55, 1977

Goldberg BBM, Ostrum BJ, Isaro HJ: Ultrasonic aortography. JAMA 198:353, 1966

King DL (ed): Diagnostic Ultrasound. St. Louis, Mo, CV Mosby, 1974

Lee KR, Walls WJ, Martin NL, Templeton AW: A practical approach to the diagnosis of abdominal aortic aneurysms. Surgery 78:195, 1975

Leopold GR: Ultrasonic abdominal aortography. Radiology 96:9, 1970

Leopold GR, Goldberger LE, Bernstein EF: Ultrasonic detection and evaluation of abdominal aortic aneurysm. Surgery 72:939, 1972

Maloney JD, Pairolero PC, Smith BF Jr, et al: Ultrasonic evaluation of abdominal aortic aneurysm. Circulation 56 (suppl II):II 80, 1977

Segal BL, Likoff W, Asperger Z, Kingsley B: Ultrasonic diagnosis of an abdominal aortic aneurysm. Am J Cardiol 17:101, 1966

Real-Time Ultrasonic Arteriography

Green PS: Real-time, high resolution ultrasonic carotid arteriography system. In Bernstein EF, et al (eds): Noninvasive Diagnostic Techniques in Vascular Disease. St. Louis, Mo, CV Mosby, 1978, p 29

Green PS, Taenzer JC, Ramsey SD, et al: A real-time ultrasonic imager for carotid arteriography. Menlo Park, Cal, Stanford Research Institute, 1977

Hobson RW, Lipp J, O'Donnell JA: Real-time ultrasonic arteriography of the extracranial carotid artery. In Dietrich EB (ed): Noninvasive Cardiovascular Diagnosis: Current Concepts. Baltimore, University Park Press, 1978, p 29

Lipp J, O'Donnell JA, Hobson RW: Real-time arteriography of the carotid artery. Clin Res 25:235, 1977

Mercier LA, Greenleaf JF, Evans TC: High-resolution ultrasound arteriography: a comparison with carotid angiography. In Bernstein EF, et al (eds): Noninvasive Diagnostic Techniques in Vascular Disease. St. Louis, Mo, CV Mosby, 1978, p 231

THE VASCULAR LABORATORY

Barnes RW: Noninvasive diagnostic techniques in peripheral vascular disease. Am Heart J 97:241, 1979

Cranley JJ, Mahalingam K, Ferris EB: Extending the vascular examination by noninvasive means. Am J Surg 134:179, 1977

Fronek A, Johansen KH, Dilley RB, Bernstein EF: Noninvasive physiologic tests in the diagnosis and characterization of peripheral arterial occlusive disease. Am J Surg 126:205, 1973

Hirsh J, Hull R: Comparative value of tests for the diagnosis of venous thrombosis. World J Surg 2:27, 1978

Kempczinski RF, Rutherford RB: Current status of the vascular diagnostic laboratory. Adv Surg 12:1, 1978

Lambeth A: Statistics in the vascular laboratory. Bruit 3:9, 1979

Lee BY, Toden WR, Trainor FS, Kavner D: Noninvasive detection and prevention of deep vein thrombosis in the geriatric patient. J Am Geriatr Soc 28:171, 1980

Lee BY, Thoden WR, Trainor FS, Kavner D: Noninvasive evaluation of peripheral arterial disease in the geriatric patient. J Am Geriatr Soc 28:352, 1980

Raines J, Larsen PB: Practical guidelines for establishing a clinical vascular laboratory. Cardiovasc Dis, Bull Texas Heart Inst 6:93, 1979

Raines J, Darling RC, Buth J, et al: Vascular laboratory criteria for the management of peripheral vascular disease of the lower extremities. Surgery 79:21, 1976

Sasahara AA, Sharma G, Parisi AF: New developments in the detection and prevention of venous thromboembolism. Am J Cardiol 42:1214, 1979

Strandness DE Jr: The use and abuse of the vascular laboratory. Surg Clin North Am 59:707, 1979

van de Water JM, Laska ED, Ciniero WV: Patient and operation selectivity. The peripheral vascular laboratory. Ann Surg 189:143, 1979

VASCULAR SURGERY AND NONINVASIVE DIAGNOSIS (GENERAL)

Abramson DI: Vascular Disorders of the Extremities, ed 2. Hagerstown, Md, Harper & Row, 1974

Barker WF: Peripheral Arterial Disease, ed 2. Philadelphia, WB Saunders, 1975

Bergan JJ, Yao JS (eds): Gangrene and Severe Ischemia of the Lower Extremities. New York, Grune & Stratton, 1978

Bergan JJ, Yao JS (eds): Venous Problems. Chicago, Yearbook Medical Publishers, 1978

Bernstein EF, et al (eds): Noninvasive Diagnostic Techniques in Vascular Disease. St. Louis, Mo, CV Mosby, 1978

Cranley JJ: Vascular Surgery. Vol 1: Peripheral Arterial Diseases. Hagerstown, Md, Harper & Row, 1972

Cranley JJ: Vascular Surgery. Vol 2: Peripheral Venous Diseases. Hagerstown, Md, Harper & Row, 1975

Dale WA (ed): Management of Arterial Occlusive Disease. Chicago, Yearbook Medical Publishers, 1971

Dietrich EB (ed): Noninvasive Cardiovascular Diagnoses: Current Concepts. Baltimore, University Park Press, 1978

Haimovici H (ed): Vascular Surgery: Principles and Techniques. New York, McGraw-Hill, 1976

Hobbs JT (ed): The Treatment of Venous Disorders. Lancaster, England, M.T.P. Press, Ltd, 1977

Holling HE: Peripheral Vascular Diseases: Diagnosis and Management. Philadelphia, JB Lippincott, 1972

Hume M, Sevitt S, Thomas DP: Venous Thrombosis and Pulmonary Embolism. Cambridge, Mass, Harvard University Press, 1970

Kappert A, Windsor T: Diagnosis of Peripheral Vascular Disease. Philadelphia, FA Davis, 1972

Madden JL, Hume M (eds): Venous Thromboembolism: Prevention and Treatment. New York, Appleton, 1976

Mannick JA, Coffman JD: Ischemic Limbs: Surgical Approach and Physiological Problems. New York, Grune & Stratton, 1973

Rutherford RB, et al (eds): Vascular Surgery. Philadelphia, WB Saunders, 1977

VENOUS IMPEDANCE PLETHYSMOGRAPHY

Deuvaert FC, Dmochowski JR, Couch ND: Positional factors in venous impedance plethysmography. Arch Surg 106:53, 1973

Dmochowski JR, Adams DF, Couch ND: Impedance measurement in the diagnosis of DVT. Arch Surg 104:170, 1972

Hull R, vanAcken WG, Hirsh J, et al: Impedance plethysmography using the occlusive cuff technique in the diagnosis of venous thrombosis. Circulation 53:696, 1976

Johnston KW, Kakkar VV: Plethysmographic diagnosis of deep vein thrombosis. Surg Gynecol Obstet 139:41, 1974

Johnston KW, Kakkar VV, Spindler JJ, et al: A simple method for detecting deep vein thrombosis. An improved electrical impedance technique. Am J Surg 127:349, 1974

Lee BY, Thoden WR, Trainor FS, Kavner D: Noninvasive detection and prevention of deep vein thrombosis in the geriatric patient. J Am Geriatr Soc 28:171 1980.

Mullick SC, Wheeler HB, Songster GP: Diagnosis of deep venous thrombosis by measurements of electrical impedance. Am J Surg 119:417, 1970

Nadeau JE, Demers R, Skinner B, MacLean LD: Impedance phlebography: accuracy of diagnosis in deep vein thrombosis. Can J Surg 18:219, 1975

Steer ML, Spotnitz AJ, Cohen SI, et al: Limitations of impedance phlebography for diagnosis of venous thrombosis. Arch Surg 106:44, 1973

Wheeler HB, Mullick SC: Detection of venous obstruction in the leg by measurement of electrical impedance. Ann NY Acad Sci 170:804, 1970

Wheeler HB, O'Donnell JA, Anderson FA, Benedict K: Occlusive impedance phlebography: a diagnostic procedure for venous thrombosis and pulmonary embolism. Prog Cardiovasc Dis 17:199, 1974

Wheeler HB, O'Donnell JA, Anderson FA, et al: Bedside screening for venous thrombosis using occlusive impedance phlebography. Angiology 25:199, 1975

Wheeler HB, Mullick SC, Anderson JN, Pearson D: Diagnosis of occult deep venous thrombosis by a non-invasive bedside technique. Surgery 70:20, 1971

Wheeler HB, Pearson D, O'Connell D, Mullick SC: Impedance phlebography: technique, interpretation, and results. Arch Surg 104:164, 1972

Index

F

G